MULTIPLE CHEMICAL SENSITIVITY

A SURVIVAL GUIDE

PAMELA REED GIBSON, PH.D.

New Harbinger Publications, Inc.

Publisher's Note

This publication is designed to provide accurate and authoritative information in regard to the subject matter covered. It is sold with the understanding that the publisher is not engaged in rendering psychological, financial, legal, or other professional services. If expert assistance or counseling is needed, the services of a competent professional should be sought.

Distributed in the U.S.A. by Publishers Group West; in Canada by Raincoast Books; in Great Britain by Airlift Book Company, Ltd.; in South Africa by Real Books, Ltd.; in Australia by Boobook; and in New Zealand by Tandem Press.

Copyright © 2000 by Pamela Reed Gibson
         New Harbinger Publications, Inc.
         5674 Shattuck Avenue
         Oakland, CA 94609

Cover design by Blue Design
Photo © TSM/Kunio Owaki, 1999
Edited by Jueli Gastwirth
Text design by Tracy Marie Powell

Library of Congress Catalog Card Number: 99-74375
ISBN 1-57224-173-X Paperback

All Rights Reserved

Printed in the United States of America

New Harbinger Publications' Web site address: www.newharbinger.com

01   00   99

10   9   8   7   6   5   4   3   2   1

First printing

To my charming husband and friend, Royce Gibson.

To those who struggle with poorly understood illnesses, and all those who have tried to help.

To the environmental visionaries who have laid the groundwork for understanding toxicants and health.

To groups such as Greenpeace and Pesticide Action Network who take a stand for people's safety every day. To the MCS support groups who educate and care for those at risk of falling through the cracks of a chemical-dependent society.

To all those with broader paradigms who understand the earth better than does western industrial culture.

Contents

Acknowledgments

With the help of my students, I have collected an extensive data bank of relevant information from more than 300 people with MCS. I thank my students for their diligent help, particularly those who remained with me for long periods of time and contributed to MCS work by researching, writing, and presenting papers. Thanks to Margie Warren, Jennifer Cheavens, Marnie White, Amy Earehart, Kelli Jones, Carrie Hood, LaQuisha Stephens, Valerie Rice, Elizabeth Placek, Darcy Stables, Kerri Spence, Lisa Engel, Jennifer Lane, Laura Milin, Sacha Ostroff, Elizabeth Dowling, Michael Keen, Maureen Adler, Colleen Crowley, and Dana Heller. It has been my privilege to work with all of you. Also thanks to Amy Rey, Kathy Palm, and Erin Deal for being such terrific examples of "studenthood" even though you didn't work directly on the MCS research.

I am grateful to Laura Brown, Ph.D., past president of Division 35 (Psychology of Women) of the American Psychological Association (APA), for appointing me the chair of a task force on New Chronic Health Conditions and Women. Under this title, and with the help of others, I was able to study multiple chemical sensitivity, chronic fatigue, and fibromyalgia, and present two symposia at the 1997 annual meeting of the APA. I am grateful also to Judy Worrell, Ph.D., and Melba Vasquez, Ph.D., who, as Division presidents, allowed the task force to continue with a focus on chemical exposure and women's health. The meetings of the Executive Committee of Division 35 are all fragrance-free to enable participation by those with sensitivities. Additionally, I was able to publish three papers on MCS in feminist journals. To my amazement, they actually had sent my papers to reviewers with chemical sensitivities and/or CFIDS.

I am also grateful to the nursing profession, which has shown some interest in this issue by publishing two of my papers in their journals—*Research in Nursing & Health* and the *Journal of Clinical Nursing*. The pervasive resistance to the topic of MCS makes the open-minded attitude of the nursing journal editors, such as Marilyn Oberst, all the more remarkable.

The sample of people who participated in my research were gathered from requests printed in the N.E.E.D.S. newsletter, through the National Center for Environmental Health Strategies (with the help of Mary Lamielle), from support groups, from physicians' offices, through newsletters, and from a random sample of the membership of the Chemical Injury Information Network. I thank Mary Lamielle, Lynn Lawson, Alice Osherman, Cynthia Wilson, Elaine Tomko, and all the other support group leaders and physicians who helped spread the word about the study.

The following people provided very helpful consultations and feedback on particular chapters: Dr. Ann McCampbell, Lynn Lawson, Susan Killian, Dr. William MacDonald, Susan Molloy, Alice Osherman, Toni Temple, and Cynthia Wilson. Diana Kaye of Terressentials provided detailed feedback on Chapter Four, "Making Your Environment Safe," and provided me with vital information on cosmetic and food ingredients. I particularly am grateful to Dr. Ann McCampbell who spent hours reviewing and giving me very detailed and comprehensive feedback on several of the more research-oriented chapters, and to Susan Molloy who read and commented on the entire manuscript. It is a better book because of them.

I thank Kristin Beck, acquisitions editor from New Harbinger Publications, for approaching and asking me to submit a proposal for a self-help book on MCS at the 1997 American Psychological Association convention after hearing our task force symposium. I also thank my editor Jueli Gastwirth for her detailed help and her enthusiasm in bringing this project to completion. Developmental editors Farrin Jacobs and Kayla Sussell helped to organize and to make the more academic portions of the book accessible to all readers. I thank Kirk Johnson for his attention to and flexibility in cover design.

My fabulous mentors Drs. Bernice Lott and Kathryn Quina set wonderful examples and I thank them for their presence during my doctoral education and subsequently. My commitment to understanding the disenfranchised was nurtured by them, and they continue to support and encourage me as my academic "mothers."

I am grateful to Drs. Laura Brown and Paula Caplan, my "distant" mentors for the inspiration I have derived from their work, their professional and personal support, and their understanding of the importance of studying MCS, a topic that is "off the beaten track."

My thinking about western industrialism, imperialism, and environmentalism has been guided by the illuminating works of writers such as Chellis Glerdinning, Gerry Mander, Ward Churchill, Vandana Shiva, Maria Mies, Noam Chomsky, and ecofeminists such as Greta Gaard, Janis Birkeland, Lori Gruen, Carol Adams, Marti Kheel, and others.

I also thank my colleague and friend Arnie Kahn for his personal and professional support. His encouragement in my writing and extensive use of the red pen have helped me to be a better writer. He has also helped me to weather negative feedback from the skeptics and made me laugh in the workplace. I also thank my colleagues and friends JoAnne Brewster, Michael Stoloff, Anne Stewart, Joann Grayson, Antoinette Thomas, Susie Baker, Sharon Lovell, and Arlene Lundquist for their supportive presence that makes work and life in general better.

I thank the members of my family who have been supportive of me, and especially my husband, Royce Gibson, for his long-suffering support that has helped me to develop both personally and professionally and to carry out my research and writing. He not only is the highest quality of spouse, but is a sounding board for my articles and chapters, and allows me to have a collection of animal companions who lower my blood pressure, force me to take breaks and walks, and provide endless, much-needed distraction and humor.

My children "facsimiles," Ben, Jodi, and Carmen, have added meaning and joy to my life for many years. Nothing would be the same without them.

I thank my personal friends Susan Rossi, Sheila Badal, and Jane Comtois for their friendship and personal support, and Chris and Charlie Moore for their compassionate help in a long-standing personal emergency. I thank Alice Christensen for contributing immeasurably to my personal growth.

William MacDonald, D.C., Beverly Sweetman, and John Glick, M.D., have made very valuable contributions to my overall quality of life.

Most of all, I thank the study participants, many of whom struggled with the printed questionnaires in spite of our efforts to make them as "clean" as possible. Many people spent hours providing me with data and detailed written responses to open-ended questions. Their desire to help people without MCS understand the illness, and people with MCS to cope, is admirable, and is the driving force of my work.

Introduction

Since 1992, I have been involved in researching how multiple chemical sensitivity (MCS) and chemical injury affect people's daily lives. As a result, I have an extensive data bank of pertinent information about MCS. I feel a sense of responsibility to share this research with other people suffering from MCS as well as with those who want to help them, i.e., family members, friends, and professionals.

Between 1992 and 1997, I collected data from more than 300 people whose lives have been significantly affected by MCS. The research, both quantitative (examining averages) and qualitative (examining individual answers in-depth), may be the most comprehensive work done to date on the impact of MCS, although there is no way to prove that my research participants are representative of the entire MCS population.

I wrote this book with the twin goals of helping people whose lives are affected by MCS—directly or indirectly, personally or professionally—and conferring academic respect to the condition. The book is meant to assist those who suffer from MCS in practical, physical, psychological and, hopefully, even spiritual ways.

It has not always been easy to publish helpful, credible information about individuals living with MCS. Often, my research articles were met with hostility by psychology, rehabilitation, and women's health journals. Initially, criticisms revolved around methodology—how I gathered my samples, etc. When I justified my methods and cleaned up what could be changed in the writing, the denials/protests took something like this form: "Although this article is well written and interesting, we cannot publish it in our journal because it addresses a condition often treated by psychologists as a psychological problem." The editor of a rehabilitation journal said, "The rehabilitation journals are waiting for the American Medical Association to give them direction on this condition." I wrote him back that, "Meanwhile people with MCS are seeking help from rehabilitation counselors who find no guidance in your journal." He did not respond.

Another critique from a somewhat hostile reviewer suggested (about a social support article now published in *Research in Nursing & Health*) that my respondents had previously "known that I was measuring social support and had purposely scored low in order to draw attention to their plight." I have read over one hundred articles on social support in various health conditions, and nowhere has *any* writer ever suggested this in reference to *any* other condition. For other conditions, the survey instruments are assumed to be valid; for MCS they often are not. These are just a few of the ways that resistance to the topic of MCS has manifested.

Almost every participant in my studies is included in this book. Their stories will increase your understanding of what it means when someone becomes chemically sensitive and will illustrate how to confront and live with chemical sensitivity.

Data Collection

Participants in my research provided information about how they became chemically sensitized/injured; the medical help they had received; how they were treated by medical and psychological practitioners; who supported them personally; and what happened at home, at work, and to their finances once they developed MCS. They answered my questions regarding whether they had applied for disability benefits and what the results were; how they felt their sense of self had changed as a result of having MCS; what they thought needed to be done to help people with MCS; and in what kind of activism (if any) they had engaged. For those of you who are interested in my methodology, more detailed descriptions of it, the results, and the papers that resulted can be found in Appendix A.

How to Use This Book

Part I of the book, "What We Know About MCS," provides a basic overview. Chapter one describes what MCS is, its symptoms, and who is most susceptible. In chapter two, I have tried to provide a user-friendly review of the major physiological and psychological theories about what causes this specific illness/disability. Part I ends with chapter three, which reviews how life often is affected by MCS, including finances, housing, career, family relations, and other quality of life issues.

Practical Matters, Research, and Personal Testimony

Part II, "Physical Issues" (chapters four through seven), discusses physiological and lifestyle issues, including creating a safe home, balanced nutrition, and a well-informed medical team. If you currently are in great distress, you may want to read chapter four first. It is a crash course on how to clean up your environment so you will be able to think more clearly and encourage your body to heal. It provides specific suggestions for making yourself healthier, safer, and more comfortable in your immediate environment. Diet and nutrition are addressed in chapter five, which includes a summary of a number of special diets as well as guidelines for avoiding toxicants in food. Chapter six discusses medical help, including who treats MCS and how. Alternative treatment methods are explored in chapter seven.

In Part III, "Psychological and Personal Growth" (chapters eight through twelve), there are discussions of psychological issues and personal growth, interweaving practical matters with research and personal testimony. Included are sections on living with chronic illness, loss of identity, lack of social support, psychological issues, and miscellaneous suggestions for personal growth.

Chapter eight will help you understand and normalize some of the difficulties of living with a chronic illness. It describes the common disruptions—such as altered relationships and diminished physical ability—that are a common part of having a chronic health condition. Chapter nine focuses on the role of psychological practitioners and discusses the MCS controversy, often found within the psychological community. That is, some people believe MCS is psychosomatic. As a result, their suggested methods of healing are frequently inappropriate and ineffective. If you have a therapist, you can share this chapter with them, especially the section entitled, "Suggestions for Treating Clients with MCS." In chapter ten, identity and growth are discussed in relation to the upheaval that may be taking place in your life. The chapter reviews the kinds of personal and emotional difficulties experienced by those with MCS, and illustrates how some people are able to triumph over the often isolating and devastating experiences caused by this illness. Chapter eleven continues to discuss the problems surrounding social support and provides some suggestions for evaluating and strengthening your own support network. Chapter twelve offers creative and supportive techniques for staying healthy psychologically, some of which are suggestions from individuals currently living with MCS.

Part IV (chapters thirteen through fifteen) is entitled "Disability, Politics, and Activism." Accommodations in the workplace are one focus of chapter thirteen, which also reviews how to qualify and apply for disability benefits, including personal examples from those who have gone through the process. Activism, education, and political work are discussed in chapter fourteen, including suggestions on how you can find and share your expertise in this regard. This chapter also gives special attention to the inspiring work currently being done by many MCS activists. Chapter fifteen, the last chapter of the book, is my final plea for greater understanding and acceptance of MCS on the part of the larger culture.

Further Resources

To live successfully with MCS and not succumb to despair, it is best to stay abreast of emerging research, treatment options, safe products, and available organizational support. Appendix A describes the research methodology used, provides some tabular results, and lists journal and conference papers from my five-year MCS research project. Appendix B is an extensive list of chapter-specific, MCS-friendly products. Appendix C contains chapter resources and further reading suggestions. Appendix D provides a list of helpful organizations. Appendix E provides references for readings in toxicology.

In the following pages, I have tried to blend much of what is known medically and psychologically about MCS into a self-help context. As a result, this book serves as both a self-help guide and a report on current research that gives voice to what people with MCS are saying. I hope you will find it a helpful tool as well as an informative book to share with others.

PART I

WHAT WE KNOW ABOUT MCS

Chapter One

It's More Common Than You Think

What Is MCS and Who Gets It?

Five years ago, Jane's workplace installed and glued down new carpeting. Following this she became ill with severe flu-like symptoms, headache, and nausea. She also developed bleeding ulcers and suffered from weight loss, confusion, forgetfulness, and ultimately, serious depression. She noticed she was becoming sensitive to odors from a variety of chemicals, but particularly formaldehyde. Within one hour of entering the workplace or of being exposed to new furniture, fabric or clothing stores, and some houses, she would develop the symptoms listed above.

As the carpet installation progressed and Jane experienced the above-described symptoms, she sent for a list of chemicals being used. It initially made no sense to her that she would suddenly become mentally unbalanced just because carpeting was being installed. Yet, this seemed to be the opinion of a number of others. At the time, she received no testing or verification for her own conclusions, which were that the carpet itself was making her ill. She tried to tough it out, hold on to her job, and keep a "normal" life by tolerating the odors.

Each time she said to herself, "I will be okay—the smell is not that bad." But her symptoms continued and even worsened, and she became frightened after she fell asleep while driving. Simple exposures to perfume and pest spray brought on such dire symptoms that she was forced to seek emergency medical treatment for vomiting and headaches. Unfortunately, just when Jane was dealing with these problems, she nearly died from a gas leak in her house. When the leak occurred and she felt faint, she attributed the symptoms to her usual sense of feeling unwell and tolerated them. Later, her daughter found her asleep in her bedroom with the entire house smelling strongly of propane. It took her two weeks to recover, after which she noticed she had become even more sensitive.

The propane heating system has now been removed from her house. In her attempt to avoid chemical exposures, she has sealed off all the plywood in the house, and she uses no scented products. She cannot tolerate the smell of her appliances, particularly new ones, and she can barely tolerate the natural smells of blooming flowers. Her joints are so inflamed and swollen that she can hardly use her hands. What sort of illness could cause such a myriad collection of symptoms?

What Is MCS?

Multiple chemical sensitivity (MCS) is also referred to as chemical injury (CI), environmental illness (EI), chemical hypersensitivity, total allergy, twentieth-century illness, and other names. There is some controversy about which name is most appropriate. Those who prefer the name "chemical injury" believe that the name should reflect a chemical cause for the problem. Those who prefer "environmental illness" believe that since patients often react to pollens, dust, molds, and animal dander, the broader term is more appropriate. Although I understand and agree with the arguments for using other terms, I will use the term "multiple chemical sensitivity" (MCS) because it is used most often in the professional literature.

Defining MCS

Defining MCS has stirred its own controversy. Simply put, people seem to undergo some poorly understood systemic damage that causes them to react negatively to common chemicals in ambient air. Jane's health has somehow changed such that she experiences violent—even life-threatening—illness from a number of chemicals that others seem to tolerate. Finding an "official" definition of MCS, however, is more complicated. Ashford and Miller (1998) propose an operational definition, claiming that an MCS patient "can be discovered by removal from the suspected offending agents and by rechallenge, after an appropriate interval, under strictly controlled environmental conditions." For example, if Jane was removed from her work atmosphere, placed in a clean environment, given time to recover, and exposed to formaldehyde, and then the formaldehyde triggered symptoms, by this definition she would be a chemically sensitive person.

A group of thirty-four researchers and clinicians with experience in the "study, evaluation, diagnosis, and/or care of adults and children with chemical sensitivity disorders" has published a consensus statement supporting a definition of MCS adapted from Nethercott, Davidoff, Curbow, et al. (1993). The consensus includes the following six criteria:

1. The symptoms are reproducible with repeated chemical exposure

2. The condition is chronic

3. Low levels of exposure (lower than previously or commonly tolerated) result in manifestations of the syndrome

4. The symptoms improve or resolve when the incitants are removed

5. Responses occur to multiple chemically unrelated substances

6. Symptoms involve multiple organ systems (added in 1999)

(Multiple Chemical Sensitivity: A 1999 Consensus)

Jane meets all of these criteria, assuming that no other medical explanation is found for her constellation of symptoms. Cullen (1987) would add that the problem must be initiated by one identifiable episode or event. However, some object to this criterion because not everyone with MCS can identify a single episode that caused their problem

Describing MCS

The first comprehensive description of patients with MCS was by Theron Randolph, who was doing research on "allergic" reactions to chemicals as early as the 1950s. He was a loved mentor and friend of practitioners in environmental medicine, and a physician to people with MCS for many years. His book with Ralph Moss, *An Alternative Approach to Allergies* (1982), describes his practice, his theories, the symptoms he believed are caused by chemicals, and the chemicals that elicit those symptoms. Randolph traced some of his patients' difficulties as they (and he) discovered their sensitivities to exhausts, cooking gas, perfumes, formaldehyde, and other chemicals. The book includes his patient questionnaire and many valuable case histories.

Chemicals eliciting illness in people with MCS fall into many classes, but often they are solvents. In Phase IV of my research, respondents rated pesticides, formaldehyde, fresh paint, new carpets, diesel exhaust, perfumes, and air fresheners as being particularly troublesome. (See Appendix A for more details.)

MCS and the Body

MCS symptoms can affect any bodily system, including respiratory, digestive, neurological, musculoskeletal, endocrinological, immunological, and others. Of the symptoms reported by respondents in a study of 191 MCS patients by the Canadian Ministry of Health (Report of the Ad Hoc Committee, 1985), forty-five affected the central nervous system, twenty-six were gastrointestinal, twelve were respiratory, eight were musculoskeletal, sixteen were genito-urinary, thirty-two affected the ear/nose/throat, seventeen irritated skin, and twelve were cardiovascular.

The five most common symptoms in my research were tiredness/lethargy, difficulty concentrating, muscle aches, memory difficulties, and long-term fatigue. This suggests overlap with chronic fatigue syndrome.

Sometimes symptoms caused by chemicals are more unusual or frightening. Some respondents reported experiencing memory loss, nervousness, bleeding from the lips, water retention, heart palpitations, hair loss, and other alarming reactions to exposures. The cerebral effects may be some of the most frightening and debilitating symptoms experienced, as described here: "I don't know what triggers it, but I'm normally quiet and easygoing. Sometimes I have temper and anger management problems along with the feeling that I am really out of control."

Another person said, "My symptoms are largely mental. I begin to have memory problems and can't think, then my face turns red and I become very irritable. Also some slowing of my speech. In traffic I'm dangerous if I've been exposed to a lot of exhaust."

Because we know so little about MCS, nothing is known about the long-term effect of actually experiencing the reactions to chemicals. As one person said: "Who knows what harm is occurring in one's head due to repeated migraines?"

Total Load

People with MCS may also demonstrate food, mold, pollen, and animal allergies/sensitivities that complicate life and increase the "total chemical load" on the person's system. The concept of *total load* says that the body can tolerate only so many insults/exposures/stresses before they start to exact a heavy toll. The body is seen as "filling up" with exposures and stressors such that one's *daily* ability to tolerate exposures may fluctuate depending on how many exposures already have been endured on that given day.

According to this concept, if you have food allergies and are eating the foods that are triggering those allergies, you may have less tolerance for chemicals than you had just a week ago when your system was dealing with fewer assaults. Similarly, if it is hay fever season and you are already reacting to pollens, you may be less able to tolerate chemicals. Conversely, anything you can do to reduce your total load may help you give your body the time it needs to heal and thus increase your ability to face future exposures without falling apart.

MCS and Electromagnetic Frequencies

Sensitivities to electromagnetic frequencies (EMFs) also may complicate people's lives, because electrical fields are emitted by high tension wires, transmitters, and other large sources of electricity as well as electrical appliances and other "small" sources found in the home. Although this is the least understood and least accepted aspect of MCS, there are some studies now that show that EMF can alter the permeability of neurons, thereby affecting the levels and circulation of brain chemicals (neurotransmitters).

In a number of these studies, EMFs also have been linked to cancer (particularly in children) (Pinsky 1995).

MCS and Allergies

More than half of the people with chemical sensitivities in a study by Meggs, Dunn, Bloch, et al. (1996) also had common allergies, such as to dust, pollen, and weeds. In addition, food sensitivities can be a major obstacle:

> "Sitting down to a meal was like dining in a minefield. Whether in a restaurant or at home, I would take one small bite, stop, and see if I reacted. If my breath didn't stop, or my head didn't pound, or my stomach didn't rebel, I would eat a little more. I did this with every bite. Experience taught me not to bother with the water. I always reacted to that."

> —Forty-seven-year-old woman with
> MCS for twelve years

Adaptation

One interesting and important dynamic to understand in relation to chemical sensitivity is that of *adaptation*. Randolph and Moss (1982) drew parallels to the addictive process in that the initial exposure to a chemical may actually cause an excitatory response. That is, you may actually feel temporarily better or more energized after an exposure when you are in the process of becoming sensitized to a chemical.

The workaholic, for example, who cannot leave the office actually may be getting an unhealthy "high" from a work exposure that excites the nervous system by producing a temporary high. However, as the exposure wears off (withdrawal), the person experiences the opposite reaction—that of energy depletion, and so forth. Over time, exposure to the chemical in question ceases to have the excitatory effect (much as alcohol does for the alcoholic), and the person feels poorly all of the time. At any one point in time we are involved in a number of cycles of exposure and withdrawal with all of the cycles overlapping. This is adaptation.

For example, you may be beginning to become sensitized to a new chemical in the workplace that makes you feel high. But this may be counterbalanced by a withdrawal reaction you are having due to not having eaten eggs for two days. You can see that with several cycles simultaneously overlapping, it would be impossible to tell exactly what is causing your reactions. This is why practitioners of environmental medicine have urged the construction of environmental hospital units where patients can be tested for reactions in a clean environment after fasting for several days on pure water. This puts patients into a de-adapted state, and makes it more likely to pinpoint precisely what is causing their reactions. Patients are challenged (tested) with one substance or food at a time, and the substances most harmful to them can then be identified.

Induction and Triggering

Miller (1994) describes the two-stage process of induction (when the person develops a sensitivity to a substance) and triggering (when future exposures to the substance bring on negative reactions). Induction may be caused by one large exposure or by a series of low-level exposures, or possibly by severe stress or physical illness (although this cause is less clearly understood).

An international study of MCS found in at least three countries that all of the following were associated with the onset of the illness: organic solvents, pesticides, amalgam/mercury, formaldehyde, renovated buildings, paints/lacquers, pentachlorophenol/wood preservative, and stress/psychological factors (Ashford, Heinzow, and Lutjen, et al. 1995). Scandinavian studies of "sick buildings" have found that being female, having preexisting asthma or rhinitis, having a history of atopy (allergy), working in particular job categories having the most exposures as part of the job, i.e., photocopying, visual display terminal use, and handling carbonless paper all increase the risk of developing symptoms in "sick buildings" (Ashford, Heinzow, and Lutjen, et al. 1995). Therefore, any preexisting vulnerabilities seem to "set us up" for chemical insult. One woman who had been sick with MCS for four years said:

"I had a minor case of asthma for about ten years and never really got too sick until they added the chemical methyl tertiary butyl ether to the gas tanks. As a result when it is used in Colorado from November to March, I develop asthma and bronchitis over and over. After five years of the irritation to my lungs I have chemical sensitivities. I am very bothered by pesticides, paint, perfumes, newspapers, copy machines, and hair sprays. I correspond with people in Alaska and Montana and they are having the same effects from the fuel."

How Many People Have MCS?

Three prevalence studies to date have looked at the incidence of MCS in the general population. In one study, Meggs, Dunn, Bloch, et al. (1996), surveyed a representative rural household sample of people. This means that the population sample selected by the university represented as closely as possible the area population. Of 1,027 people, one-third reported chemical sensitivity, with the major incitants being perfumes, pesticides, cigarette smoke, and fresh paint. Chemical sensitivity without allergy was almost as common as allergy without chemical sensitivity (16 percent versus 18 percent), was present in all age, income, race, and education groups, and caused 3.9 percent of respondents to become ill every single day.

Two additional studies were done by the State Departments of Health in New Mexico and California. In New Mexico, Voorhees (1999) found that 16 percent of people reported being sensitive to chemicals, 2 percent had been diagnosed with MCS, and 2 percent had lost a job or career because of the sensitivities. Kreutzer (1999) found that of a random sample of California adults, 15.9 percent of respondents reported being "allergic or unusually sensitive to everyday chemicals," and 6.3 percent had been diagnosed with the problem. According to these studies, chemical sensitivity seems to be fairly evenly distributed by age, educational level, marital status, job, and geographic location.

If approximately 4 percent of the U.S. population is becoming ill every day from chemicals, this extrapolates to over 11 million people having moderate to severe MCS, a formidable number of people to be ill without so much as an agreement as to what to call their condition. If 2 percent have lost their jobs because of the problem, then the productivity of five and a half million people has been compromised. If this many people are sick from chemicals, why is Jane receiving feedback that she has psychological problems?

At least two papers document MCS as a global concern. An international team of researchers found reports of chemical sensitivity in Denmark, Sweden, Norway, Finland, Germany, Holland, Belgium, the United Kingdom, and Greece (Ashford, Heinzow, Lutjen, et al. 1995). Cynthia Wilson (1995) compiled data that suggests that MCS is a global, albeit an unlabeled and insufficiently researched problem.

Who Gets MCS?

Ordinary people get MCS. Variables that increase your chances for developing MCS seem to be large single exposures to chemicals, low-level chronic exposures without adequate ventilation, being female, having a family history of chemical sensitivity, and other possible insults to your body that reduce its ability to detoxify chemicals, such as serious illness or damage to your enzyme systems. (Enzyme systems are important components of the body's detoxification pathways.)

People from all walks of life develop MCS including professionals, office workers, homemakers, and farmers. My data sample contains large numbers of homemakers, clerical workers, students, teachers, and nurses. Other represented occupations include chemists, engineers, professors, hairdressers, and accountants. Having a "good job" does not protect you from getting MCS. In fact, more than half of those in my data sample who reported an initial known exposure that had damaged their health said that it had occurred in the work environment. For most people, MCS appears to be a long-term chronic condition. The volunteers in my sample had been sick with MCS for an average of fifteen years. For seven and a half of those years their problem was undiagnosed. (See Appendix A for the demographics, occupations, and other data from my research sample.)

Gender

Most study samples consist of 80 percent women. Although no one knows for certain why women appear to be more susceptible to MCS, there are several hypotheses that may explain these percentages. Some simple explanations may be that women are physically smaller on average than men and, therefore, may be less able to metabolize chemicals. Women also have a greater total percentage of body fat, which stores chemicals. There is an enzyme called alcohol dehydrogenase that detoxifies not only carbohydrates, sugar, and alcohol, but also chemicals. Men have much more of this enzyme than women do (Freeza, Padova, Pozzato, et al. 1990; Rogers 1990). Also butylcholinesterases, which scavenge chemicals, are lower in females over the age of ten than in males, and decline further in women over the age of thirty (Wilson 1997).

Our culture also encourages women to use many chemically based cosmetics filled with hundreds of ingredients for which Material Safety Data Sheets (MSDS) say, "Do not inhale vapors" or "Avoid contact with skin." Women are then exposed to one another's fragrances in small working spaces.

Recent information about the importance of hormone mimickers may also explain some of the gender disparity. Many commonly used chemicals contain known estrogen blockers or mimickers (i.e., "xenoestrogens"), which may disrupt endocrine functioning in women differently than they do in men (Colborn, Dumanoski, and Myers 1997). These "xenoestrogens" may enter the body and activate estrogen receptors, thus simulating a high estrogen content in the body (mimicking), or may fill, but fail to activate, a receptor, thus disrupting the body's estrogenic processes (blocking). Cynthia Wilson (1997) explains that the P450 enzyme system, which is responsible for removing toxins from the blood, can be inhibited or even inactivated by these estrogen-mimicking chemicals. Because permissible levels for chemical exposure set by the Occupational Safety and Health Administration (OSHA) are based on young, healthy, 154-pound white men, women, children, and minorities are probably not being adequately protected (Wilson 1997).

It is possible, however, that the gender difference in MCS is exaggerated as a result of using volunteer and medical samples. In Meggs, Dunn, Bloch, et al.'s household population study (1996), the ratio was much smaller, with 24 percent of men and 39 percent of women reporting illness due to chemicals. Although still favoring women, this is a much smaller differential than has been found in other studies. It is also possible that women have better support networks, and thus find their way to studies or to medical treatment more easily.

Another possibility is that men may call their symptoms something else. In our culture we teach men that they must endure. A friend of mine returned home one day to find the man who had been hired to paint the inside of her house walking around in circles in her yard. When she asked him what was wrong he said that this "always happened" when he painted. This man probably did not use the term "MCS," yet clearly, he was experiencing reactions to chemicals on a regular basis.

Race

Race is certainly a variable in how much of a toxic load a person is expected to bear. Our industrial culture puts poor and minority people at risk for much greater exposures in their neighborhoods because of environmental racism. Minority groups inhabit neighborhoods close to polluting facilities after these neighborhoods have been depopulated by middle-class families who have improved their "standard of living" and moved to the suburbs. In other cases, minority neighborhoods are purposely targeted by industry for facilities that contaminate air, earth, and water because industry expects less resistance in communities where people have little political power, few resources, and are more desperate for jobs. The result is often serious illness, decimated communities, and the destruction of family life. Nowhere is this more evident than in the African-American communities in Louisiana between Baton Rouge and New Orleans, an area that has earned for itself the name "Cancer Alley." I am not aware of any studies of MCS that have specifically surveyed African-American inhabitants of such areas.

There were no African-American participants in my study. However, Meggs, Dunn, Bloch, et al. found that African-Americans reported MCS in the same percentages as Caucasians (33 percent).

Certainly, Native Americans endure the level of contamination found in Cancer Alley. There are several reports that MCS is prevalent among Native Americans. The environmental contamination on reservations is high due to the presence of radioactivity, waste dump sites, pesticide use, contaminated water, and the high consumption of fish (which accumulate toxins in the food chain) (Hall 1994; Hansen and Lurie 1995). Factories have been and still are allowed to contaminate drinking water for Indian nations (Hall 1994), and radioactive dump sites are situated on their lands. These and other forms of industrial contamination take their toll on Native American health. Hansen and Lurie (1995) described the pesticiding of Lurie's neighborhood on the Rosebud Reservation in Mission, South Dakota. The scenario is a chemically sensitive person's worst nightmare with trucks repeatedly spraying malathion and leaving a sticky residue in the interiors of people's homes and on their possessions (including food and clothing). Without air-conditioning, residents were forced to keep their windows open. When Lurie and his pregnant wife were trying to detoxify their belongings and cope with their symptoms, which included splitting headaches for themselves and breathing difficulties for their two-year-old daughter, even fans were absent. The spraying also sickened all fourteen neighbors who had been home on the night of the spraying. The sprayings continued with the mayor refusing to provide notification or to turn off the spray when the truck passed the Lurie home.

Clearly, we are all exposed to unsafe levels of many chemicals. Nonetheless, the less powerful and more oppressed members of the population are most at risk for harm from decisions made by those in power who subject them to unsafe substances. As Lois Gibbs says, "Pollution begins in the boardroom."

Chapter Two

What Causes MCS?

Physiological and Psychological Hypotheses

Many people with MCS associate one large chemical exposure with their decline in health. Others who report sensitivity to chemicals are not able to cite one specific exposure, but report a series of low-level exposures; and still others do not know what triggered their problems. Many people with MCS know only that they seem to become ill from common chemicals.

What People with MCS Say About the Cause

One person with MCS said, "I was aware that I arrived at work feeling well and after exposure to people smoking I experienced headaches that lasted the remainder of the day, and nausea, as well." Some suspect but can't be sure of exactly which chemicals caused their problem. For example, one woman who has coped with MCS for six years said, "I do not know the names of chemicals—just that they were the chemicals in a copy machine. I sat four to five feet from a copy machine for three years. I then became sensitive to certain colognes and petro [petroleum]-based products."

When I asked respondents from Phase II of my research study what they thought had caused their problem, more than half said they suspected that they had been made sensitive by one identifiable exposure, one-quarter said that they had not, and another quarter did not know. The most commonly cited exposures thought to cause MCS were pesticides, remodeling, and workplace renovations. (See Appendix A for a full list of exposures thought to cause MCS.)

The remainder of this chapter will review various scientific hypotheses as to what causes MCS. I have tried to review theories in such a way as to condense academic findings into understandable language. Theories are broken down roughly into physiological and psychological causes; however, many feel that this is an artificial distinction because the brain and behavior are so intricately intertwined. For practical purposes, the division here is into theories that assume MCS is a physiological/medical condition versus those that describe it as a psychological problem.

Physiologically Based Theories

Probably the most general theory regarding the cause of MCS is that people's bodies are breaking down in response to chemical insults, much as animals have been found to develop tumors, suppressed immunity, and reproductive problems in response to contaminated habitats.

Systemic Breakdown in Response to Pollution

To many, it makes sense that humans would become weaker in the face of increased environmental contamination. This is the canary down the mineshaft theory. It suggests that increasing numbers of people will experience MCS and other toxic injuries as more and more people are subjected to chemical contamination. This is a generalized hypothesis and does not specify exactly how people's bodies break down and become damaged or hypersensitive. But nervous system damage figures prominently in a number of theories.

Limbic Kindling

One hypothesis receiving serious attention is that of limbic kindling through the olfactory-limbic system (Bell 1994; Bell, Miller, and Schwartz 1992). There is a direct pathway from the nose into the central part of the "old" animal brain, or limbic system, which is involved in governing sleep, mood, eating, aggression, and other very basic survival behaviors. It is called "kindling" because kindling in biology refers to the process of sensitizing nerve tissue. For example, if you put a frog's nerve in a petri dish, and stimulate it with electrical impulses that individually are too mild to fire the nerve (called "sub-threshold" impulses), eventually, due to the repeated stimulation, that nerve will fire.

Some individuals are thought to have sensitized or "kindled" to low-level chemicals, which trigger serious reactions mediated through limbic pathways. In other words, very small amounts of chemicals can induce reactions that normally would not be expected. Because the limbic system is connected to and involved in regulating so many body systems, its disruption could easily cause many of the symptoms reported by MCS patients. This theory also explains the "spreading" phenomenon where people acquire more and more sensitivities even without further chemical exposures, which has been demonstrated in animal research. Iris Bell (1994) and her colleagues (Bell, Miller, and Schwartz 1992), and Claudia Miller (1992) suggest that limbic kindling is one possible explanation for the development and worsening of MCS. John Rossi (1996) reviewed the kindling research in a technical but very comprehensive and informative paper and made suggestions as to what type of kindling might be operating in MCS.

Studies show that many areas of the brain can be sensitized, but that the limbic system kindles more easily than any other area. Although there are several types of chemical kindling, Rossi (1996) believes that IntraCerebral-Localized (ICL) kindling is the most probable model for MCS. In ICL kindling, a chemical is introduced into the brain of an animal through a narrow glass tube at frequent intervals until localized seizures result. Future chemical infusions cause seizures that are longer and more severe, occur farther away from where the chemical was introduced (causing other parts of the body to be affected), and eventually involve the whole organism. Doesn't this sound like MCS reactions? Rossi suggests that because chemicals can stimulate the brain via the olfactory system, and olfactory bulbs are sensitive to chemical kindling, that repetitive inhaled exposure to low-dose chemicals may trigger responses in the brain's limbic area. He suggests that although animal researchers have not directly investigated kindling and MCS, they easily could.

Enzymatic Damage/Depletion

Xenobiotic (chemical compounds foreign to living organisms) detoxification pathways are responsible for responding to toxicants that enter the body, but because of genetic or acquired variability their effectiveness differs from person to person. Sherry Rogers' book, *Tired or Toxic* (1990), explains some of the workings of the detoxification system, reviews some of the problematic pathways specific to MCS, and makes suggestions for testing and for replacing nutrients and nutrient precursors (substances that your body uses to make nutrients). (See Appendix C for further reading.)

Toxicants that enter the body through breathing, eating/drinking, or are absorbed by the skin must be detoxified or biotransformed. This means that for excretion, chemicals must be made into less toxic compounds. If your detoxification system is damaged, the excretion process could be too slow with the resultant buildup of poisons; or it could be pathological, and you might actually manufacture compounds that are more—rather than less—toxic.

Although many water-soluble compounds are excreted in the urine without metabolizing, fat-soluble compounds must be processed by the body. Rogers (1990) cites studies that show deficiencies in zinc, iron, and molybdenum are common. If you are deficient in one or more of these minerals and thus cannot process toxicants through your detoxification pathways, you may shunt to an alternative pathway to make chloral hydrate instead. This can contribute to your own continued poisoning, since another name for chloral hydrate is "Mickey Finn" or "knockout" drops. One problem is that the same pathways that detoxify environmental chemicals also metabolize alcohol, sugar, and endogenous hormones. So these substances may accumulate if these pathways are not working properly.

Inherited enzyme deficiencies may predispose some groups of people to particular weaknesses with respect to detoxification. For example, inherited porphyria is a deficiency in the enzyme system that synthesizes heme, a component of hemoglobin that carries oxygen to all tissues. Porphyria can also be acquired, or caused by drugs, chemicals, infections (including hepatitis C), and malnutrition. Baker (1994) reported that about half of his chemically injured patients tested positive for porphyria.

Another example of an inherited deficiency is that of the enzyme G-6-PD (glucose-6-phosphate dehydrogenase). G-6-PD predisposes 16 percent of African-American men to greater risk from environmental oxidants, such as ozone and nitrogen dioxide (Rios, Poje, and Detels 1993), much as the sickle cell trait makes African-Americans more vulnerable to aromatic amino and nitro compounds, carbon monoxide, and cyanide than other racial groups.

Many chemicals are capable of inactivating or impairing enzymes, including enzymes that metabolize toxicants. In fact, pesticide manufacturers take advantage of this either by designing active ingredients to wreak havoc on the enzymes themselves, or by adding an "inert ingredient" that harms enzyme pathways and thus keeps the active ingredient in the body longer. Examples of the first strategy are found in organophosphate insecticides that knock out acetylcholinesterase (AcE). Normally, AcE breaks down the neurotransmitter acetytlcholine so there is not too much stimulation at once at the nerve junction (the site where chemicals cross from one nerve to another and cause the receptive nerve to "fire"). When AcE is depleted, acetytlcholine builds up at the nerve site and the targeted bugs die of convulsions after exposure to the pesticide. Since humans have the same neurotransmitters as bugs, these chemicals also affect us. People may experience a great many symptoms from too much acetylcholine including convulsions, nervousness, excess salivation, nausea, vomiting, abdominal cramps, headache, weakness, tremors, noise sensitivity, and many others.

An example of the second strategy is seen in the addition of piperonol butoxide to the biological insecticide rotenone. By itself, rotenone is very toxic. With the addition of piperonol butoxide to knock out liver enzymes, the poison stays longer in the body, and is thus even more toxic.

The upshot of this is that there is a strong suggestion that people with MCS may have damaged detoxification pathways from environmental insults, but we don't have much detail regarding which exposures are likely to knock out which pathways. There are studies that show some people are poor sulfate metabolizers and some do not metabolize through the pathway at all. Reduced sulfate metabolism has been found in Parkinson's, Alzheimer's, systemic lupus erythematosis, as well as in MCS. McFadden (1996) focuses on Phase II sulfation and points out that sulfation also metabolizes neurotransmitters such as adrenaline, noradrenaline, and dopamine; steroids; bile; progesterone; DHEA; and other drugs and chemicals. Thus, poor sulfation alone can impair many bodily functions and create the poorly understood collection of symptoms called MCS.

Immunological Insults

Some researchers believe that MCS is primarily the result of immunological damage (Meggs 1992a; 1992b). Many chemicals including formaldehyde, solvents, hydrocarbons, and organochlorines have been shown to suppress immune system functioning in humans (Thornton 1993; Vojdani, Ghoneum, and Brautbar 1992, as cited in Duehring 1993a). Other researchers think that the immune problems may be secondary to neurological or other damage.

Helper and Suppressor Cells

The helper/suppressor ratio is often used as one index of immune system health. Helper cells fight pathogens or turn *on* an immune response, while suppressor cells turn *off* or prevent a response. Too *few* helper cells are present in conditions such as AIDS, while too *many* helper cells are present in autoimmune conditions, such as systemic lupus and multiple sclerosis. Immunological findings in MCS include elevated, normal, and depressed helper/suppressor ratios (Heuser, Wojdani, and Heuser 1992; Levin and Byers 1992). Although a few studies have found too high a ratio of helper/suppressor cells in MCS, more have found the opposite—a reduced ratio.

Levin and Byers believe that this may be because immune profiles for those with MCS are unstable early on, but that the profiles stabilize to low helper/ suppressor ratios as the disease progresses.

MCS patients may generate antibodies to chemicals, or even to their own tissues, which may activate an autoimmune response where the immune system acts against its own body. Levin and Byers report finding antithyroid and antismooth muscle antibodies in MCS patients, and some chemically sensitive patients may eventually develop full-blown autoimmune disease (Heuser, Wojdani, and Heuser 1992; Levin and Byers 1992). Levin and Byers found that some of their patients developed cancer, lupus, multiple sclerosis, or adult onset diabetes. The authors say, "In our opinion, these patients have a genetic propensity to a specific illness, which was triggered by an insult from an environmental agent. The first symptoms of this triggering were MCS."

Airway Inflammation and Neurogenic Inflammation

William Meggs (1995a; 1995b) believes that MCS may be mediated by neurogenic inflammation, and develop in a fashion similar to reactive airways dysfunction syndrome, where an airborne insult such as fumes or smoke initiates chronic asthma. In reactive upper-airways dysfunction syndrome, people experience rhinitis (inflammation of the mucous membrane of the nose) following a chemical exposure. Meggs and Cleveland (1993) found that patients with MCS do have nasal abnormalities including increased nasal resistance, cobblestone-like appearance of the pharynx and base of the tongue, swelling, abnormal mucus, and pale mucosa with prominent blood vessels.

Meggs explains that we know that chemicals cause receptors on sensory nerves to produce substance P and other chemicals that mediate neurogenic inflammation. Epithelial cells form the top layer of cells of the mucous membranes and protect the underlying nerve cells. But if the epithelial layer is damaged, nerve cells are more likely to suffer damage from contact with irritants such as chemicals.

We know that MCS also involves symptoms such as confusion and fatigue that are not directly connected with airways. Meggs proposes that these symptoms occur because impulses can travel from inflamed mucous membranes to the central nervous system, where they are rerouted to distant locations to produce neurogenic inflammation at the new site. He refers to this as "neurogenic switching."

Cynthia Wilson (1993) believes that neurogenic inflammation, mediated by substance P, can cause damage in many parts of the body including the digestive system and the brain. For example, Wilson says that neurogenic

inflammation will activate mast cells (connective tissue cells that are important in blood coagulation) in the digestive system and thus be responsible
for some kinds of food intolerances. She also believes that some people feel
badly from yeast because it forms acetaldehyde, which in addition to being
directly toxic to some cells is a porphyrinogenic substance. In Wilson's view,
MCS is a three-pronged problem that includes neurogenic inflammation,
chemical toxicity, and porphyrin abnormalities. She thinks that MCS is
mediated by aminolevulinic acid crossing the blood-brain barrier to interact
with inhaled chemicals.

Candidiasis

With candidiasis, allergies and chemical sensitivities can be caused by
an overgrowth of candida albicans and related yeasts that compete with
healthy digestive bacteria for space in the gut. Pathological yeasts may
become overpopulated in the digestive tract including the mouth and colon,
in the vaginal tract (causing repeated yeast infections), and even eventually
in internal organs. The yeast growth is seen as being caused by a high sugar
diet; the use of antibiotics, steroids, birth control pills; and the elevated hormones that occur during pregnancy. The yeasts are problematic because
they manufacture toxins, such as acetaldehyde, which may cause adverse
reactions in any number of organs, and may also suppress immunity.

In their mycelium form, the yeasts may grow completely through the
intestinal lining creating an opening for undigested food to enter the bloodstream (hence the term "leaky gut"). This presence of undigested food in the
bloodstream is thought to trigger allergic reactions to foods. Yeasts are also
said to cause headaches, depression, menstrual difficulties, and autoimmune
problems. There are a number of tests for this condition, many of questionable accuracy. Often a sugar-free, yeast-free diet is prescribed along with the
use of oral acidophillus to add beneficial bacteria to the gut. People with
conditions unresponsive to these measures may be prescribed antifungal
medications such as Nystatin that kill yeast in the gut, or Nizoral, Diflucan,
or Sporanox, which are absorbed into the general system to eliminate yeast
in blood and internal organs. The anticandida diet is summarized in chapter
five, and suggestions are offered for further reading.

Carbon Monoxide Poisoning

Albert Donnay (1999) of MCS Referral and Resources believes that carbon monoxide may be a causal factor in MCS, and has noted numerous
descriptions of MCS-like symptoms dating back to Edgar Allen Poe. Donnay
believes that historical cases of MCS may have been caused by illuminating
gas poisoning. In fact, some physicians are now experimenting with oxygen
treatment in order to clear the body of carbon monoxide.

Additional Brain Changes

Chemicals certainly affect brain activity, function, and even structure. Brain activity can be measured by an electroencephalogram (EEG) where electrodes are attached to the person's head, and brain waves are measured either in the resting state, or when "evoked" by some stimulus (sound, chemical, etc.). People with MCS have demonstrated abnormal EEGs in the resting state and abnormal evoked potentials (purposefully elicited in the lab) during chemical exposure (Dudley 1993).

Those who believe that MCS is caused by changes in the brain often cite the research done with people who had large occupational solvent exposures. People exposed to solvents have demonstrated slower brain waves (which means slower cognitive processing) (Morrow, Steinhauer, and Hodgson 1992); decreased activity on a positron-emmission test (PET) scan (a measure of brain activity); problems with learning, memory, attention; and indicators of psychological problems (Morrow, Ryan, Hodgson and Robin 1990). In one study, painters were shown to have more neurological problems in areas such as mood, concentration, sleep, and fatigue than did people in the study's control group (Hooisma, Hanninen, Emmen, and Kulig 1994).

Tests that show how the brain is working, e.g., brain wave tests (EEG), measures of metabolism (PET scans), and blood flow (Single Photon Emission Computed Tomography (SPECT) scans), can indicate problems even when tests that measure brain shape/structure (i.e., magnetic resonance imaging [MRI] and computerized tomography [CT] scans) do not. Therefore, a SPECT scan is more likely to provide evidence of brain damage/dysfunction in people with MCS than is an MRI or CT scan, although some people with MCS do show abnormal MRI results as well (Heuser, Wojdani, and Heuser 1992).

Psychological Theories

There are researchers and writers who believe that MCS is a psychological illness, although they are in the minority and don't seem to understand the experience of people who have MCS at all. I have included these theories not because I believe they should be taken seriously, but because familiarity with them reduces the likelihood that they can be used against you effectively (forewarned is forearmed). (See chapter nine for a critique of these theories.)

Psychological and Behavioral Conditioning

MCS patients are sometimes said to blame chemicals for the angst of modern civilization as well as for their illness. Brodsky (1983) believes that media attention to toxins contributes to patients' heightened health concerns or "ecofear." He says, for example:

> [U]ncertainty about the presence of toxic substances in the workplace makes intoxication in the workplace a likely projective target for those who feel unwell and in whom physical illness cannot be diagnosed. It is an explanation that places the cause and the responsibility in the environment and avoids the stigma of mental illness that they fear (p. 463).

In some cases, avoidance of chemicals is seen as leading to agoraphobia since people are advised by doctors to avoid crowds, malls, and other places where they would encounter perfumes and chemical vapors. Black (1996) describes a patient who developed reactions that included anxiety, fear, shortness of breath, and dizziness in places such as malls, which would remit soon after she left. This patient is seen by Black as having behaviorally conditioned herself to avoid malls. In other words, she came to believe that she was sensitive to odors, avoided these, and thus conditioned herself to have a more and more restricted life. Black suggests that treatment should include desensitization where "the patient is gradually given increasing exposure to odors and fumes in typical home and work situations."

Odor Conditioning

Odor conditioning is related to behavioral conditioning, but it is able to actually train physiological responses. To understand odor conditioning, you must understand classical conditioning in psychology. As an example, if I gave you an avocado, and every time you tried to eat it, I whacked you upside the head, you would eventually get nervous when you tried to eat an avocado. Why? The avocado did not cause the knock on the head. I did. But the avocado would become associated with the knock on the head. A fear of avocados would be a conditioned response to being hit whenever you tried to eat one.

Simon (1994) points out that animal studies show that physical processes, such as immune response, can be classically conditioned. The proponents of odor conditioning believe that people with MCS may have had one experience that caused *true* symptoms in response to a chemical, but that *future* reactions to the low levels of the same chemical are a conditioned (learned) response to the odor of the chemical and not to any harmful properties of the substance. When repeated encounters with the odor provoke symptoms, and the response has become strengthened, the person has been classically conditioned to experience symptoms when exposed to the odor. *Generalization* occurs when the conditioned response takes place to stimuli that are similar to, but not identical with the original stimulus. One common example of this is seen when assault victims come to fear people who resemble their attackers. The same model applied to chemical sensitivity posits that someone who has an initial reaction to diesel fuel eventually will come to react to all petrochemicals. Proponents of the odor conditioning theory, such as Bolla-Wilson, Wilson, and Bleecker (1988), believe that this explains why people with MCS respond to more and more chemicals over time.

Preexisting Psychological Vulnerability— Anxiety and Depression

Donald Black (1996) has said:

> . . . many individuals who receive a diagnosis of EI (environmental illness) suffer from common emotional disorders, such as depression, anxiety, and somatization, and that these illnesses are, in fact, responsible for the high level of symptoms of psychological distress that they exhibit; in these cases, a diagnosis of EI represents a misdiagnosis.

Simon, Katon, and Sparks (1990) found that plastics workers who developed sensitivities tended to have a history of anxiety, depression, and unexplained physical symptoms, but no current psychological symptoms. They concluded that "development of environmental illness related more to an underlying trait of symptom amplification and prior psychological distress than to current psychiatric symptoms or diagnoses." In other words, previous psychological distress, particularly depression or anxiety, is seen as predisposing people to develop MCS, which is considered to be a different manifestation of psychological illness.

Symptom Amplification

Part of the preexisting pathology for MCS is sometimes said to be symptom amplification. People are seen as amplifying (or exaggerating) any negative sensations or as being more disturbed than others by noxious odors. Simon (1994) says chemically sensitive patients may exaggerate symptoms from low-level exposure, or normal subtle sensory phenomena, and then attribute those sensations to chemical exposures.

Negative Affectivity

People high in negative affectivity experience more negative moods and emotions, such as anxiety, dissatisfaction, and pessimism. They are more introspective and focus more on negative aspects in regard to themselves and other people. Regardless of health status, people with high negative affectivity report more symptoms than those with low negative affectivity. They pay more attention to their bodies, worry more about symptoms and, because of this, are seen as being at risk for MCS (Pennebaker 1994).

Personality Disorders

Personality disorders are a category of mental illness and are seen as being long-term exaggerated personality styles. They are not generally understood as intermittent like acute bouts of anxiety and depression, but are said to appear in late adolescence and to continue throughout life. Personality disorders are seen as being difficult to treat and requiring long-term psychological care. Black (1996) labeled three-quarters of a sample of twenty-three people with MCS as having at least one personality disorder.

Somatization Disorder

Another viewpoint is that people with MCS are somaticizers, that is, people who project their psychological problems onto their bodies and experience them as physical symptoms. The idea of somatization has its roots in Freud's work. He coined the term "somatic compliance" (cooperation from the body) and said that if a person had somatic compliance, they could place their mental symptoms and conflicts onto the body and then develop hysteria rather than another mental illness.

People who are diagnosed as having somatization disorder are said to have a number of complaints for which no physical cause can be found. Complaints begin before age thirty, persist long term, and impair functioning. At some time during the course of the disturbance, the person must have four pain symptoms, two gastrointestinal symptoms, one sexual symptom, and one pseudoneurological symptom, according to the *Diagnostic and Statistical Manual of the American Psychiatric Association (DSM IV)*. Diagnosticians are ten times more likely to give this diagnosis to women than to men, and four times more likely to give it to African-Americans than to Caucasians (Nevid, Rothus, and Greene 1997).

In a culture that generally discounts women and denies decent health care to minority people, there may be all sorts of biases operating here. Donnay (1997) has cited studies that show that MCS symptoms have only slight overlap with somatization disorder criteria.

Childhood Trauma

Another writer, J. C. Selner (1988), believes that symptoms in response to odors are "traceable to identifiable psychotrauma frequently experienced in childhood, but often continuing into adult life." Selner says that psychotrauma affects more women than men and that the coping mechanisms that were developed for keeping the trauma at bay tend to deteriorate between the ages of thirty and fifty. Hence, the large numbers of middle-aged women who are diagnosed with MCS.

This is refuted by population studies, such as those done by Meggs, Dunn, Bloch, et al. (1996), where MCS was found to be fairly evenly distributed by both gender and race. Selner and Staudenmayer (1992) describe "universal reactors" as fragile personalities who feel unsafe in the world due to early childhood trauma. People are seen as having repressed (unknowingly buried) or suppressed (consciously placed out of awareness) memories of childhood abuse. As adults, these individuals are left with depression, anxiety, and poor coping skills; they project the trauma onto external factors, such as chemicals.

Thought Patterns/Cognitions

The premiere issue of the *Journal of Health Psychology* published an article on MCS that said that all of the cognitions/thoughts of people with MCS revolve around chemicals (Gomez, Schvaneveldt, and Staudenmayer 1996):

> Psychologically, EI/MCS patients differ from normal patients in personality, attitudes, affect and, most relevant to this research, strength of belief about toxicogenic attribution. We hypothesized that if psychosomatic illness is mediated by belief, then methods for representing beliefs should show systematic differences between psychosomatic patients and other populations (p. 119).

There were many sophisticated schematics, but the bottom line was that the thought processes of people with MCS have erroneously placed chemicals in a more central position than they belong or than they have in the schemas of "normal people."

Controversy Affects Treatment Protocols

There is tremendous controversy around the nature of MCS, which ends up as vehement disagreement regarding its treatment. Practitioners who treat MCS as a *physiological* disorder prescribe chemical avoidance to prevent further deterioration in their patients' health. Those treating MCS as a *psychological* disorder advise treating the underlying psychological problem, discourage chemical avoidance, and advise altering patients' beliefs that toxicants are making them ill. These practitioners have been criticized on ethical grounds by physicians who treat MCS as a physiological problem (Levin and Byers 1992; Ross 1992; Ziem 1992). Ziem (1992) reported that several of her patients were made worse by following advice not to worry about chemical exposures. Practitioners who believe that MCS is psychological in nature criticize avoidance for worsening social isolation and reducing mobility and productivity in people with MCS.

Levin and Byers (1992) believe that MCS has a psychological "overlay" that can distract health providers from the physical nature of the condition. We also know that chemical injury can cause psychological symptoms. For example, Morrow, Ryan, Goldstein, et al. (1989) showed personality disturbances in solvent-exposed workers, and Dager, Holland, Cowley, et al. (1987) describe panic disorder resulting from exposure to organic solvents. Heuser, Wojdani, and Heuser (1992) note that patients with systemic lupus erythematosus often exhibit psychiatric symptoms; they believe that any psychiatric symptoms exhibited in MCS may be neurologically based. In an attempt to separate physiological from psychological indicators, Bell, Peterson, and Schwartz (1995) examined self-reported illness from chemical odors in a nonclinical population and found that people who became ill from chemicals tended to have close family members who had physiological—but not psychological—illnesses. (See chapter nine for more information on the psychological symptoms as well as criticisms of the psychological research.)

Chapter Three

How Lives Are Affected by MCS

With all the medical controversy about whether MCS is "real" or not, the people who suffer have been left to fend for themselves. People with MCS are falling through the cracks and becoming an "invisible" disabled minority whose lives are no longer compatible with any of our medical, educational, or social institutions. For some, the suffering is immense. Others, who are more mildly affected, are able to make minor or moderate changes that allow them to live more or less "normal" lives (Gibson, Cheavers, and Warren 1996).

The story of those who are falling through the cracks must be told for several reasons. First, it is important to label the suffering and thus raise awareness about this hidden minority in the hope of drawing support for those who are suffering. It also is important for higher functioning people with MCS to understand the importance of preserving their current level of functioning. Knowing that you may become totally disabled without chemical avoidance and proper self-care can cut through denial and may help you to take your condition seriously.

Also, a commentary on our society has to be made when it permits a substantial portion of its people to become disabled from toxicants to preserve the economic status quo. This chapter discusses the many impacts on everyday life that result from having MCS, including the areas of work, finances, housing, family planning, public access, and quality of life issues.

Although it can be depressing to think about these issues, this introduction might be an excellent summary to share with therapists and with friends and family members who are trying to understand what you are up against. If you are already too familiar with the difficulties of MCS patients, you might want to skip to chapter four and begin working on cleaning up your home.

Another point should be made about the impact MSC has on daily life: The research and reports on the difficulties of living with MCS are very real and, for some, are devastating. However, the summary statistics are just that—summaries of information from many people. The statistics do not predict anything about any *particular* person. There are many people with MCS who function well in spite of the condition. They maintain relationships with friends and lovers, have satisfactory jobs, live in safe houses, and feel satisfied with their lives. As you will see in chapter fourteen, some even believe that having MCS has contributed substantially to their personal and spiritual growth. Therefore, keep in mind when you read the information in this chapter that it does not necessarily predict anything about your present or future experience.

What Happens When You Are Chemically Injured?

There is no aspect of life that is totally immune to the impact of MCS. People with MCS report that it affects their work, finances, housing, physical access, social relationships, and future plans. The remainder of this chapter reviews these changes. (See chapter eleven for more on social relationships.)

On the Job

Depending on your level of chemical sensitivity, work is likely to be very affected when you develop MCS. People with mild or moderate sensitivities often can make minor adjustments and continue to work. As a rule, however, there is some stress involved in obtaining the needed accommodations in the workplace. Often, people who are very sensitive are unable (at least temporarily) to continue in their present jobs. This is especially true if the person was first injured in the workplace. In my research, more than half of those who reported an initial known exposure, which damaged their health, said that it occurred in the workplace. Fewer than one-third of Phase I participants were still working outside of the home. Unfortunately, three-quarters of those who *had* been working had to quit their jobs to avoid further chemical exposures.

For example, one woman who worked as an advertising consultant often had to conduct her business in office buildings, graphic arts departments, and printing plants. With the onset of MCS, she became reactive to "almost everything" she "ate, breathed, or touched." Having to avoid the chemicals in print shops and offices meant losing all of her clients. Her computer and electronic devices had to be removed from her home as well; the only electronic appliance she was able to tolerate was a very small, old black-and-white TV. All her attempts to keep working failed.

In another instance, a man went from working as a chemist with a large salary to being disabled, unable to work, homeless, powerless, and ostracized by his family. Fortunately, he did find a safe apartment eventually. Only about one-fifth of Phase I participants who worked were working under conditions they considered safe for their health.

Trying to avoid chemicals in the workplace can lead to increased stress in relationships with co-workers because they may not be cooperative when asked to discontinue using fragrances or other personal care products that are sources of difficulty for those with MCS. Eventually the consequences for the MCS worker are major, as they were for this woman:

> "Working near smokers, perfume users, in moldy, dusty areas, and the refusal of everyone involved to understand or moderate behavior has determined my life course. [This has been] very unsatisfactory to me and has left me destitute financially. Limping along, struggling from exposure to exposure, from job to job, has created an insurmountable obstacle to my accomplishing what I wished I could carry out."
>
> —Sixty-two-year-old woman with MCS
> since childhood

Many respondents were devastated by the thought of giving up work in a culture that so emphasizes "productivity." One woman with MCS said:

> "I have found it very difficult to hold up without the outside reinforcement that the working environment provided me. Without the reinforcement that I got at work, I began to feel resentful and even worthless."

Consequently, some people pushed themselves far beyond what their bodies could endure, unable to accept the loss of employment. One woman with MCS said:

> "I was interviewing for new jobs and wondering at each interview how I was going to work in this particular building when my body was going into spasms. I was having trouble breathing, and I was

having trouble tolerating the place for the hour or two of the interview. In today's lingo, I still hadn't 'gotten it.'"

It seems that chemical injury can occur in almost any job context, although homemakers, clerical workers, students, teachers, nurses, and social workers were most heavily represented in my study. (See Appendix A for the occupations of Phase III participants at the time of chemical injury.)

The accommodations that they were able to obtain at work differed. Obtaining the necessary accommodations mostly depended upon the sensitivity of the employer. Some people received no help and were even ridiculed for asking. Others were allowed to work in safer parts of buildings, at off-hours, or partly at home. Some were even able to create ways to earn money at home. For example, one woman did child care for children whose clothes were washed in safe soaps without fabric softener. Some started small businesses relating to MCS, such as consulting; or they made or sold useful products like masks, supplements, purifiers, or other chemically safe items.

Finances

Multiple chemical sensitivity has been described as a "rich person's disease" because of the tremendous financial demands it places on people. The need to avoid chemicals often means replacing clothing, furniture, bedding, even homes, as well as purchasing purifiers and nutritional supplements. Conventional medical care for MCS at this point is seldom described as helpful and often as downright harmful (see chapter six), and alternatives are often not covered by insurance (see chapter seven). So, for the sufferer, just as income may be declining, costs are escalating.

Income declines drastically for anyone who can no longer engage in full-time work. Although *household* annual income for my research sample averaged about $35,000, average *personal* income for participants was just a little more than poverty level (about $12,000). People suffered sharp declines in their income after losing jobs, and much of their income after leaving work was from disability payments. People with partners who had good incomes suffered the least as they were able to stop work without completely devastating their finances. Others pushed themselves to keep working in spite of their illness because their families depended on them. One man described dragging himself to work to support his family, and spending virtually all of his off time recovering from exposures. Some people were caught in a downward financial spiral and were afraid of becoming homeless. One woman lamented, "It has been very hard on my children. They cannot understand why we don't have what we used to when I worked or why we've lost our car, cable TV, and next will be the telephone. It's worse for the thirteen-year-old."

Those who became sensitized later in life seemed to suffer less financial devastation because they had time to build up some savings. One woman explained:

"I came down with MCS later in life so we were able to live a great lifestyle most of our married life. For this I am grateful—I feel I missed very little and am not terribly discontented staying home. We have a lovely home, and more than adequate friends—good friends. Although once in a while I feel sad to have [MCS]. Our HEAL support group has been a lifesaver."

People who are chemically injured while young never have a chance to build up a financial cushion, and thus are hit very hard. It is important for those with MCS to consider this information when planning for their future. For example, the $10,000 you may spend on a new therapy must to be considered in the context of your overall financial health. Consider whether you have a large enough nest egg to experiment so that you won't be financially devastated if the therapy doesn't work.

Housing

People try to avoid chemical exposures by replacing household items, such as carpets, formaldehyde board, plastics, and other items. But many are unable to afford these replacements. Consequently, some people reported either continuing to live in unsafe conditions, or spending their life savings redoing their homes and purchasing air purifiers or other necessities. Some spent almost $28,000 to clean up their homes, and only two-fifths were living in homes rated as safe. Some respondents reported being unable to tolerate *any* traditional housing due to chemicals used in construction, and they lived in very unusual conditions.

For example, one respondent had lived in her horse trailer for a year. Others described being homeless or living in their cars, in RVs, in one purified room in their house, or in tents. Many did stints on their friends' porches or in the homes of their parents. In Phase II, two-thirds of the participants had lived in highly unusual conditions at some point to avoid chemical exposures. It seems MCS brings out the survival instinct and forces one to be unusually resourceful.

"I live in a tent all summer (May to November). I can tolerate [temperatures] to twenty degrees, so [I] stay as long as possible. In winter, I have [a] room that only has a bed, wood floors, and no heat for my safe room."

—Forty-seven-year-old man with
MCS for five years

Many people wrote to me asking if I knew of safe housing. I know of none. People with MCS are trying to find niches for themselves with very little help from our society. Many have already fallen through the cracks, and others fear that they will too. Probably no one has brought this home to us more so than Rhonda Zwillinger (1997) in her photo-essay of homeless people with MCS entitled, *The Dispossessed: Living with Multiple Chemical Sensitivities.*

Although there are some projects on the table for creating safe housing, this is extremely difficult because people vary so much in regard to their sensitivities. Constructing housing that is safe for all people with MCS is almost impossible. Some people move to the country to avoid city industries only to face agricultural chemicals. Others move to suburbs and then must confront their neighbors' lawn chemicals. Renting an apartment is difficult because you cannot control chemical use by your neighbors or the proprietor, and thus may be exposed to smoke, propane cooking, herbicides or pesticides, and fabric softeners. Some people were fortunate to be able to construct safe houses with some buffer against others' pollution, but it takes considerable resources to do this. Some moved almost continually in search of a clean area only to find that pollution is virtually everywhere.

On the other hand, moving into a safer setting helped a lot of people considerably. One woman had suffered a series of environmental insults including beauty school, and formaldehyde exposures in multiple settings. She had endured two ineffective sinus surgeries prescribed for chemically induced nose, head, and shoulder pain. She wrote, in Phase II of my research: "I try to be positive but there were only sixty days from January through November that I was without pain in 1993." A move to a cleaner area and discontinuing a job with formaldehyde exposure set her on a healthier course. By Phase III of the follow-up study, she was traveling in a converted van to visit family (13,000 miles in one year) and said, "I am very lucky to be as well as I am. I don't have 'the old pain' anymore. But I do have to be on guard for smells every day."

I believe that housing is *the* single most important issue regarding MCS. A safe zone can help prevent further health deterioration, and provide a place to detoxify after exposures received from the outside community. In my estimation, even research is not as crucial as safe housing. After all, it already seems clear that environmental contamination causes illness. Do we have to wait until we know exactly how the body breaks down in laboratory animals before we allow people to live in safe homes?

Family Planning

In some cases, MCS had a profound influence on family planning. For the more than half of the women in Phase II of my study who did not have children, MCS was the reason for their childlessness. Reasons included the inaccessibility of medical offices, poor health, financial problems, and fear of passing on MCS to a child.

Public Access

Being housebound to some degree was a common experience for people with MCS. Some research respondents were able to construct or arrange safe housing, but then felt like prisoners in their homes while trying to avoid outside exposures. Some respondents reported becoming ill from taking walks outside their homes due to outdoor chemicals, such as petrochemical exhausts and pesticides. A number of people reported staying inside to avoid their neighbors' use of pesticides and herbicides, paints, fabric softeners in dryers, construction chemicals, or other contaminants.

At the time of our study, 8 percent of all respondents were totally housebound. Even if the immediate area around the safe house was safe, venturing into the larger community was risky. Churches, movies, malls, and restaurants were off-limits for many respondents. Almost half of the sample said they were unsafe in any public areas in which perfume was likely to be encountered; and many reported being so sensitive to personal care products that they were unable to have perfumed visitors in their homes. The following comments were fairly typical in regard to public access:

> "I am extremely limited, I can drive on unheavily traveled roads with my car air cleaner. I can get myself to the doctor and to food shop. Not much else. I have a recovery period of up to two days after exposure, for example, to perfumes. I have to use a mask, pick times and places very carefully, and be ready to leave or change plans at any time."
>
> —Forty-seven-year-old woman with
> MCS for four years

> "I have learned I can't go everywhere I want to go or do everything I want to do so I pick and choose carefully. Before a special outing I rest up for a few days, enjoy the event, then plan a couple of rest days afterwards. I know full well in advance what reactions to expect. I don't do anything that would result in serious harm. I used to sit at home (afraid to go out), but realized this was only making me worse emotionally and physically. Because of my 'outings' there is a little more fatigue—but it's *happy* fatigue. I no longer feel trapped or controlled by this illness. I enjoy the quality—not the quantity—of outings."
>
> —Forty-four-year-old woman with
> MCS for eight years

Personal Distress

Many respondents reported that they had experienced severe stress and trauma because of the life changes and losses that took place as a result of their chemical sensitivities. Many were living without necessities, such as housing, medical care, and public access. Others had access to necessities, but reported other kinds of losses, such as career advancement, education, travel, hobbies, and community involvement. Further personal distress was reported as a result of the lack of attention and concern for this health problem by the medical profession and the general public. For some, the stresses had become overwhelming. One-fifth of the Phase I respondents had seriously considered suicide, 8 percent had made a suicide plan, and 3 percent had actually attempted it. The following quotations describe severe suffering as a result of severe loss:

> "Toxic chemicals [have] ruined [my] life . . . Plus [losing my] husband, social life, [and] inheritance. I'm going to end up alone in a nursing home with rheumatoid arthritis and chemical sensitivity. All my friends and family are busy with their own lives."
>
> —Woman with MCS for thirty-five years

> "My dreams have been shattered. Life has merely become a matter of survival, as if I'm in a prison camp. My self-esteem has been damaged due to hostility and ridicule from co-workers and management. I was formerly optimistic and confident in my ability to overcome obstacles. Years of poor health and increasing persistent obstacles have made me sad and bitter . . . the future is bleak. As my health worsens and money continues to dwindle, I fear I will end up with only one option."
>
> —Thirty-six-year-old man with MCS
> for six years

Quality of Life Measures

Instruments commonly used to assess the quality of life demonstrated the suffering of respondents in all phases of my study. Note that these are not measures of psychopathology, but variables associated with happiness and fulfillment. We gathered measures of hope, social support, life satisfaction, and disability-induced dysfunction, and the sample scored very low in comparison with people who were sampled in other research.

I think that if any other more "legitimized" group scored this low on *any* of these variables, it would be cause for great alarm among helpers and researchers. But the MCS population, being invisible and delegitimized, does not draw support. These measures may give you an indication of how much this population is suffering. (Of course, most of you already know that.) And remember, again, these are means (averages) and, as such, obscure the fact that some people actually scored very well on some or *all* of the measures. (See Appendix A for published articles and for more detail about the quality of life research.)

Hope

With *legitimized* illness, such as cancer or diabetes, there is the understanding that it is important for a person to maintain some sense of personal well-being despite the illness. With the aim of extending this concern to MCS, my students and I measured the hope of Phase I respondents. During the study, we used the Herth Hope Scale (HHS) (Herth 1991), which is a respected instrument used to measure hope as an index of well-being. We found that MCS respondents had lower levels of hope than several other populations tested by Kay Herth.

Levels of hope in MCS respondents surpassed the hope level only of elderly widowed people. Interestingly, a higher level of hope was associated with a perceived safer home. This information provides support for the instructions to clean up your home environment (see chapter four). Younger people had lower levels of hope than did older people. Adjusting to the loss of lifetime ambitions and the inability to become financially secure may be more difficult than finding out later in life that you have a disability. (For more detail about the hope study, see Gibson 1999).

Social Support

One important area of study in relation to any chronic health problem is that of social support. We know that for the chronically ill, lower levels of social support are associated with more symptoms and greater mortality. A high level of social support is a good predictor of psychological well-being. Phase I respondents scored lower than healthy people on Part II of the Personal Resource Questionnaire 85 (PRQ85) (Weinert 1987), which measures how much support the test takers feel they have. They scored slightly lower than a sample of women with diabetes who were tested by a fellow researcher, and quite a bit lower than a sample of people with multiple sclerosis. (For more detail about social support, see chapter eleven, and Gibson, Cheavens, and Warren 1998).

Life Satisfaction

During Phase III, we used three popular tests that measure satisfaction with life. MCS respondents scored much lower than did medical outpatients, elderly respondents, and people with other chronic illnesses and handicaps, and residents in all countries except for China. (See Gibson, White, and Rice 1997 for more details.)

The Impact of Illness on Daily Functioning

The Sickness Impact Profile (SIP) (Bergner, Bobbit, Kressel, et al., 1976; Bergner, Bobbitt, Pollard, et al. 1976) looks at respondents' assessment of the limitations in daily functioning caused by illness. Phase IV respondents' scores were somewhat alarming in that they were indicative of more dysfunction than is experienced with a large number of other illnesses. MCS respondents had particular trouble in the categories of work, alertness, and recreation and pastimes. Considerable impairment was also shown on the measures for Sleep and Rest, Social Interaction, Home Management, Emotional Behavior, and Mobility. (For more information, see Gibson, Rice, Stables, et al. 1997).

Limitations and Thwarted Goals

The severe limitations and losses that people with MCS often experience are two good reasons for such low scores on quality of life measures. Rippere (1983) showed that people with allergies reported substantial limitation and impairment in their quality of life, and it was expected that people with chemical sensitivities would report even more impairment. We asked Phase I respondents, "Is there any goal or activity that you have really wanted to pursue but haven't been able to because of chemical sensitivity?" Responses here included the categories of work, education, hobbies, travel, visiting family, and attending church. Remember, access to public buildings is contingent on the ability to tolerate exposure to smoke, petrochemicals, perfumes, and pesticides. Because MCS respondents cannot be near these chemicals without serious health consequences, their work and educational lives are jeopardized.

One-quarter of all participants in Phase I had their education interrupted or denied due to chemical sensitivity. One-third had to discontinue their involvement with their hobbies (e.g., painting) because of their inability to use artistic materials. Others missed travel, socializing, and visiting family. Respondents' comments were indicative of the severe and even catastrophic impact of coping with their sensitivities. One person wrote, "It has been my 'goal' to be self-reliant, but this appears to be impossible." Another wrote, "I have endured losses and heartbreak to degrees that have nearly devastated me." Still another said, "I've stayed out of (romantic) relationships because I didn't think anyone would understand my needs. I've not had children because of this illness. These have been hard [decisions] to deal with. Sometimes I grieve for the many losses I have had; it never seems to end."

Clearly, as a group, people with MCS do not have access to the benefits of normal work or social lives. Rippere (1983) pointed out that her respondents (many of whom were allergic to foods) missed out on many occasions that provided others with pleasure and socializing. Chemically sensitive people miss out not only on pleasure, but on the necessities for independent living. When people are unable to work, further their education, or enter public buildings, serious quality-of-life issues are raised.

Neurological symptoms, for some, added to people's isolation and were cause for embarrassment. Although one woman expressed anxiety regarding what others might think of her, she explained that those who know her well understand her slurred speech, unsteady gait, and lessened cognitive abilities. Cumulative losses of people with MCS were more than most any "normal" person would be able to bear without experiencing severe distress.

> "I don't think about goals anymore. For the past thirteen years, I have had hopes that were destroyed. I used to work. . . . I counseled people. I gave up my job, used to direct groups at home, but slowly I couldn't be with people. I moved . . . and started groups again, but I got sick. I loved cats—had to give them up. I joined groups. I gave that up. Each time my world got smaller, I cried and mourned my loss. Then, I accepted my life and made the best of what I have left. I don't think about tomorrow. I'm grateful for each moment that I survive. I'm overjoyed for each 'good day' when I'm able to accomplish something I want that day."

> —A woman with long-term MCS

It is important to understand that personal distress in the face of chronic illness/injury is normal and understandable. (See chapter eight for more about adjusting to chronic illness.) Sometimes goals became simple and survival-related. One person's goal, for example, was "not to get migraine headaches that incapacitate me for days." It may be that for a time your goals will be that basic; but for most people, this is temporary.

Not one respondent in any phase of my research gave up easily. People struggle against insurmountable odds to better themselves. The accusations that those with MCS are experiencing "secondary gain" or somehow "milking the system" are ludicrous when one listens to descriptions of effort and loss as in this account of one woman's attempt to attend college:

> "I was diagnosed with chronic fatigue syndrome and again was told it was temporary and to continue with my plans to go to college. My doctors told me I was doing better even though it now took me an entire day to do a half day's work. I could no longer do yard work or cook meals, thought processing was extremely erratic and I was having difficulty walking. I actually attended one class.

The first half was a struggle to keep up with mentally, and the last half was just a blur. Fortunately, I had arranged for someone to pick me up after this class. I was disoriented upon leaving the building and, after walking in circles, finally reached the prearranged place to be picked up. It was extremely difficult for me to accept that not only would I not be going to college, I was unable to do anything else. I knew that I was getting worse, but had so wanted and hoped to make this change I believed the doctors."

—Woman with MCS for eighteen years

Fortunately, almost everyone had some blessings in their lives. Some were almost totally housebound, but had loving and supportive families. Some were ostracized by family, but had found support and strength through helping others. Some could still use computers; some could leave their homes. People seemed to take, use, and develop whatever resources they could to make some semblance of a reasonable life. Some described riding horses, gardening, writing books, heading support groups or organizations, supporting others with MCS, writing poetry, and starting MCS-related businesses. (See chapter fourteen and Appendix C for further resources along these lines.)

Every aspect of one's life can be impacted by MCS. For many, the condition is more of a hurricane than a redirecting wind. It takes resourcefulness, patience, and fortitude to confront the challenge of MCS. The remaining chapters in this book are designed to help you with this undertaking.

PART II

PHYSICAL ISSUES

Chapter Four

Making Your
Environment Safe

If you are newly diagnosed as chemically sensitive, or are living in a home that still needs some cleanup, probably the most important thing you can do to protect yourself is to reduce your chemical exposures. By making a safe haven for yourself, you will suffer *fewer* reactions and have a safe place to clear out your body from exposures that occur outside of your home.

This chapter will help you clean up your home environment quickly so you can function better and so you can avoid the MCS tendency to develop more chemical sensitivities. The chapter does not cover every safe product available, but you can go for quite a while using a few safe cleaning products, personal care items, and clothes. (See Appendix B for product sources.)

When you feel better and have the time, you can explore a wider variety of options. Keep in mind there are hundreds of products on the market that are designed more to make money than to help you with your health *regardless of what advertisers say*. Michael Lax (1998) warns about "entrepreneurial activities without patient welfare in mind" (p. 734). For example, any product rubbed into the skin is absorbed through the skin and can be detected in the blood in minutes. (This is how nicotine and estrogen patches work.) Therefore, you need to exercise particular caution with personal care products.

Be sure to investigate all products before purchasing them. The rule "Buyer beware" applies as much to health food stores and alternative mail-order catalogs as it does to mainstream products. In fact, health food stores are becoming mainstream; large companies are buying out the smaller ones, and more and more toxic products are appearing on their shelves.

It is very difficult to market truly safe products because most very clean products are made by small companies, don't have a long shelf life, and the ingredients must be purchased in small quantities. Because distributors want to earn a high profit, it is virtually impossible for most small companies to market through the usual distributor channels. Note: When new products are introduced in distributors' catalogs, no ingredients are listed and busy buyers may assume products are "natural." Products with toxic ingredients commonly are given names with "earth" and "natural" in them and are marketed as though they were chemically or environmentally safe. This practice is called "green-washing." My friends who own a health food store learn the ingredients in their products the same way you do—by walking around their store and reading labels.

In the Home: The Big Stuff

Some of the accommodations that are needed to make a home chemically safe are so extensive that they may involve structural change and may be so costly that it becomes necessary to move. You will have to assess your location and house structure before you can decide if your home is safe enough to not further jeopardize your health.

Can This House Be Saved?

The following questions may help you to sort out what works from what doesn't:

Outside Your Home

- Is your home located near polluting traffic or industry fumes that will make it impossible to go outside or to open your windows, even if the inside of the house is made safer?

- If you are gas-sensitive, are you subject to neighbors' heating fuel smells, gas from propane cookers or dryers, or fumes from neighbors who do their own auto work?

- Do close neighbors use lawn treatments that will expose you to dangerous herbicides and pesticides?

- Does the local county do aerial spraying for mosquitoes, gypsy moths, or other insects?

- Is your home downwind or downstream from any large polluting agencies most of the time? (Wind directions vary, but they have common patterns.)

- If electromagnetic frequency (EMF) radiation is a problem (or even if it isn't), is your house near large sources of EMF? That is, are there high-tension electrical wires or power stations close by? You can acquire a meter to measure magnetic fields for both outside and inside sources. (See Appendix B for product sources.)

Inside Your Home

- Is your home heated with gas or oil? If so, is the cost of a changeover to electric heating worth it because the house is otherwise safe?

- Is your house so full of formaldehyde-offgassing materials, such as particleboard, that you could never adequately reduce the emissions? Both plywood and particleboard have formaldehyde in their contents. Particleboard is a bigger concern because it contains both a larger percentage of formaldehyde-containing glue, and a more toxic form of formaldehyde (i.e., urea formaldehyde).

  The highest levels of offgas occur in the first year after construction; but offgassing may continue for a number of years. If you live in a prefabricated or mobile home, chances are that particleboard makes up much of your flooring, external walls, and roof panels. However, you can seal cabinets, paneling, and other particleboard with sealants made to prevent offgassing from porous surfaces, such as mortar, plywood, concrete and others. If you can tolerate the product, it may be worth sealing some of the surfaces that are offgassing (See Appendix B for product sources.)

- Does your house have a stubborn mold problem that cannot be remedied? For example, an old house with a lot of shade or a wet basement will expose you to more mold.

If none of the problems is insurmountable, then it may be worth cleaning up your current home. Note: If a problem really is not fixable, it's better to face it and change location than to continue living in a place you are attached to, which is making you ill. It is imperative to avoid a further decline in your health, and denial will not serve you well here. It is much easier to prevent further decline than to recover from more serious injury. Sometimes it can be a judgment call, but we usually know when we are kidding ourselves. On the other hand, relocation, either locally or long-distance, should be well thought out as it is full of snares.

The following suggestions are some of the more permanent kinds of changes you may need to make to clean up your home:

Petrochemicals: Appliances and Heat

Appliances. If your home has natural gas or propane appliances, such as a stove, dryer, or water heater, you will want to replace them with electric ones. Although some environmentally aware people advocate the use of gas because it is cheaper than electricity, health effects also must be factored into the cost. Gases are sensitizers and rank high on the list of chemicals to which people with MCS react. As early as the 1950s, Dr. Theron Randolph (Randolph and Moss 1982) discovered that people have allergic-like adverse reactions to petrochemicals, including gases and heating oil.

There is also evidence that women who use gas stoves have more respiratory problems than those who use electric ones (Jarvis, Chinn, Luczynska, et al. 1996). The nitrogen dioxide from cooking gas is a home pollutant. Although you should probably replace your appliances with electric ones, you will have to consider the cost involved. (And for some, EMFs may be a problem. An acquaintance has tested electric stoves with an EMF meter and found them to be very high.) You can consider buying used appliances, but washers and dryers in particular may be problematic because of lingering odors from previously used fabric softeners and detergents.

Note that when constructing his inpatient unit for people with chemical sensitivities, Randolph found that some patients did not become cleared of symptoms until the wood floors were replaced, as the floors had absorbed petrochemicals from previous gas heating. But certainly you would be reducing your exposures tremendously by replacing appliances.

Heat. A larger obstacle is heat. If you have forced air oil or gas heating, combustion products are entering your house air. Some of the newer heating units are self-contained in a sealed combustion unit, with the heating fuel located in a sealed chamber and vented to the outside. With the sealed combustion unit, the air that heats your house does not mix with the fuel source. If the unit is vented to the outside, then you may be able to keep petrochemicals out of your indoor air altogether.

Some people put their heat source in a garage or other separate building. In both scenarios, you still have petrochemical emissions very close to you, and you will be exposed to them when you go outside. If you use diesel oil, it is 95 percent as heavy as air and will rise very slowly. Propane is actually heavier than air and, therefore, lingers in low areas unless blown away by the wind.

Without adequate breezes, propane will remain around your house and you will be exposed when you go outside or open a window. In addition, you will have to worry about potential spills when you receive deliveries. Even one drop of oil can smell for days, and cleanup can be difficult. If a tank leaks, it could contaminate the area around your house and render it unlivable for you.

For these reasons, my own bias is that people with MCS have no business living with petrochemical heat of any kind. Ideal, safe heat sources, of course, are the renewable sources such as wind and solar power. These energies have not received the research funding or attention that they deserve because of the petrochemical industry's political clout.

We all know that there are environmental problems with every other energy source. For example, some of our electricity comes from nuclear-powered plants that pose devastating risks, including potential and actual accidents and the storage of permanently radioactive waste.

Even hydroelectric power often destroys habitats when dams are built and flood people's land (often Native American land). So, if you are resourceful enough to find a truly safe energy source, you not only will improve your own health, but help to preserve the health of many others. Sometimes you can receive a lot of benefit by doing something small, such as installing south-facing windows for passive solar heating.

Some people can use wood stoves, although wood burning also generates a considerable number of pollutants likely to irritate sensitive people. Marinelli and Bierman-Lytle (1995) suggest looking for a stove that burns cleanly with a high-efficiency rating. They believe pellet stoves are the cleanest because they use waste wood and burn efficiently. There are some beautiful masonry heaters available; however, they are quite expensive. Before making such a large investment, I suggest finding someone who has such a heater to see how well sealed it is, and to see if you can tolerate it. Small ceramic heaters may be more affordable, but be sure your electrical system can tolerate the load.

You may decide you need to replace your gas furnace with an electric one. If you do and the heat is forced air, you can take advantage of the opportunity to install a whole-house dust filter or an electrostatic precipitator to reduce the amount of energy you put into dusting. Electrostatic precipitators use static electricity to trap oppositely charged molecules. They generally use synthetic materials, however, that pose some concern for people with sensitivities.

If the ducts are cleaned in the changeover process, be careful, as professionals will often use solvents for this purpose. Specify that solvents or chemicals of any kind cannot be used. If your house has no furnace, or if you don't want to use ducts that previously carried petrochemicals, you can install individually controlled electric baseboard heating units in each room. These will be more expensive to operate than gas or oil, but individual units allow you to adjust or turn off heaters in unused portions of the house, thus saving you some expense. If you install electric heating in a house that has not previously had it, you will need to be sure the electrical system can handle the load and has a 200-ampere board in the electrical control box.

Carpeting

Conventional carpet may emit dangerous volatile organic compounds (VOCs), dyes, formaldehyde and, worst of all, 4-phenyl cyclohexane (4-PC). The 4-PC appears to be directly associated with causing illness and MCS, and often is found in the styrene-butadiene latex backing of carpeting. Formaldehyde, which is commonly used in carpeting, is a respiratory irritant, is classified by the Environmental Protection Agency (EPA) as a probable human carcinogen, causes cell mutation, and produces metabolites that appear to be toxic to the human nervous system.

There are many documented cases of people, particularly children, becoming ill following the installation of new carpeting. For example, the dangers of toxic carpet were very much brought to public attention in October 1987 when the EPA (of all agencies) began installing carpet in its Waterside Mall headquarters in Washington, D.C. Although the EPA received 1,141 health complaints from employees, it took them two years to remove the toxic carpet (Duehring 1993b). Consequently, some employees became permanently sensitized from the experience: some are unable to work in the building and some are unable to work at all. Terese Svoboda made a video about the incident entitled "EPA Poisons EPA." (See Appendix C for chapter resources.)

In April 1991, New York State Attorney General Robert Abrams petitioned the Consumer Product Safety Commission (CPSC) to add warning labels to carpeting. Although twenty-five other state attorneys general signed the petition, warnings have not yet been issued. Despite admitting to union employees that the carpeting caused the illness, the EPA's public statements denied it, and the carpet industry mounted a public relations campaign to convince consumers of the safety of carpeting (Duehring 1993b).

This occurred despite the fact that when Anderson Laboratories tested carpet samples by exposing mice to the carpet, they found the mice had neurological damage and even died (Duehring 1993b). John Bower (1997a) said that some of the carpet samples that killed mice were as much as twelve years old.

Hirzy and Morison (1993) report that as little as five parts per billion (ppb) of 4-PC induced illness. They believe that a metabolite of 4-PC found in the carpeting is "capable of attacking DNA and of affecting detoxifying enzyme levels, processes hypothesized to be involved in induction/expression of multiple chemical sensitivity." (Remember that enzymatic damage/depletion is one of the hypothesized causes of MCS discussed in chapter two.)

Anderson Laboratories collected health information from 110 families who had lived with toxic carpets, and found their symptoms overlapped with MCS. Symptoms that were reported include fatigue, limb or trunk pain, central nervous system (CNS) problems affecting concentration or memory, skin rash or hair loss, tremors, irregular heartbeat, swollen glands, diarrhea, constipation, blurred vision, paralysis, respiratory dysfunction, headache, weakness, and eye, nose, and throat complications. The average person suffered seventeen symptoms (Anderson 1997). Anderson Laboratories created a videotape demonstration of mice reacting to carpeting, air freshener, and school air. (See Appendix C for chapter resources.)

Some people question whether there is any such thing as truly safe carpeting. An owner of one popular carpet store said that yarn used for New Zealand wool carpets often has been treated with synthetic pyrethrin, as moth proofing is required for some imported wool.

Wes Conneley (1998), technical manager for a company that promotes imported wool, said that moth-resistant treatment is not an import law, but rather a company-specific requirement. To bear the label "New Zealand Wool," carpeting must be moth proofed. Most carpets are treated with either pyrethrum or Mitin-FF (sulcofenuron) as a way of making the carpet resistant to moth larvae. Conneley stressed that the treatment is at a very low level (.025 percent) and is delivered during the dyeing process. It is not very effective because the moths have to actually eat the carpet before they die.

Given this information, if you want carpet that is truly pesticide-free, I suggest you ask a lot of questions. (To date, the only truly pesticide-free carpeting is produced by Nature's Carpet. See Appendix B for product sources.) For people with severe chemical sensitivity, wall-to-wall carpeting may not be an option at all. That is, flooring may have to be tiled using nontoxic grout, and covered with truly nontoxic area rugs. Other options for carpetlike floor coverings include jute, sisal, and coir (all made from plants). (See Appendix B for product sources.) Be aware, however, some sources say that customs regulations require plant materials such as these to be fumigated at the port of entry if they are not in sealed containers to prevent infestation by Mediterranean fruit flies. To test carpeting (or any product that will be in your living space), try sleeping with a sample next to your bed and see if you feel any worse from the exposure.

Wall Covering

It is not recommended that chemically sensitive people use conventional wallpaper. It often is made of or coated with vinyl (which offgasses considerably), coated or treated with fungicides, and requires glue for application. Alternatives are available, including recycled and/or chemical-free paper, cork, and fabrics. Traditionally, adhesives were made from simple wheat paste mixed with water. Although wheat paste has little or no chemical additives, without fungicides there is the possibility of mold buildup behind the covering, particularly in moist areas such as bathrooms and wooded settings.

For patterned or textured walls, alternatives to wallpaper are decorative painting techniques and faux finishes with nontoxic paints.

Chemical-Free Wallpaper Paste Recipe

Place 1 cup white flour in a double boiler. Add 1 tablespoon of alum or borax (as a natural fungicide), and 1 tablespoon water. Bring to the consistency of heavy cream. Stir out lumps, and heat until thickened to the consistency of thick gravy. Cool. Stir in an optional 10 drops of oil of clove as a natural bactericide. Paste will keep for two weeks in the refrigerator.

—Annie Berthold-Bond, *Our Toxic Times*, 105.

Paints and Finishes

All paints, both oil- and water-based, contain the following four components:

- *Solvents* keep the paint liquid and evaporate while drying (enamels may contain up to 50 percent).

- *Binders* harden the paint into a durable coating. These can be resins in oil-based paints and acrylic latex in water-based paints.

- *Pigments* for color.

- *Additives* such as dryers (can include ether), preservatives, fungicides, and mildew preventatives.

(Marinelli and Bierman-Lytle 1995)

Although you can test paints to determine which ones you tolerate best, be sure to buy low VOC paints and, before occupying a room, allow the paint to offgas for several days.

There is no good reason to coat an entire living space with a layer of toxins. Alternatives to toxic paint are not plentiful, although natural paints and citrus-based solvents are available. (See Appendix B for product sources.) My recommendation is to use old-fashioned milk-based paint, which comes in powder form, is totally solvent and chemical-free, and can be pigmented to your color choice. Milk-based paint is a little harder to work with as it must be mixed (you can use an electric hand-mixer) and needs two or more coats. It allows people with MCS, however, to safely do their own painting, and it dries to a hard surface with no odor. The drawback to milk-based paint is that it may collect mold in humid areas like bathrooms because it does not contain fungicide. You can experiment with adding alum, borax, and/or cloves as natural antifungal and antibacterial agents.

Additional safer alternatives include paints low in biocides, fungicides, and VOCs. These paints emit lower levels of pollutants than traditional paint, but still contain petroleum solvents and other substances. (See Appendix B for product sources.)

John Bower (1997b) suggests testing products with samples provided from the manufacturer: Paint a 2 ft. x 4 ft. piece of drywall, let it dry for two weeks, and then sleep with it next to your bed. If you sleep without symptoms (i.e., without restlessness, nightmares, etc.), you probably can tolerate the paint.

The Building Question

Many people will suggest that you build your own safe house. If you can afford it, the potential exists to create a beautiful and environmentally sound home which may help you to heal. Unfortunately, building a home has many snares and involves considerable expense.

Before making any decision, you need to learn about safe materials and the general building process, as well as to decide whether you can afford to hire an architect and/or a builder who specializes in environmentally safe housing. This is the best route, as you will not have to work as hard to ensure that no toxic products enter the work site.

On the other hand, specialists can be expensive, and you have to decide what you can afford. If you act as your own general contractor, you will have to be on the work site most of the time to ensure that no toxic materials are used. Your presence will also guarantee that the materials being used are the ones you ordered. If you want a big challenge, and are healthy enough to take it on, it might be a worthwhile project. However, to educate yourself about the process, including the challenges, I suggest you speak with several people who have built their own homes, and read available books on the subject. (See Appendix C for further reading.)

In the Home: The Portable Easier Stuff

Unlike outside exposures, the products you use in your home are entirely under your control. It is easy and less expensive to find and use alternative products for cleaning, pest control, and personal care.

Cleaners

You probably will want to stop using most or all of your commercial cleaning and bleach products. Commercial cleaning products contain petrochemicals, dyes, fragrances, phosphates, and bleaches, all of which may initiate adverse reactions in people with MCS. They also contribute to environmental degradation (e.g., phosphates pollute water supplies; chlorine is a hormone-disrupter), and are frequently tested on animals. (It would be wise to find alternative safe products and discontinue the use of any questionable ones. See Appendix B for product sources.) If you are unsure whether this step is worth the trouble, a walk down the cleaning aisle of your grocery store (no fair holding your breath) should convince you that it is. So first, dispose of or give away any product you suspect is unsafe for you. Keep in mind that many commercial and household cleaning products are considered hazardous waste and should be disposed of accordingly.

Chances are you already possess two or three safe products you can use while you are obtaining catalogs and exploring a wider variety of options. Baking soda can be used for cleaning sinks, tubs, clothing, and even glass (if you rub off the film with a cotton cloth). Some people are able to tolerate vinegar (although its odor can be a problem for many), which can be used to wash floors, walls, and windows, as well as to kill mold and remove chemical odors from new clothing. You also can clean mold with grapefruit seed extract, which is available both as a nutritional supplement and a household-cleaning product.

Several companies specialize in alternative cleaning products. I suggest you make a list of your needs and priorities and then screen items to see if they meet your requirements. For example, you might decide you need products that are free of petrochemicals, phosphates, dyes, artificial fragrances, and animal products. Although you may determine that you need completely fragrance-free products, there are several very good options that have natural citrus or herbal scents. It is important to keep in mind, however, that even citrus products can be irritants to many people, probably because of the limonene, which is a natural ingredient in citrus. Read labels and sniff products until you find the ones you can tolerate.

There is a lot for you to learn and make adjustments to once you have developed MCS. Finding the perfect product for every household function, however, does not need to take up a lot of your time and resources. There is nothing wrong with using one tolerable product for a number of tasks, e.g., using one safe shampoo for washing hair, clothes, floors, and your dog; or using dish soap for dishes, laundry, floors, and toilets. Still, be careful not to use a harsher product for a gentler job.

Pesticides

Pesticides need to be avoided inside the house. Commonly used roach, flea, and ant poisons are the reported cause of many cases of MCS and many other health complaints as well.

Pesticide companies will assure you that their formulas are safe for you and your children. I suggest, however, that you speak to people who were told the same thing and still developed MCS after home pesticide applications. There are many safe alternatives for indoor pest problems. Diatomaceous earth (DE) (not the swimming pool type) is very effective in the house or garden for killing, via dehydration, flea larvae and other soft-bodied larvae, insects, and slugs. (DE is like tiny glass shards to bugs. It will also irritate human mucous membranes—so don't breathe it in.) Boric acid powder will kill and discourage ants, roaches, and other insects (be sure not to put it down where children or pets can get into it). Safer alternatives include traps, fly swatters, and many others. Some people use ground-up natural pyrethrum (not the synthetic pyrethrins) from chrysanthemums, but I recommend you use it with caution because, although it is natural, it is toxic. If you do want to use it, you can grow your own chrysanthemums and grind them.

Pets

Don't forget your pets (if you have them) when switching to all natural pesticides. Conventional flea shampoos, dips, and sprays contain highly toxic ingredients. Most flea collars, for instance, contain Dursban. In a letter from EPA Administrator Lynn Goldman to DowElanco's chief executive officer, the EPA ruled that Dursban must be removed from flea collars and not be used as an indoor flea spray (Goldman 1997).

Flea combs, vacuuming, and possibly herbal flea collars (if you can tolerate them) are alternatives. You can purchase natural animal supplies and homeopathic medicines. Also, you can wash your animals with mild scent-free shampoos (with large pets this can be expensive). (See Appendix B for product sources.)

Personal Hygiene

Personal hygiene and body care products contain a number of controversial ingredients that are both natural and synthetic. Even in health food store products, you usually will find questionable ingredients, including cocamide diethalanomine (DEA), sodium laurel sulfate, and hydrolyzed proteins. Although cocamide DEA is from coconut, topical applications of it may cause cancer in laboratory animals. (DEA has the potential to be contaminated with nitrosamines, some of which are powerful carcinogens.)

Sadly, many manufacturers of chemical ingredients have lobbied successfully for legislation that assists them in marketing toxic products.

Currently, there are no legal definitions of the words "pure" or "natural," and most chemical companies use this to their advantage. Additionally, companies are not legally required to disclose anything about their manufacturing processes. If pressed to make information known, many companies will rely upon the phrase "proprietary trade secret" to withhold important information and protect themselves.

Ironically, most cosmetic ingredients are never screened for neurotoxic effects, despite the fact that many Material Safety Data Sheets (MSDS) specifically cite them. The use of MSDS was instituted by the Occupational Safety and Health Administration (OSHA) in 1985. The data sheets provide safety and health data and are required for every chemical used in the workplace.

Many MSDS for common perfume and cosmetic ingredients specifically warn: "irritant," "do not inhale vapors," and "avoid contact with skin." These same ingredients are then mixed together and sold as creams, lotions, and perfumes.

Lynn Bower (1995) explains that it is not required that cosmetics be registered with the FDA. Instead, they are overseen by the industry's Cosmetics Ingredient Review Board.

Be warned: Even if you are reading labels carefully, it still may be impossible for you to determine all of the ingredients in a product. Note that the vast majority of cosmetic and body care manufacturers do not prepare all of the ingredients in their products themselves. Rather, they buy individual ingredients from many different manufacturers and combine them. For example, a company that makes vitamin A may be using butylated hydroxytoluene (BHT) to preserve their product. The preservative BHT can cause allergic reactions and toxicity, and may convert some ingested substances, such as oral contraceptives, into toxic or cancer-causing chemicals (Winter 1994). The body care item that has vitamin A in it, however, does not have to list BHT as a product ingredient.

Similarly, plant extracts are carried in propylene glycol (commonly used as a solvent or antifreeze), which also does not have to be listed on a label. Given this state of affairs, it is best to avoid all synthetic scents. You probably will want to clean out all of your chemically formulated cosmetics and start from scratch with truly natural products. Because sensitivities tend to increase, I recommend doing this even if there are perfumed products that you can still tolerate. (Besides, you risk offending others with sensitivities if you wear artificial scents.)

To ensure the personal hygiene products you use are made from the very purest ingredients, you may have to make your own, refer to consumer dictionaries, and/or order from small manufacturing companies. There are companies listed in Appendix B that manufacture or sell safe products, including soap, shampoo and hair conditioners, toothpaste, moisturizers, and makeup.

Soap

Surprisingly, it is quite difficult to find fragrance-free soap at many health food stores, although many sell natural fragrances. Detergents and soaps contain many antibacterial agents that technically are classified with the EPA as pesticides.

Two safe options are castile and coconut soap. Castile soaps are made from vegetable oils and come in liquids and bars, although a true castile is made from olive oil, water, and wood ash. You may find coconut oil soap in your health food store.

Hair Products

At the very least you need a safe shampoo and conditioner. Unfortunately, as I've previously mentioned, most products, even at health food stores, are full of natural and/or synthetic fragrance. Keep in mind, if you have fragrance residues on your hair or clothing, they may prevent you from identifying other fragrances you are sensitive to, and make it difficult to convince others that you would appreciate them being fragrance-free. You can always use an unscented castile soap to wash your hair and make your own rinses from natural ingredients. A few recipes are listed later in this chapter.

Toothpaste

Until you find the right toothpaste—or just for simplicity—you can brush your teeth with baking soda. There are, however, numerous alternative toothpastes you can buy. Remember, if you are taking homeopathic medicines, you will have to avoid any tooth product with mint or strong fragrance (natural or otherwise), as strong smells are thought to disturb the subtle action of homeopathic medicines.

Moisturizers

For moisturizer, you can use any natural oil that agrees with you, although it may be greasy. An oil that is not greasy and which dissolves nicely into the skin is called African Shea butter.

Makeup

Natural makeup has progressed to the point where conventional chemical products have virtually no advantages. If you use makeup, the safest choices are those products that are free of coal tar dyes (which cause cancer in laboratory animals), heavy metals, such as aluminum (which has some relationship to developing Alzheimer's disease), and other toxicants.

A walk down your drugstore makeup aisle should convince you that changing to natural products would be worthwhile. Count how many eye makeups list aluminum as an ingredient. All of the dyes listed are made from coal tar. Additionally, many companies test on animals and use countless animal ingredients.

Homemade Personal Care Recipes:

Astringents: hot water; apple cider vinegar; and lemon juice in cool water

Blackhead Therapy: lemon juice; equal parts baking soda and water

Dental Care: brush with baking soda or salt. As a tooth whitener, mix baking soda with a 3 percent dilution of hydrogen peroxide

Deodorant: baking soda or cornstarch

Hair Conditioner: egg yolk beaten with a few drops of oil; rub into hair and leave on hair for twenty minutes; and then rinse

Hair Spray: cook one unpeeled lemon with 2 cups water; boil down to 1 cup; cool; strain through cheesecloth and pour into spray bottle. Store in the refrigerator

Hair-Setting Solution: dissolve 2 tablespoons of superfine sugar in 1/2 cup warm water; apply to hair while still warm (be forewarned, this is also a yellow jacket or wasp lure)

Shaving Cream: use a tolerable unscented soap and lather; or, dissolve 4 tablespoons of baking soda in 1 pint of hot water; apply

—recommended by Lynn Bower, 1995

Household Items

Most people don't have the option to spend thousands of dollars to clean up their homes. Because of this, I recommend simplifying rather than replacing. Buying all new furniture, for instance, might be nice, but there probably is a less expensive alternative for most of your concerns. One woman living with MCS explains it this way:

"I got to the point where I wanted nothing except my health. Eventually I learned to simplify my life. I realized I didn't need gobs of money to buy fancy [environmental illness] products. I took the vacuum cleaner and hung it out the window. I sewed my own crude quilts until I had enough to comfortably sleep on. I took washable cloths and stuck them in pillowcases for cushions. I just let go of wanting things—all I wanted was to get better.... The things, products, methods, techniques, etc., just didn't matter."

Clothing

You may want to go through your clothing and decide what to give away based on the materials used, whether they are contaminated with fragrances from fabric softeners and detergents, or they have been dry-cleaned. There may be particular materials that you can tolerate better than others. For instance, for some people, polyester, a petrochemical product, may be troublesome, but acrylic (closer to plastic) may not be.

Cotton and hemp are probably the soundest choices, but cottons can become contaminated in laundering or through the use of perfume. If some of your clothes have picked up odors, you can try washing them in vinegar or baking soda to remove the smells. Vinegar should not cause the colors to bleed, while baking soda may.

New clothing is often a long way from tolerable for people with MCS, so don't give away most of your clothing before ensuring that you have something to wear. Although you may find some untreated clothing in stores, it is rare, and you will have to come up with a strategy for acquiring safe clothing. If you can afford it, there are some beautiful natural cottons and hemps available through catalogs and in some alternative stores. They are generally priced similarly to upscale conventional clothing.

Cotton can be unbleached, organically grown, and dyed with vegetable color-grown dyes. Organic color-grown cotton or hemp are probably your soundest choices.

There are a few new companies that specialize in mail-order hemp clothing. Hemp can be grown with less water than cotton and without pesticides, and is a durable fabric for clothing. Since it is illegal to grow hemp in the United States, it has to be imported.

Other clothing options exist. You can buy commercial clothing and wash it to remove chemical treatments. First, you can soak and wash a commercially bought garment in vinegar, and then in baking soda. Do not mix them, as they will neutralize one another and become ineffective. The problem with this approach is that it takes a while.

According to Lynn Bower (1995) vinegar may corrode parts of your washing machine if clothing is left to soak. Further, extended soaking still may not make the clothing safe. (Note: You are washing harmful chemicals down the drain into the environment, including dioxins and pesticides.) In addition, some clothing from India and Asia has a turpentine-like smell that never comes out. Apparently there is a petrochemical used in Asian processing that does not break down in washing.

Another option is to buy used clothing. However, you have to be sure previous owners did not use perfumes, mothballs, fabric softeners, and dry-cleaning products. Dry-cleaning odors will not become apparent until you wet the fabric, so it is impossible to tell in the store whether a piece has been dry-cleaned. Dry cleaning is usually done with trichlorethylene or perchlorethylene and residues remain in the clothing. If you avoid clothing likely to have been dry-cleaned (such as suits, skirts, and better fabrics), and if you screen for perfume odors, resale shops may be an option for affordable clothing.

Bedding

Making a safe bedroom can be a challenge. There are various degrees of safety you can create. If you awaken with symptoms, your bed or something in your bedroom may be unsafe. Ideally, to create a safe oasis in your bedroom, you would have only the necessities in there, such as a bed and a dresser. There would be no carpet to collect dust or odors; a high quality air purifier would clean floating dust, pollen, mold, and chemicals from the air; clothing would be stored in a closed space, such as closet, to minimize dust; and no books would be stored in the room. If your bedroom is safely heated, not recently painted with a toxic paint, and not carpeted, the major item left to clean up would be your bed. You are exposed to your mattress, sheets, pillows, and blankets for one-third of your life and are breathing in their emissions. Therefore, they should be as clean as possible.

It is fairly easy to acquire sheets, blankets, pillows, and even mattresses made from organically grown materials, although it is not always easy to afford them. If your bedding is old, it may be safe for you, although bleached cottons can continue to emit dioxins for years. I suggest deciding how much you can afford and then making the most of your resources. Safe sheets and pillowcases are a priority. If you cannot afford a new mattress one lower-cost option would be to cover your own mattress (assuming it is not too contaminated) with a barrier cloth cover. Barrier cloth is woven so densely that it is thought to stop dust and synthetics from offgassing; however, some people dispute this. You can make your own barrier cloth cover, or purchase one from a store or catalog. (See Appendix B for product sources.)

When choosing bedding materials, you should know cotton that is labeled as "green" is not necessarily organic, but is processed without bleaches, dyes, and other chemicals, such as formaldehyde. The growing process, however, may include pesticides. For the purest product, ask for cotton that is organically grown and processed without chemicals.

Furniture

A lot of furniture is made of polyester, foam that contains formaldehyde, and other synthetics. Because of the buildup of dust mites in the fabric and cushions, even cotton furniture can be a problem. Most furniture fabrics are treated with stain repellents and other finishes. Furthermore, new furniture (even all-wood furniture) may offgas stains and glues (and even formaldehyde if particleboard is used). Therefore, safe furniture for one person with MCS may differ completely from what is safe for someone else.

Wooden furniture that has aged and has not been refinished is probably fairly safe. There are many sources of all-wood furniture. Many varieties can be purchased at secondhand stores or garage sales. Some options for soft furniture include futons for sofas and pullout beds. Many shops sell futons made from untreated cotton, although with some futons, there is still an odor. If you want to keep cotton furniture that may have become dusty, you can put smaller items like pillows in the electric dryer for thirty-five minutes on high heat to kill the mites. You can also cover the larger pillows with barrier cloth. Pillows of unsafe materials, such as foam, can be replaced or restuffed with organic cotton (although they will not have their previous shape or resilience).

If you can afford to invest in some clean furniture, some companies have totally organic furniture pieces, including chairs, love seats, sofas, bedding, futons, and crib mattresses. For a nominal fee, you may be able to acquire and test samples of all items used in the furniture you are considering buying. You can put each sample item in a glass jar, set it in the sun to heat for several hours, then open the jar and breathe the fumes to test your reaction. If it seems okay, you can then sleep with it by your bed to test it further.

Furniture delivery should be considered as well. One store's delivery process deserves special mention: The company, *furnature*, has a very MCS-conscious delivery process. Many stores could learn from their example. All items delivered from the company are wrapped in zippered bags of organic canvas, then wrapped in paper, and then shrink-wrapped as a third layer to protect from pesticides in trucks or any other toxins used in shipping. When the delivery arrives at your house, the wrapping is removed outside, the driver then puts on a white gloves that have already been sent to the purchaser for this purpose, and the item is carried inside. (How's that for careful?) (See Appendix B for product sources.)

Air

You may decide that you need air filters in certain parts of your home, or even a whole-house air filter. (See Appendix B for product sources.) Filters are not a substitute for cleaning up your indoor air, but depending on what type you purchase, they can offer extra help against certain pollutants. A filter can reduce dust, pollen, dander, smoke, gases, formaldehyde, and biological elements depending on its specific purpose. All filters have drawbacks, but some can clean an airspace reasonably well and reduce contaminant loads. One caution: Many filters are not very effective, and some (particularly those with HEPA filters) are made of the same contaminants (polyester, polypropylene, etc.) that you are trying to take *out* of your house. So, carefully research any filter before you purchase it, and talk to the manufacturer to find out exactly what materials are used to make it. I suggest you make a list of those contaminants you need help with, and purchase the appropriate filters for those substances. For example, you may need a filter that specifically removes dust and pollen.

The following sections describe various air filters:

Activated Carbon and Activated Alumina

Activated carbon, made from coconut shell, wood, or coal, has a pitted surface that adsorbs many pollutants, including gases, benzene, perfumes, pet odors, phenol, solvents, paints, and many others. Lynn Bower (1995) cautions that activated charcoal may adsorb pollutants during times of high contamination and release them back into the air during times of lesser contamination. This medium reacts with so many pollutants, however, that many people with MCS use it successfully both in home and auto air purifiers, and find they can tolerate the coconut shell charcoal. Activated carbon does not clean formaldehyde very well, and therefore is often combined with activated alumina, which is aluminum oxide impregnated with potassium permanganate.

Activated alumina (sold as Purafil, Purapel, and other brand names) reacts with many chemicals, including alcohols; aldehydes; aromatics, such as paint solvents; ethers; oxides, such as carbon monoxide; nitrogen and sulfur dioxides; phenols; and others. By combining charcoal and alumina, you can filter a large number of pollutants. Products must be changed periodically. You can tell if your alumina needs replacement, as it will change its color from purple when it is new to a darker brown when it has adsorbed to its capacity. If you purchase a filter that can be refilled, you can save money by ordering it in bulk. (See Appendix B for product sources.)

HEPA Filters

High efficiency particulate-arresting/accumulator (HEPA) describes a type of filter that can either stand alone or be combined with charcoal and alumina. HEPA filters remove particulates, such as dust, pollen, mold, and viruses, but do not affect gases. The problem with HEPA filters is that many are made of polyesters and glues that have no business being in the home of a person with chemical sensitivities. To me, this is an example of prescribing more chemicals to cope with chemical sensitivity. How can using a chemical purifier be good for anyone, especially people with MCS? I suggest that if you use a HEPA filter, you find out exactly what is in it, and get the purest one available. Also, be aware: If activated charcoal is downwind from the HEPA filter, it may adsorb problematic emissions from the toxic elements found in the filter.

Extended Surface Filters

Extended surface filters have a large pleated/folded surface made of polyester or fiberglass for maximum air contact. They filter particulates, not gases, and need replacing periodically. There are the same concerns about synthetic materials here as with HEPA filters, but Lynn Bower (1995) says that to reduce odors some people bake filters in their ovens at low temperatures for about two hours. (She cautions that you should ask the manufacturer if the filter can tolerate this. Also, be sure to close off your kitchen from the rest of your house, open the windows, and use your hood fan to reduce the chance of smells spreading through your house.)

Electrostatic Filters

Electrostatic filters use static electricity to trap pollutants that have opposite charges of the (generally) plastic filters. They trap molds and pollens, but not gases. The filter can be vinyl, polyester, or polystyrene, all substances of concern for those with sensitivities, and to those concerned with environmental sustainability.

Electrostatic Precipitators

Electrostatic precipitators use live electrical current—much as electrostatic filters use static electricity—first to charge, and then to collect the molecules of pollutants. Metal wires charge the molecules, and then electrical plates collect them. The plates need washing when debris collects on them. Sometimes, the molecules end up being re-released into your air.

Ozone Generators

Ozone as an air cleaner is a controversial topic. Although ozone is a pollutant, some people use generators to create ozone to react with VOCs and to kill bacteria and molds. Although ozone can break down some pollutants, it may also combine with chemicals to create other pollutants. Bower (1997a) reports that the FDA says ozone paralyzes the olfactory nerve, thereby deadening smell. Just because you can't smell something doesn't mean it can't affect you. Look very carefully into ozone before exposing yourself to it.

Ozone is an irritant that reduces lung function and increases "airway reactivity, permeability, and inflammation." Studies show that ozone generators may reduce levels of some chemicals, such as 4-PC, but that they are ineffective with formaldehyde. Further, the generators will change other pollutants into formaldehyde and VOCs. They also cause olfactory fatigue, so you will not smell the pollutants (Johnson 1996).

There is some question of danger when operating ozone in a place that has previously been treated with pesticides. One person with MCS reported becoming extremely ill after doing this and said that her physicians finally came to the conclusion that the ozone had actually fused the pesticide residues into her tissues. Johnson (1996) published a statement from John Banta, an environmental consultant, who said the following:

The only way I ever will use or recommend ozone is as a fumigation technique with no people, pets, or plants present while the ozone is being used. A window should be left open slightly to allow some fresh circulation into the area being treated. The area should be allowed to air out for a while after treatment before reoccupying the area . . . there is always the possibility that the ozone treatment will ruin the area for occupancy for some people.

Johnson also points out that ozone breaks down natural rubber through destroying double carbon bonds. This means that if you use ozone generators, you could destroy the electrical wiring in your house (if it's older and the wiring is made of real rubber), or damage important car parts, such as hoses.

Negative Ion Generators

Negative ion generators create negatively charged ions that attach themselves to particles, giving them a negative charge. Negative ions are thought to be healthier than positive ones. In fact, negative ions may be the reason that the air near mountains and larger bodies of water has a positive effect on people. Once they are negatively charged, particles tend to cling to surfaces that have positive charges, such as walls and ceilings. Although the air will be cleaner, particles may build up on surfaces and eventually reenter the environment once they lose their negative charge. However, if the ionizer has a built-in filter that is able to trap the particles, then this problem is not as much of a concern. Some people with MCS have used ionizers in automobiles or as personal portable devices to create a small, clean airspace in polluted settings.

Water

Unfortunately, drinking water, regardless of its source, may contain a number of dangerous contaminants. Municipal water contains pharmaceutical drug residues, chlorine, fluoride, household chemical residues, and possibly biological elements. Well water is at risk for containing bacteria, nitrates, pesticides, and VOCs. You may want to test your water for the following pollutants:

Biological Elements

Biological pollution can result from agricultural runoff, a septic system field that is less than 100 feet from a well, and other sources. Harmful biological elements include fecal and total coliforms; bacteria, such as salmonella, molds, viruses; and other living organisms. Labs often test for coliforms, because their presence in water indicates other dangerous biological elements may be present.

Nitrates

Nitrates often can be traced to chemical fertilizers that have run off into water supplies. However, they may also occur as the natural product of organic matter breakdown. In well water, nitrates indicate that pesticides and herbicides may be present. In the adult body, a small portion (about 5 percent) of nitrates is converted into nitrites, which can interfere with oxygen transport and cause a condition called methemoglobinemia. The hemoglobin in the blood, which normally carries oxygen, becomes methemoglobin and can no longer function properly. Infants are most susceptible to methemoglobinemia, as they are able to convert almost all ingested nitrates into nitrites. It is especially dangerous, therefore, to have an infant in a house that has nitrite pollution (Harte, Holdren, Schneider, and Shirley 1991).

Pesticides

The presence of pesticides in water is cause for serious concern. They easily are absorbed by the skin and, in fact, are often more dangerous through this dermal route than when otherwise ingested. Pesticides are contaminating wells throughout the United States due to the continued use of aerial and ground spraying in agriculture. If you live in an agricultural area, you should definitely test for pesticides. Further pesticide hazards are discussed in the gardening section, page 71.

Particulates

Suspended particulates in water can be dirt, sand, mold, or other matter. They make water cloudy and the water is said to have high turbidity. Turbidity can be tested by passing a beam of light through a water sample to see how much light is deflected by particles.

VOCs

VOCs are chemicals that easily can evaporate and include some pesticides and chlorine, gasoline, PCB, and solvents such as trichloroethane and trichloroethylene. Most have serious health effects and thus are dangerous contaminants of groundwater.

Radon

Radon is a radioactive, colorless, odorless gas that is a carcinogen. It is present in particular areas of the country that have certain geological characteristics (e.g., rock and shale formations) that promote its formation and release from the ground.

Radon enters inhabited spaces through cracks in basements, and can be found in high concentrations in water as well. If radon is in your water, it will enter your airspace whenever the faucet (particularly hot water) is turned on. You can test for radon yourself with a separate kit, or have it included as part of a more comprehensive test.

Metals

Lead and copper can leach into drinking water from local or municipal pipes. Lead was used in the past to make water pipes, which often still exist in older homes. Additionally, lead was used as solder for copper pipes until 1986 (Bower 1995).

Because of lead's widespread use, you should always test your water for lead content. Lead can poison every system in the body, especially the central nervous system, and its effects on children include learning disabilities, mental retardation, and emotional disturbance. In adults, lead is linked to fatigue, irritability, insomnia, nervousness, headache, weakness, and depression (Schottenfeld and Cullen 1984).

Copper and mercury are metals that should be tested for, as well. Too much copper can damage the myelin sheath of nerve tissue (Bryce-Smith 1986). Excess mercury has been found to cause respiratory, gastrointestinal, and skin problems, as well as anxiety and personality disorders (Perez-Comas 1991).

Water Filters

There are a variety of filters—both whole-house and individual units—that treat home water. A water test will help you to determine which type is best for you; each filter has strengths and weaknesses. Additionally, the level and type of pollutant also determine whether you need a whole-house purifier, or if simply filtering your drinking and cooking water will suffice. If a well is contaminated with gasoline or pesticides, simple filtering is not enough because your skin will absorb these pollutants when you shower, and vapors will be released into the air. As mentioned earlier, radon also is released into the air when water is heated. So, at the very least, a shower filter is needed. If you use municipal water, the local county agency tests it periodically for some contaminants. If you have a well, testing for coliform bacteria may be free.

You may be able to purchase a simple test kit locally to test your water. However, to get a detailed look at your water, you might have to pursue professional testing.

The following section describes some of the filters that are available and the types of pollutants that they address. It is particularly important for you to do personal research and reading regarding water filters as Ingram (1991) warns that there is a lot of false and exaggerated advertising. (See Appendix C for further reading, and Appendix B for product sources.)

Activated Charcoal Filters. This is the same material that is used in air purifiers, and comes in granular and block form. Because block form is denser, it is more efficient. Some block filters are made with a plastic that may cause problems for people with MCS (L. Bower 1995).

Granular activated charcoal will remove chlorine, gases, VOCs, radon (but not all of its radioactive particle emissions), tastes and odors, and some sediment. Solid block activated charcoal will remove chlorine, gases, VOCs, sediment, pesticides, radon, and some fluoride. Charcoal filters do not remove biological elements, and may even build up bacteria. Combining them with reverse osmosis or kinetic-degradation-fluxion (KFD) devices is often suggested.

Carbon block will last longer and remove more pollutants than granular because water may channel through the granular without enough contact with the medium. However, the carbon block needs a sediment prefilter to prevent it from becoming blocked. Ingram (1991) warns also that pollutants can break away from the carbon due to water pressure changes and be ingested. To prevent this, he suggests using a slow flow rate and allowing the water to flow for thirty seconds before drinking it whenever the filter has not been used for several hours. Carbon block, but not granular, will remove some asbestos. Lynn Bower (1995) says it removes heavy metals, while Ingram says that it does not unless it is combined with reduction oxidation filtering. Because carbon does not remove biologicals, Ingram further recommends that it not be used in private water sources (e.g., wells) without adding a method of disinfection.

Reverse Osmosis. In these units, water is forced through a synthetic membrane that will not allow pollutants to pass through. The size of the pores in the membrane determines the size and type of contaminants that will be removed. These units may be slow, and they are expensive to operate because they use several gallons of water to make one gallon of purified water. They will remove minerals, nitrates, fluoride, sediment, heavy metals, and asbestos, and will lessen salt and some harmful biological elements. Unfortunately, reverse osmosis does not remove gases such as chlorine or radon, and the membrane can become contaminated with bacteria. Also, be aware that these filters may remove too many of the minerals, leaving you with drinking water that is demineralized, and thus capable of leaching minerals from your body. Reverse osmosis does not accumulate pollutants as carbon does. Membranes are made of cellulose acetate (CA) or thin film composite (TFC). Ingram (1991) says that TFC performs better and lasts longer than CA, but cannot be used with chlorinated water without a chlorine prefilter.

Distillers. Water distillers boil water, turning it into steam, and then recollect it as the steam condenses. Contaminants are separated out in the process and harmful biological elements are killed in the boiling. The units will remove sediment, minerals, nitrates, metals, asbestos, fluoride, and dangerous biological elements. Distillers do not remove VOCs or gases such as chlorine and radon. They tend to be slow, eliminate too many minerals, create heat, and are expensive. On the positive side, they are very reliable and have no parts that need replacing.

Kinetic-Degradation-Fluxion (KDF) Devices. KDF devices use an alloy of zinc and copper to cause oxidation (the loss of electrons) and reduction (the addition of electrons) to the molecules of contaminants in water. As contaminants come into contact with the zinc and copper filter, they are transformed into safer substances. In addition, heavy metals are removed by becoming attached to the device; and oppositely charged zinc and copper disrupt bacteria with a small electrical current. KDF devices will remove chlorine, sulfur dioxide, methane, some heavy metals, and most bacteria. They do not remove VOCs and gases.

In the Car

Driving can be one of the most problematic ventures for people with chemical injuries and sensitivities. To travel by car, you have to expose yourself to the interior and exhaust of your own car, the exhaust of other vehicles, and any other industrial/chemical smells en route. However, there are some strategies you can use to minimize exposures and thus retain your ability to drive.

Seal It from the Outside

Before attempting to clean up your car, you might want to see if it is even safe for you to sit in. If you feel sick before you even turn the car on, you may want to replace it with a safer car you can tolerate. If sitting in your car causes only mild health problems, you can close all the doors, bake it in the sun, and then open and air it out repeatedly, each time cleaning off the film from the windows that accumulates from the vinyl and other materials that are offgassing. You can also wash the interior with baking soda, or seal it with a safe sealer. In addition, scouring powder or solvents, such as citrus, will remove vinyl treatments that emit troublesome odors.

Once the vehicle is tolerable, parking it in the shade will prevent further unwanted offgassing.

If your car is safe to sit in, then the interior is tolerable for you. In this case, it may be worth attempting to seal the car to minimize your exposure to outside fuel emissions. Most cars with air-conditioning have a recirculate option. This means that the air is not drawn from outside, but rather from the interior of the car. Using the recirculate option will minimize outside odors from other vehicles and other exposures you may encounter while traveling. It would be beneficial to use the recirculate option for the heating unit as well. Ask your mechanic if the outside control vent is manual or automatic when you turn on the car. (For example, some cars have a manual vent that can be closed for air or heat.) If the vent is automatic, ask your mechanic how to bypass and fix the switch so it will stay closed while you are driving. With the vent closed all of the time, however, mold may build up. To air out the heater coils and air conditioner, you can open the vent while your car is not operating. If the vent is pneumatic, however, it will close automatically when starting the car, and open when the engine is turned off. The windows fogging up in the winter may also be a problem. (You may be the only person on the road using the air-conditioning to clear your windows in 20-degree weather.) It is difficult to generalize from one car to another, and mechanics will not be familiar with this request. You will have to explain exactly what you are trying to do. For example, you may have to say, "I am trying to avoid breathing outside pollution when I drive." If you don't have air-conditioning, you will have to open the windows in the summer. This can be a problem even in sparsely traveled areas because cars take in their own exhaust aerodynamically.

Other openings to the outside environment also will have to be sealed. Try to find all vents by looking at the doors (especially the bottoms of doors), near the rear window, above the rear windshield, and any other place that seems likely. Sometimes a vent is identified by a rubber flap. You can seal vents with foam, silicone, or any other tolerable material that will block air. One person with MCS used sheets of aluminum, caulk, and tape to make cutouts that fit all of her air intakes on her vehicles. She rated sealing these intakes as the second most important strategy in avoiding further deterioration (living in the country was first). Be aware that sealing your car will not protect you from exhaust leaks. If you seal off outside "fresh" air, yet have an exhaust leak, you could be doing yourself more harm than good.

Introduce No New Contaminants

Of course you will not want to use any upholstery treatments, cleaners, or preservatives in your car that may leave odors. Do not allow anyone to smoke or wear perfume in your car. Perfume can linger and become absorbed into the upholstery. Air fresheners should be avoided. If you have your car professionally cleaned, be sure they know that no air fresheners are to be used, and that no one is to get in the car wearing fragrance. It is probably safer to wash your own car.

Another caution is that you should never transport anything in the passenger compartment that could contaminate your interior. If you must transport something, place it in the trunk and put it into a second sealed container in case of a leak.

Maintenance

You probably will need help from others to maintain your car. It is very important to have the exhaust checked regularly. A muffler leak the size of a pinhole may negatively affect you, even if you have sealed your car to the best of your ability. The mechanic who checks the exhaust or performs other functions must know not to use *any* chemicals or air fresheners inside the car. Also, mechanics should be sure not to bring any oils or gasoline into the car on their hands or shoes. One participant was made sensitive when workers at a body shop spilled a whole gallon of air freshener in her car. (They did not have her consent to apply the freshener in the first place.) You or a friend can explain that you are extremely sensitive to chemicals, and that even a little oil from shoes can make the car intolerable to you. As a precaution, put down newspaper on the floor and cover the seat with a towel. If any oils get on the steering wheel they can be washed off.

You may need someone to pump your gas. If this is not an option, you can try parking upwind from the pump. Tying a small flag or piece of yarn on your antenna can help you to determine wind direction. Simply stop the car and observe in which direction the flag or yarn is blowing. Try not to step in any gas. Pick up the nozzle with a disposable paper towel or plastic bag in case it has gas on it from previous use. Be careful not to overfill the tank, as gas will spill on your car and on the ground. If someone else pumps your gas, or if you go to a full-service station, be sure and stress that it is important not to overfill the tank.

Driving

While driving, some strategic moves may minimize your exposures. Avoid driving closely behind diesel or very smelly vehicles. I do not advocate kamikaze tactics such as passing at any risk. Rather, pull off the road and let the polluter get far enough ahead so that you can safely drive again.

It is possible that you may have a limit to how long you can be in the car before you get sick, e.g., twenty minutes or so. You may be able to extend this amount of time by taking a break in a clean area or simply by pulling off the road, turning off the car, and breathing from your air purifier for a few minutes. If your reaction is triggered by a threshold effect, try stopping a few minutes before you will feel ill, turn off the engine, and breathe the cleanest air you can for five to ten minutes. If this works for you, you may be able to then drive for another period of time before stopping again.

If you have passengers riding with you, ask them to wait a minute or so after you shut down the engine before opening the doors. This will allow the exhaust to dissipate and will reduce your exposures. Also, explain to people that you cannot pull up next to them, open the window while the car is running, and chat.

Parking

At home, you may want to arrange for a place to keep your car that minimizes your exposure to it. If you have an attached garage, for example, I suggest not using it, as cars emit odors when cooling and starting up. Likewise, parking your car right next to your window or your porch may not be a good choice, as you will be breathing whatever it offgasses. If cars have leaks, they may emit odors all of the time. Of course, if you have a car with a leak, it needs to be fixed or sold.

Purifiers

Even if you seal your car as much as possible, you still will get some outside air along with its accompanying exposures. An auto air purifier may help to further reduce these exposures if you can find one that is of good quality. Many companies that produce room air purifiers also produce auto air units that can be plugged into your cigarette lighter. (You won't be using it for anything else, after all.) (See Appendix B for product sources.)

Lawns and Gardens

With limited energy, you may not be anxious to grow your own food, but gardening can provide you with exercise, organic food, increased contact with the earth, and a healthy hobby. If you have little time, you could begin by growing something easy that requires little space, such as lettuce. It is possible to grow all of your own organic salad greens in a very small space, and you will have the satisfaction of knowing what went into your food when it was grown.

The Problem with Pesticides

Conventional garden techniques often include the use of pesticides (including herbicides or weed killers). Although your own gardening practices may be no different, once you have developed sensitivities, the use of garden chemicals is one of the most important practices to discontinue.

Pesticides are ubiquitous in our air and water; they are poorly tested and understood, highly toxic, and, when combined together, even more toxic. They are named by a large number of people with MCS as the initial cause of their illness, and are implicated in a myriad of other diseases including cancer (especially breast cancer and non-Hodgkin's lymphomas), reproductive disorders, and Parkinson's disease.

The active ingredients in pesticides often comprise only one to five percent of a preparation. The rest of the product is often labeled as "inert ingredients." The implication is that inert ingredients are inactive. However, a lawsuit by the Northwest Coalition for Alternatives to Pesticides (NCAP) against the EPA forced the EPA to reveal a long list of hazardous substances that may *legally* be added to pesticides as inert ingredients. The list includes industrial sludge, other pesticides, and even radioactive waste (*Toxic Secrets* 1998).

All pesticides are toxic by some mechanism as they are designed to eliminate living organisms. Organophosphates deplete acetylcholinesterase, increasing acetylcholine in the nervous system, and thus kill bugs with convulsions. In humans, they can cause reactions that include ringing in the ears, nervousness, nausea, vomiting, cramps, weakness, seizures, and more. Lieberman, Craven, Lewis, et al. (1998) found that home use of organophosphate pesticides can cause chromosome damage.

Children and pets are particularly vulnerable to poisoning and long-term health effects from pesticides. A study by Davis, Brownson, Garcia, et al. (1993) found an association between childhood brain cancer and the use of pesticides, including termite treatment, diazinon in the garden, lawn herbicides, Kwell shampoo (used to eliminate lice and nits), indoor pesticide treatment, pest strips, and even flea collars.

Likewise, Gold, Gordis, Tonascia, et al. (1979) found that family insecticide use was one of five variables associated with the development of childhood brain tumors. For some reason, indoor pesticides are likely to migrate to children's plastic toys and thus end up in children's mouths (Guranathan, Robson, Freeman, et al. 1998).

Adult women also may be harmed by long-term pesticide exposure. Women with breast cancer have higher levels of pesticides in their breast tissue than do women with benign breast disease (Moses, Johnson, Anger, et al. 1993; Thornton 1993).

Men are not exempt either. Farmers have a higher incidence of cancer than do nonagricultural workers, and Parkinson's disease is associated with rural living and pesticide exposure.

If you poison yourself with pesticides you are unlikely to get proper medical treatment, as most providers are uneducated regarding proper testing and intervention. Sherman (1995) found that forty-one patients with organophosphate poisoning were misdiagnosed, endured costly and ineffective treatments and, because of this, did not improve.

Pesticides poison the environment in myriad ways. They degrade soil and groundwater, kill beneficial organisms, poison wildlife, create long-term dioxin residues, and leave poisonous breakdown products in your soil. Given all this, there is no sane reason to continue using these chemicals. You may have to sacrifice the perfect green lawn (which is nowhere near natural anyway), and some seemingly quick solutions to bug problems, but many safer alternatives and strategies are available. Be aware, however, some organically derived pest poisons also have inert ingredients that include petrochemicals and other toxins. There is evidence that with healthy care and feeding of the soil, pest populations decrease each year. There are books available that cover low-maintenance, organic, edible gardening, including design, planting, and pest management. (See Appendix C for further reading and Appendix B for product sources.)

"Pressure-Treated" Lumber

As its name would imply, pressure-treated lumber used to be strengthened through pressure. Presently, however, it is dipped in chromated copper arsenate, a source of arsenic. Arsenic is a human carcinogenic nerve poison, and can cause harmful cardiovascular changes. Chromated copper arsenate comes with warnings to avoid inhaling the dust, to wash thoroughly before eating, and to launder clothes separately after working with it. Pressurized lumber is a source of arsenic to those who touch it, to the soil around it, and to the children and pets who play and walk on it.

Pressurized lumber may be present around your flower beds, in your food garden, or on your deck. Most decks are constructed of pressure-treated lumber because insects will not eat it (which says something about the common sense of insects). Although there are alternative woods that are insect-resistant, pressure-treated lumber is the industry standard. People are generally uninformed about its toxicity as evidenced by its widespread use on decks, in gardens, and even on playgrounds.

I suggest removing all pressure-treated lumber from your yard and garden. Do not burn it, but take it to the landfill for hazardous waste disposal. At the very least, it should never be where rain could cause arsenic to leach into your food plants or into soil you will work with your hands. If your deck is made from treated lumber (it has a greenish cast and is unfinished), you may want to seal it with a low-toxicity, outside-use sealant to contain the arsenic.

Your Mailbox

It is amazing how many fragrances can invade your home through the mailbox. If you are sensitive to fragrances, your mail can become contaminated and therefore unreadable from magazine inserts, special mailers, and samples. However, now there is a postal code on your side. United States 39 Code 3001g was listed in the April 9, 1998 *Postal Bulletin* (*Bulletin* no. 21969, p. 26) and reads:

> A fragrance advertising sample, i.e., any matter normally acceptable in the mail, but containing a fragrance advertising sample, is permitted in the mail only if it is sealed, wrapped, treated, or otherwise prepared in a manner reasonably designed to prevent individuals from becoming unknowingly or involuntarily exposed to

the sample. A sample meets this requirement if it uses paper stock with a maximum porosity of twenty Sheffield units or 172 Gurley Hill units treated exclusively with micro encapsulated oils, and if the sample is produced so that it cannot be activated except by opening a glued flap or binder or removing an overlying ply of paper.

You may be able to use this code to stop unsealed samples from reaching you in your mailbox. One person got her post office to send a letter to the offending company ordering them to cease and desist from any further violations. When another person tried to get her post office to do the same, they attempted to pass the buck. They asked her to bring in the sample, suggesting that it was the problem of the company, and offered to send the sample to the specific arm of the post office that deals with meeting code. It is not unreasonable, however, to expect the post office to comply with its own code, and this ruling eventually will help.

At Work

If you work outside of the home it also is crucial to clean up your work environment as much as possible. Workplace cleanup and accommodation is discussed in chapter thirteen on workplace accommodation and disability issues.

For Further Help

If you need additional assistance about safe products and cleaning up your home, there are consultants available for this purpose. Fees vary, but if you learn as much as you can on your own and prepare your questions ahead of time, it might be useful to get specific help from experts. (See Appendix C for chapter resources.)

Chapter Five

Facing Food

Nutrition and Diet

Attempting to consume a healthy diet is difficult enough for anyone nowadays when most food is contaminated with pesticides, herbicides, bovine growth hormone (BGH), artificial colors and flavors, preservatives, or aspartame.

For chemically sensitive people with food allergies and severe food intolerances, eating can be a veritable land mine, as even pure, organically grown foods may not be safe. In general, the issue of food intolerances is poorly understood, even by those who treat MCS. For example, even people who advocate for a yeast-free diet disagree as to exactly what foods are to be avoided.

There is much disagreement regarding MCS and the testing and treatment of food allergies. Allergy testing is expensive and often yields conflicting results. One woman reported spending money on three different types of food allergy testing, all of which provided contradicting reports. In the end, she relied on her own judgment, eliminating those foods that seemed to make her feel the worst, but retaining as many foods as possible to sustain decent nutrition. Some people would disagree with her, in the belief that she should attempt to eliminate all foods that tested bad regardless of the test used. The problem with this approach, however, is that it would have left almost nothing for her to eat. At one point, this woman had a list of only twelve foods that did not give her a twelve-hour negative reaction. She later discovered that her petrochemical heating system was causing her to become intolerant of chemicals and foods. By moving to a safer living environment, she gained back her tolerance for most foods.

This chapter will help you to eliminate some of the most toxic types of foods, and will familiarize you with some of the popular diets that have been tried for MCS, including the rotary diversified, macrobiotic, anticandida, and Atkins diets. It is not, however, an exhaustive resource for any of these topics, and further reading is suggested in Appendix C. Being informed about how food is produced or transported will make you a safer consumer. Not many people, for example, know that the same trucks that transport toxic liquids may later be filled with food products, making for dangerously contaminated food (Lawson 1994).

The importance of diet for people with MCS was evidenced by the fact that ninety people in Phase II of my research responded to the question "If you have improved, to what do you attribute the improvement?" by listing vitamin and mineral supplements. Other nutrition-related items that respondents reported attributing their improvement to included:

- General strict diet
- Anticandida diet
- Macrobiotic food
- Bottled water
- Antioxidants
- Garlic
- Anitfungal medications
- All natural products
- Non-fat diet
- Elimination diets

- Organic food
- Rotation diets
- Amino acid supplements
- Dechlorinated water
- Enzyme treatment
- Yeast treatment
- Tap water
- Fasting
- Eating slowly
- Acidophilus

Many people with MCS report that taking food supplements is beneficial. In Phase I of my research, 35 percent of respondents reported great benefit, 26 percent moderate benefit, 23 percent mild benefit, 8 percent no benefit, and 8 percent reported adverse reactions. I suggest learning as much as possible about basic and specialty nutrients in order to be your own nutritionist. (See Appendix C for further reading.)

Toxins in Foods

In our industrialized culture, food unfortunately has become a storable, commercial commodity that often reaches the table bearing no resemblance to its original form. In fact, often there is little or no nutritional value in packaged foods. Try going into a convenience store and finding one product that is actually good for you. You may luck out and find a piece of fruit, but it's not likely. (I have tried and been unable to do it.) Foods are processed, bleached, preserved, and colored, and contain only a small percentage of the nutrients they have in their natural state. A friend once came to a potluck party at my house, held up his packaged food contribution, and laughingly bragged that it did not contain *one* natural ingredient. He was right. How does one go about eating even a reasonably decent diet when food has degenerated into a money-making commodity?

Eliminate as Many Chemicals as Possible

For anyone with sensitivities, carefully reading food labels must become a way of life. Ingredients are listed on labels in the order that they exist in the food from the largest to the smallest amounts. For example, if the first ingredient is sugar, then the product contains more sugar than any other ingredient. You must read all of the ingredients listed. **Be aware:** Labels can be misleading. If the label says "organic whole wheat flour, enriched wheat flour," then the product contains some organic whole wheat flour, but it also contains nonorganic, nonwhole wheat flour. When wheat flour is processed, the wheat germ (the inner part containing the vitamin E) and the bran (the outer layer containing the roughage) are removed and sold to health food stores, and you get the leftover starchy part of the grain. To make matters worse, the grain is bleached white and the product is depleted of B vitamins to the point that only a fraction remain. As a partial remedy, manufacturers often will "enrich" their products with two to three of the seventeen or so vitamins depleted.

You want to buy foods that are in as natural a state as possible, with as few added ingredients as possible. If you have sensitivities to foods, you particularly need simple foods that are not stacked with many ingredients so that when you test yourself, you will know to which ingredient you are reacting. If you eat a packaged food with thirty ingredients and get a reaction, you will have no idea to what ingredient you are reacting. On the other hand, if you eat a meal of natural cauliflower and have a reaction, it will be clear that you are sensitive to the cauliflower. It is important to note, too, that although ingredients are required to be listed on packages, preprepared added ingredients do not have to be broken down on labels. For example, yogurt could be listed as an ingredient in a cookie, but the food label does not have to list the fact that the yogurt itself has gelatin in it. Therefore, it is possible to consume items we are unaware of despite conscientious care. In fact, with the advent of genetically engineered foods, the difficulty of knowing to which allergens you are being exposed has become even greater.

Ingredients to be avoided in a natural diet include:

- Artificial colors (derived from coal tar dyes; suspected and, in some cases, confirmed as carcinogens)

- Artificial flavors

- Preservatives (added to increase shelf life)

- Monosodium glutamate (MSG) (added as a flavoring agent; common in Chinese foods and hidden in a large number of other foods)

- Artificial additives and other conditioning agents, such as "dough conditioner" in bread

Ruth Winter's book *A Consumer's Dictionary of Food Additives* (1994) reviews more than 8,000 food additives, and examines the state of current food safety regulations. Interestingly, since the book's first edition in 1972, thirty-five popular food additives have been removed from the market because of their ability to cause cancer. Clearly, it is prudent to avoid as many artificial additives as possible. This is especially true given the constant efforts to weaken regulations that limit food carcinogens, and the lack of adequate testing for most products. Even if additives are tested, they are not tested in combination. Furthermore, regulatory bodies do not take into consideration that some populations eat certain foods in greater quantities. For example, when calculating the danger of pesticides in fruits, the fact that babies and young children eat many times the amount of fruit that adults do in comparison to their body weight is not considered. Also, food additives and other environmental toxins are most often tested exclusively for carcinogenicity. However, neurotoxicity (nervous system poisoning) and hormone disruption may be even greater concerns and may occur at much faster rates than do the carcinogenic effects (which may take twenty years to appear in humans). The following sections review additives that are best avoided.

Sweeteners

In general, the use of sweeteners should be kept at a minimum, especially if you have sensitive reactions to yeast. I suggest particularly avoiding aspartame, which breaks down into formaldehyde both in the body and during storage. A twelve-year-old girl did the research to prove that the longer Diet Coke is stored and the higher the storage temperature, the quicker aspartame turns into formaldehyde (Cohen 1997). Research supports the contention that aspartame is a neurotoxin, yet it is allowed to remain in food products because "diet food" is a multimillion dollar industry. Further, the aspartic acid in aspartame can cause MSG-type reactions for people sensitive to MSG.

Preservatives

Preservatives give food a longer shelf life and prevent mold, spoilage, and the degeneration of fat that results in rancidity. Preservatives include butylated hydroxyanisole (BHA), butylated hydroxytoluene (BHT), potassium sorbate, "food grade" waxes, and others. (See Appendix C for further reading.)

Food Coloring

Although some food colorings, such as turmeric and annatto, are natural, most are made from coal tar dyes, which have been shown to cause tumors in animals. Some colorings have been removed from the Federal Drug Administration's list of "allowed additives" because of the harm that they have caused in animal testing.

Food colors are added to butter, candies, cereals, and canned items. Even dog food has food coloring added to it. (I can only assume this is the result of marketing on the part of the chemical companies and that the color of food does not increase my dogs' culinary enjoyment.)

Flavorings and Flavor Enhancers

Winter (1994) says that of 3,000 food additives, 2,000 are artificial flavorings used to replace the natural flavors lost in processing. Flavor enhancers, such as MSG, are of great concern because they excite the nervous system and because we don't know enough about their neurological effects. Some people say that MSG causes reactions in sensitive people due to the free glutamic acid found in processed food (The Truth in Labeling Campaign, Darien, Illinois). Proteins containing bound glutamic acid or glutamic acid in unprocessed food that contains natural glutamic acid do not cause the same reaction. It is extremely difficult to avoid MSG, as it is always present in gelatin, textured protein, hydrolyzed protein, and yeast; and is often present in malt extracts and flavorings, barley malt, carrageenan (used as a thickening agent), whey protein, flavors, soy sauce, soy protein, and all fermented foods, to name just a few. Amino acids and hydrolyzed ingredients in soaps, shampoos and conditioners, and cosmetics may also trigger MSG reactions. MSG is made through protein hydrolysis. When the product is 99 percent free glutamate it is called monosodium glutamate. If the free glutamate level is lower than 99 percent, no mention need be made that MSG is present, and it can be called something else, such as sodium saxienate, calcium casientate, autolyzed yeast, textured protein, hydrolyzed protein, and others. (See Appendix C for further reading.)

Irradiation

Irradiation consists of exposing foods to ionizing radiation to kill molds and bacteria, and to slow down ripening. It was approved in 1986 by the Federal Drug Administration (FDA) for fresh fruits, vegetables, grains, nuts, teas, spices, and some meats. Although food does not become radioactive, there are outstanding questions about irradiation given that its approval was based on theoretical calculations rather than actual testing. Questions about the safety of irradiating food are still being raised. Such questions include: What effect does irradiation have on the nutritional value of the food; are there molecular changes as a result of the process; and what health risks may be present? Although irradiated foods are labeled with a logo that looks like a flower in a circle, when they are added to processed foods as an ingredient, they are not labeled.

There are environmental concerns about irradiation as well. These include the increased transport and storage of radioactive material used in food irradiation facilities and the location of the facilities. Concerned about the public's awareness of and negative response to irradiation, food irradiation technology firms have coined a new phrase for the process: "Electronic Pasteurization." Much as sugar is now called "pure cane juice crystals," irradiation has a new deceptive euphemism as well.

Pesticides

Pesticides probably represent one of the most insidious and harmful ingredients in our food and are discussed at length in chapter four, "Making Your Home Safe." One study cited in the *Nutrition Action Healthletter* (1997) showed that strawberries had more pesticides and more endocrine disrupters than any other fresh food. Also high in pesticides were United States cherries, apples, Mexican cantaloupes, Chilean grapes, blackberries, pears, raspberries, and other fruits. Fresh foods that were the least contaminated included cauliflower, sweet potatoes, onions, corn, peas, carrots, and avocados. When buying organic food, you can use this information to best spend your dollars. For example, if your funds are limited, buy organic strawberries and other fruits, and buy commercial vegetables from the less contaminated group.

Another study cited in the *Nutrition Action Healthletter* found that washing produce with water and dishwashing liquid and peeling the skins and outer leaves eliminated pesticide residues from about half of the contaminated produce. Other options are to purchase vegetable washes or to soak produce with crushed tablets of hydrochloric (HCL) acid in the water. (I have tested the HCL on pears that actually smelled of pesticide and it works.) Some foods, however, are grown with systemic pesticides that are taken up through the roots into the plant and cannot be washed off. Also used on crops are growth regulators, chemical fertilizers, and municipal sludge that contains heavy minerals and human waste. Of course, it is best to eat organically grown and organically processed food whenever possible. The problem, of course, is the cost. Another consideration regarding organic foods is that many health food stores stock organic produce, but they spray pesticides inside their facility; pesticides migrate, negating the benefit of stocking organic foods in the first place. I would not buy organic produce from any store that sprayed the very chemicals that organic growers work so hard to do without.

Most farmland is blanketed with herbicides each spring even if pesticides are not used. Corn, for example, is grown on land that is first treated with herbicides, including 2-4D, atrazine, paraquat, or other toxic substances that kill weeds. As if this is not enough, some farmers apply a "preemerge" (what I call the "Don't even think about growing here") chemical to prevent certain weeds such as redroot from germinating. One farmer I know mixes his own poisons, combining five different herbicides, one of which is 2-4D. He then provides his young son with a cotton painter's mask and takes him to spread the mixture with his own truck.

Indirect Contamination Through Animal Products

In addition to direct additives in your foods, there are a host of indirect chemicals that reach you as a result of eating meat or animal products. For example, cows graze on land that has been treated with the herbicide 2-4D (used to kill thistles). This chemical builds up in their milk and then is passed on to you. Similarly, animals often are fed steroids (for growth), antibiotics, in some cases bovine growth hormone, and are sometimes tranquilized when taken to market. Some of these drugs are used illegally (Lawson 1994). All of them are passed on to you. (See Appendix B for further reading.)

My own bias is that eating animal foods is neither healthy, nor environmentally sound. In the present world economy, rain forests are being cut down to provide grazing land to produce more beef. Beef cattle eat many, many pounds of grain to produce one pound of (often contaminated) meat. More people could be fed, fewer forests cut down, fewer chemicals consumed, and less violence done to animals if the grain went directly to people. People differ in their views of animals. In addition, they often hold romanticized views of dairy farming (thought to be less violent than beef farming). The truth is that beef cows used as breeders have longer lives that those used for milk. The average dairy cow lives three to four years, after which she is slaughtered for meat because her milk production has dropped below an artificially high standard that can only be achieved through pushing the cow's system to produce more than is natural for her to produce. Sometimes this is done with heavy graining, other times with bovine growth hormone.

Food Storage and Preparation

In addition to commercial degradation of food, storage and preparation poses further risk of contamination. For example, storage in plastic exposes food to pthalates, which are hormone disruptors. It is best to minimize the purchase and use of plastic containers; use cellulose bags instead. (See Appendix B for product sources.) This can be difficult because even health food stores provide customers with plastic bags in which to collect and store food that is to be purchased. You might want to bring your own cellulose bags when you shop. **Note:** Most yogurt manufacturers that store their product in plastic containers, are not even responsible enough to use recyclable plastic. In my mind, these companies—regardless of how they attempt to represent themselves—are no more deserving of our money than are the conglomerates that monopolize the grocery store chains.

Aluminum exposure is another toxic consideration. Cooking utensils made of aluminum are a high risk for contaminating food. The development of Alzheimer's disease has been linked with aluminum buildup in the brain. Aluminum foil, conventional baking powder, and many over-the-counter drugs also contain aluminum.

Learn to Be Self-Sufficient

Of course the best answer to avoiding chemical food contamination is to grow your own food. A patch of clean ground that has not been exposed to chemicals is a valuable treasure. If you can grow organic tomatoes, you can dry some in a food dehydrator and use them all year. With just a couple of pots on a porch, you can grow a large number of tomatoes that will taste much better than those plastic-tasting ones in the grocery store. You can grow sprouts year-round in your kitchen. It also is relatively easy to grow lettuce, mustard, chives, carrots, beans, and other important foods. (See Appendix B for product sources.) I highly suggest learning how to grow your own food. It is fun, it gets you outside, and it provides gentle exercise.

The magazine *Organic Gardening* is a tremendous resource for growing organic produce and for providing information about pesticides. The editors are committed to the issue of safe organic food and the magazine is a leader in responding to the ever-present threat of the weakening of standards for growing organic foods. In fact, the former editor, Mike McGrath, in several issues reported the ongoing harassment and threat of lawsuit by pesticide producers for speaking out in regard to toxic pesticides.

Between growing your own food and buying food from a reputable health food store, you can eat at least a partially organic diet. It is fairly easy to find organically grown staples, such as rice, barley, wheat, nuts, and seeds, at the health food store. Be careful, however, with regard to packaged ingredients; many packaged "health food" items are no healthier than items in the regular grocery store, despite their inflated costs. Proprietors have a difficult time finding companies that truly attempt to provide pure products. In fact, many companies merely change the name of an item rather than eliminate it.

Fats are another food ingredient of which to be aware. Many of the fats in health food snacks are hydrogenated, which means hydrogen is bubbled through the food molecules during processing. This process alters molecules so much from their original form that they react entirely differently in the body. Furthermore, these fats can clog cell walls and prevent the cell wall (or "keyboard" of the cell) from carrying out important metabolic functions, such as manufacturing energy and allowing nutrients in or out of the cell. Therefore, you will want to avoid any ingredient that says "hydrogenated," "partially hydrogenated," or "fractionated."

Dietary Treatments for MCS

A host of diets claim to prevent or cure disease, and some specifically have been suggested for people with MCS (e.g., the macrobiotic diet). As with any other MCS intervention, no one diet is effective or safe for everyone. Following are some of the more popular diets that people with MCS have tried.

The Rotary Diversified Diet

The rotation diet has you eat one food at a time, and consume that food or any food from the same family only once every four days. The rationale behind food rotation is that because it takes three to four days to clear a food from your system, you can unmask some of your food reactions and thus avoid foods that have been acting as hidden allergens. Because of the cross-reactivity in food families, you must isolate families of foods together. For example, since both wheat and barley are in the grass family, you would not eat wheat on Monday and barley on Tuesday. Instead, you would eat items from the grass family on Monday, and not ingest any of them again until Friday. Guides are available to help you set up a rotation diet of safe foods. (See Appendix C for further reading.) Generally, guides suggest that you start with a few foods that you know are safe, eat them every four days in very simple meals of only one or two food combinations, and then slowly start to eat and test additional foods. You must plan carefully, chart your food plan to be sure you don't get confused, and be certain that particular food items will be in the house on their "day."

Of course, there are considerable limitations to this diet. First, it eliminates any spontaneity when it comes to eating out with others. If someone invites you over for a meal on a Thursday and they aren't serving bananas and bananas alone, you'll be out of luck. And, you can guess how exciting these meals are to your housemates. However, rotating food families does help some people get a better handle on what foods they are reacting to, and it does introduce some order and discipline into eating. Of the participants in Phase I of my research who had rotated foods, 36 percent reported great benefit, 25 percent moderate benefit, 21 percent mild benefit, 18 percent found no benefit, and 1 percent had adverse reactions.

Sherry Rogers (1986) says that "only highly sensitive people, highly chemically sensitive people, universal reactors, and those on food injections need to rotate" (p. 282). She says you have severe food allergies if you cannot control your symptoms through avoidance of some foods and/or if you need injections. Rotating food is especially helpful for people who need injections because it prohibits the body from being constantly overloaded with the same antigens, and from developing new allergies by abusing other foods. Rogers says that a good way to start rotating is to pick four unrelated foods (from different families) that you rarely eat (because you are less likely to be allergic to them) and eat one of them a day until your symptoms clear. You may feel worse before you feel better because you will experience withdrawal from your allergic/addictive foods. Next, she suggests consuming two unrelated, rarely eaten foods per day, and adding one new food a day as long as you still feel okay. This will help you to build up two lists: one of foods that are safe, and one of foods that are not. Unsafe foods can be identified by negative reactions that may be immediate or delayed (even a day later). You can also use your heart pulse to identify unsafe foods. Test your pulse twenty minutes after eating a food to see if it changes. By becoming familiar with your resting pulse (seventy-two to eighty beats per minute is considered normal, but yours may vary), you will be able to identify unsafe foods by identifying which ones cause your pulse to deviate from its normal range. Once you get to the point where you have about sixteen safe foods, Rogers says to eat four different foods each day, being sure to rotate them every four days. (See Appendix C for further reading.)

Remaining Questions

One complication regarding food rotation is that we do not know enough about cross-reactivity. In personal communication, Susan Killian told me that while doing research on cross reactivity she has found that seemingly unrelated foods may contain the same antigens (protein or carbohydrate substances). Therefore, it's possible to think that you are rotating your foods, but actually not be doing so. Killian, Fretwell, and McMichael (1997) found cross-reactivity within food families, across families, and even between foods and both fungi and animals. The grass family seems to be particularly cross-reactive. For example:

- Barley cross-reacted with potato and tomato (nightshade family) as well as wheat, oat, and corn (all in the grass family).

- Corn reacted with rice and wheat (same family), and with potato, sugar, and tomato.

- Grass had fairly strong cross-reactivity with string beans, soy, orange, potato, ragweed, and rice.

- Wheat reacted with rice, rye, milk, and potato.

(Killian, Fretwell, and McMichael 1997)

Killian feels that there may be a limited number of antigens (perhaps twenty or so) that appear in a number of substances; and if we could discover which antigens these were, we could neutralize them and thus desensitize people to a large number of foods.

Anticandida Diets

The anticandida diet consists of the avoidance of antibiotics, hormones, and steroids; augmentation of the immune system; a low sugar/carbohydrate diet; and sometimes either natural or prescription agents to kill excess yeast. One hypothesis regarding the cause of MCS and of food allergies in particular is that the person's body has sustained an overgrowth of yeastlike fungi in the candida family.

Although candida is present in all bodies, it causes problems when there is an imbalance between it and the normal healthy bacteria present in the mouth, intestinal tract, and vagina. Yeasts manufacture aldehydes, which can block pathways used for detoxification, and can also produce chemicals that mimic autoimmune reactions against the body's own organs. Aldehydes also displace healthy bacteria in the digestive tract which aid in digestion and in the production of nutrients. Some people believe that yeasts can grow through the digestive walls causing "leaky gut" syndrome and exposing the blood supply to undigested food particles. Because they are not digested, the body identifies these food particles as foreign, and immune reactions or allergies may develop to the foods. Sherry Rogers (1986) says that although there are more than 200 journal articles supporting the role of yeast in illness, this theory has not received much respect or recognition among physicians or allergists. In fact, although yeast overgrowth is contributed to by antibiotic use, only rarely do physicians advise the use of acidophilus along with prescribed antibiotics. Acidophilus is a useful microorganism found in dairy products. It replenishes the "good" stomach flora that antibiotics kill. Other factors thought to contribute to yeastlike overgrowth include steroids, prescription medications, birth control pills, stress, and a diet particularly rich in sugars and carbohydrates. (See Appendix C for further reading.)

In his book, *The Yeast Connection*, William Crook (1986) says that symptoms caused by yeast include fatigue; depression; headaches; skin problems, such as athlete's foot, nail fungus, rashes; gastrointestinal symptoms, such as constipation, bloating, and abdominal pain; reproductive problems, such as menstrual pain; and other problems. Crook sees chronic fatigue, fibromyalgia, headaches, depression, and MCS as common yeast-related syndromes that afflict both men and women. Although less commonly, people with asthma, multiple sclerosis, psoriasis, and autoimmune disorders have responded to antiyeast therapy. Crook believes that yeast may cause women to experience recurrent burning vulva, premenstrual syndrome (PMS), endometriosis, cystitis, interstitial cystitis, sexual dysfunction, and infertility.

Although there are always new laboratory tests being invented to detect yeast levels, yeast problems have generally been diagnosed by an antiyeast program trial. If a person shows improvement during the trial, then it is thought that yeast played a part in their illness. Because of the mainstream attacks upon practitioners of environmental medicine, some physicians have told me in personal communication that they are now protecting themselves by insisting on a stool test to detect high levels of yeast before prescribing antiyeast medication.

The anticandida diet suggests you avoid the following foods:

- sugars
- breads
- cheeses
- coffee and tea
- mushrooms
- fruit juices
- fermented condiments, such as mustard, ketchup, soy sauce, tamari, etc.

- processed foods
- pastries
- alcohol
- malts
- melons
- dried fruits

A diet heavy in vegetables, meats, eggs, nuts, and seeds is suggested. Crook allows potatoes, sweet corn, sweet potatoes, and whole grains in lower quantities.

In her book, *Who Killed Candida?*, Vickie Glassburn (1991) describes a comprehensive program for eliminating yeast. (This book is out of print, but you may be able to find it at your local library.) It is called the "3 C Diet"— Choices Conquer Candida—and is recommended to those with candida, immunodeficiency, and MCS. The main objective of this diet is to make long-term lifestyle changes in order to:

1. Regulate the digestive system

2. Strengthen the immune system

3. Cease yeast overgrowth

Throughout her book, Glassburn stresses the importance of a strong immune system, and continually reiterates that many factors contribute to poor immunity. She believes that to be healthy, people must regulate their digestive system by putting their bodies on a strict schedule. She sees fermentation as the reason that some foods do not digest as well as others. Glassburn suggests that foods (e.g., beef) that delay the digestive process begin to ferment internally, causing alcohol-like products to accumulate. It is this process that contributes to symptoms such as fatigue, feelings of disorganization or disorientation, and confusion.

Nine important steps will facilitate regular, rhythmic digestion. According to Glassburn, all nine steps must be followed closely to absorb nutrients most effectively, avoid the slowing of the digestive process, and eliminate symptoms such as allergies, lack of energy, etc. These steps include:

1. Chew food well.

2. Eat two or three meals a day.

3. Avoid consuming liquids with meals.

4. Eliminate eating in the evenings.

5. Keep the number of foods at a minimum with each meal.

6. Learn to combine food properly.

7. Limit refined and concentrated foods.

8. Exercise.

9. Control stress levels.

Glassburn also strongly believes in the importance of water, air, sunlight, exercise, and rest to build up the immune system. She recommends large quantities of distilled water to rid the body of harmful toxins. Fresh air and sunlight aid in the rejuvenation of the body and produce more white blood cells, thus giving the body the capacity to fight off infection. Regular, sustained exercise, a minimum of one hour per day, without exception, will help to regulate blood sugar levels, reduce blood sugar, eliminate fatigue and depression, as well as bring more oxygen into the body's system allowing it to fight off illness. (Be careful: Not only must every person find the appropriate type and level of exercise for themselves, but exercising immediately before or after a meal may delay the digestive process.) Finally, the body must rest at the end of the day to repair itself. A good night's sleep enables the immune system to regenerate if the body is on a regular regimen. Glassburn warns that daytime napping may be harmful because it can detract from the quality of nighttime sleep.

Differences Between Anticandida Diets

Anticandida diets differ on several points, including their treatment of fruit and complex carbohydrates (grains). Glassburn admits that grains foster yeast growth, but she thinks that they help to heal the immune system, and therefore includes them in her diet. On the other hand, she disallows all animal products. Most anticandida diets prescribe avoidance of dairy products due to the lactose. Fruits receive differential treatment. Those that include fruits define them as natural and healthy foods that are metabolized slightly differently by the body than are processed sugars. Those who restrict fruit consumption point out that it is nonetheless sweet, and, as such, feeds yeast. People disagree on the eating of ferments also. Some believe that yeast and mushrooms need only be avoided if the person is allergic to them. Others believe that they feed the yeast directly.

Each person has to determine for themselves what seems to cause the yeast to flare, and then avoid those foods. Women may have an easier time of determining this, as they can tell fairly quickly what will cause a vaginal yeast problem to flare. Men have to rely on other indicators of yeast flare-up. The anticandida diet often is paired with substances that help to kill the yeast. Natural remedies include garlic, caprylic acid, homeopathic solutions of candida, grapefruit seed extracts, and antifungal herbs. Other remedies include nystatin, Nizoral, and/or Diflucan. Nystatin is an antibiotic substance that stays in the digestive tract and is not absorbed into the system. Nizoral and Diflucan are absorbed into the bloodstream and may help to kill yeast that has taken hold in organs other than the digestive tract. Nystatin is fairly well-tolerated, although some people report "die-off" reactions as yeast cells burst and release their contents. With Nizoral and Diflucan, you must have your liver enzymes tested regularly, as both are somewhat liver toxic and there is a danger of liver damage if enzymes become elevated.

My concern regarding anticandida treatments is that the body seems to want to override the treatment, and even becomes "addicted" to the antiyeast medication. While on a yeast program, even a tiny amount of sweetener can trigger a flare-up and, for some people, the amount becomes smaller and smaller rather than larger with treatment. Given that people don't even agree as to what constitutes an antiyeast diet, I don't think we know enough about yeast treatment. Nevertheless, some people have benefited greatly from it.

Alison Johnson (1996–1998) found that 58 percent of 200 people reported either major or enormous help from an anticandida diet, and 25.4 percent, 30.2 percent, and 37.8 percent reported either major or enormous benefit from nystatin, Nizoral, and Diflucan respectively. However, 19.5

percent, 26.7 percent, and 14.3 percent reported harm from nystatin, Nizoral, and Diflucan respectively.

Fit for Life Diet

Harvey and Marilyn Diamond, authors of *Fit for Life*, describe a basic philosophy for diet and a healthy lifestyle called "Natural Hygiene." Natural Hygiene promotes healthy living by relying on the body's natural tendency to cleanse itself of waste material. The diet tunes into the body's digestion cycles to detoxify the system. The Diamonds explain that through this organic cleansing process, the human body achieves a maximum level of wellness.

The primary goal of the Natural Hygiene lifestyle is to detoxify the body completely of increasing amounts of toxic waste material. Toxemia, which is an "abnormal condition associated with the presence of toxic substances in the blood," leads to poor health, including lack of energy, excess weight, and illness.

Inadequately digested food causes toxins to build up in the body. In *Fit for Life*, the Diamonds suggest integrating three basic principles into one's lifestyle. These include:

1. Food with a high-water content

2. Proper food combining

3. Proper food consumption

High-Water Content

Because the body is 70 percent water, the Fit for Life diet places great emphasis on consuming foods that are high in water content. In fact, high-water content foods should be 70 percent of one's food intake; the other 30 percent should consist of grains, breads, meats, dairy, etc. Fruits and vegetables are considered to be high in water content. The water in these foods provides the body with vitamins, minerals and other enzymes that aid in the digestive process and are not available in regular drinking water. It also flushes the system of harmful toxins and transports nutrients within the body.

Proper Food Combination

Proper food combining plays a key role in food digestion. According to Fit for Life principles, the body can digest only one concentrated food at a time ("concentrated" is defined as any food that is not high-water content). Thus, one may feel sluggish and tired after eating a big meal because the body is using a lot of its energy trying to digest several concentrated foods at once. The Diamonds believe that proper detoxification is dependent on the amount of available energy. If the digestive process uses all of the body's energy trying to break down improperly combined foods, toxins can accumulate. Digestive juices are another consideration of proper food combination. The stomach secretes different digestive juices depending upon the food that has to be broken down. If different foods require different digestive juices, then these juices may neutralize each other causing a delay in the digestive process. This slowing of digestion can cause food to sit in the stomach for up to eight hours and remain in the intestine for approximately twenty to forty hours. The stagnant position of partially digested food causes proteins to putrefy and carbohydrates to ferment. Fermentation can cause harmful toxins to be released within the body.

Proper Food Consumption

Proper food consumption calls for only one protein to be eaten at a time without any carbohydrates. However, two starches may be combined at one meal, provided no protein is consumed at the same time. The Fit for Life diet calls for fruit to be eaten frequently, but with great care. Fruit is cleansing to the body, takes the least amount of energy to break down, and is not digested in the stomach. The Diamonds describe most fruit as being predigested, passing quickly through the stomach to release its nutrients in the small intestine. Therefore, fruit digestion efficiently preserves energy that the body then can use to rid itself of toxins. Moreover, substances found in fruit act as blood thinners, which help to prevent clogged arteries and thus reduce the risk of heart disease. Consuming fruit also allows the digestive tract to rest. However, if other types of food are eaten at the same time as fruit it may be taxing on the digestive system. The Fit for Life diet advocates that fruit be consumed at very specific times. For example, fruit should be consumed only on an empty stomach and at least thirty minutes prior to eating any other type of food; at least two hours after eating a vegetarian meal; and at least four hours must pass after eating a nonvegetarian meal. Additionally, only fruits and fruit juices should be consumed from waking until noon to maximize energy levels.

Three digestive cycles are emphasized in *Fit for Life*.

1. The "Elimination Cycle" takes place from 4 A.M. until noon. During this cycle only fruits and fruit juices should be consumed.

2. The "Appropriation Cycle" takes place from noon until 8 P.M. Meals are consumed this time. Proper food combining is essential and of utmost importance during this cycle.

3. The "Assimilation Cycle" takes place from 8 P.M. until 4 A.M. Restful sleep allows the body to extract and absorb all nutrients as well as rebuild the body's immune system.

Like other holistic diets, the Fit for Life system includes aerobic exercise, fresh air, and sunshine as aids in the detoxification process and weight loss. It examines the importance of mental attitudes and how they may affect weight loss.

This healthy lifestyle plan is geared toward people who are interested in losing weight and/or looking for a diet and way of life that maximizes the body's energy levels and detoxifies the human system. Through proper eating habits, food combining, and exercise programs, the body can digest food properly and gain energy for everyday living. Detoxification and efficient digestive processes contribute to greater health and a stronger immune system.

The Macrobiotic Diet

The macrobiotic diet system has its origins in Japan and is a holistic life *philosophy*, rather than just a *diet*. The system espouses balancing the body in regard to yin (feminine passive) and yang (masculine active) energies so that you no longer are eating foods that are extreme in either direction. In June 1991, Sherry Rogers personally told me that the macrobiotic diet may be a good solution for those who are meant to be alkaline types.

The macrobiotic diet includes whole grains, vegetables, beans, seaweed, seeds, and condiments. It eliminates meat and fowl, but includes some fish. Whole foods are consumed during their natural season. Foods eliminated by this diet include refined sugar, meat, eggs, poultry, dairy, tropical fruits and juices, coffee, dyed tea, refined foods, colored, preserved, sprayed or otherwise treated or irradiated foods, overstimulating spices, alcohol, and sweeteners, such as honey and molasses.

This diet consists of approximately 50 percent whole grains, 20 to 30 percent vegetables, 5 to 10 percent soups, and 5 to 10 percent beans and sea vegetables. Occasional foods include fish, seasonal fruits, nuts, and seeds. Grains can include rice, barley, millet, oats, corn, rye, wheat, and buckwheat, and should be consumed whole, as opposed to the processed form, such as pasta. Vegetables should be locally grown and cooked in a variety of ways. They include cabbage, kale, broccoli, cauliflower, collards, bok choy, dandelion, onion, daikon, turnips, carrots, squash, and others. Potatoes, tomatoes, eggplant, peppers, spinach, and beets are not recommended for regular consumption. Beans can include chickpeas, azukis, lentils, tempeh, tofu, and others. Sea vegetables (seaweeds) such as nori (be careful: some nori is dyed), wakame, kombu, dulse, and arame are seen as important sources of trace minerals (I have not seen anyone address the concern about water pollution and its effect on the quality of seaweeds). Soups include vegetables, grains, beans, miso, tamari sauce, and sea salt. Beverages can be natural teas, such as bancha twig, barley, dandelion root, and cereal grains. Fish can be eaten one to three times per week, although beware of eating fish from contaminated waters. Other occasional foods can be roasted seeds, nuts, and some fruits. Condiments include gomasio (roasted sesame seeds and sea salt), seaweed powder, umboshi paste and plums, and others. Food must be chewed very well (fifty times per mouthful). (See Appendix B for product sources.)

Some nondiet lifestyle suggestions of macrobiotic philosophy include outdoor exercise, wearing natural clothing, and cooking with gas rather than electric. (For people with chemical sensitivities, I heartily disagree with the gas recommendation.)

Some people have reported great improvement on this diet, but others have not been so fortunate. I believe it is a basically healthy diet except for the lack of raw food and the almost complete absence of fruit, which contains much nutrition and many important enzymes. Some macrobiotic sources do recommend the use of some fruit, but advocate steaming it rather than eating it raw.

The Atkins Diet

The Atkins diet is a low carbohydrate diet that restricts the use of processed and refined carbohydrates, such as bread, pasta, cereal, starchy meals, and processed sugars. Instead, the diet emphasizes high protein and fat consumption, which prevents the body from producing high levels of insulin from carbohydrate consumption. In the absence of carbohydrates, the Atkins diet causes the body to burn its own fat for energy, thus cleaning out stored toxins, reducing variations in insulin levels, and reducing the risk of heart disease and stroke. Dr. Atkins uses this diet to treat patients at The Atkins Center for Complementary Medicine in New York. He disputes the claim that most major diseases are linked with fat intake and points out how processed carbohydrates contribute to diseases, such as diabetes, cancer, cardiovascular disease, and other conditions. (See Appendix C for further reading.)

No One Diet Is Right for Everyone

You can see that the diets discussed in this chapter fundamentally differ from one another. There is no one diet that seems to be correct for all people. You may want to spend some time learning more about the diets that interest you and then experiment to see which has the most beneficial effect on your unique body.

Chapter Six

The Dilemma of Medical Help

If the Treatment Doesn't Kill You

The sociologist Michael Bury (1982) said the following about getting medical help for chronic illness:

> The realization that medical knowledge is incomplete, and that treatment is based on practical trial and error, throws individuals back on their own stock of knowledge and biographical experience. The search for a more comprehensive level of explanation, a more certain basis of coping with the illness is often a long and profound one (p. 174).

If disillusionment with the help-seeking process is a normal part of dealing with "established" illnesses, getting help for MCS is even harder. In Phase II of my research, participants who provided medical care information saw an average of 8.6 medical practitioners. Of these practitioners, only 27 percent were described as being helpful. Respondents had spent an average of $5,784 on medical care in the previous year, and an average of $34,783 over the course of their illness.

More than one-quarter of the participants still did not have a doctor who was knowledgeable about chemical sensitivity. Because few physicians receive adequate training in toxicology or environmental causes of disease, few are prepared to help those with MCS. Perhaps this is why so many people with MCS are self-diagnosed. For example, in Phase I of my study, 47 percent were self-diagnosed; physicians diagnosed 32 percent, other professionals identified 1.3 percent; 3.3 percent of respondents were diagnosed by others with MCS; and 13 percent reported that their diagnoses were made by a combination of methods. The additional 3.4 percent of respondents did not answer the question.

In addition to physicians' lack of training, chemical barriers in offices often make it impossible even to meet with a medical practitioner. MCS patients frequently do not seek help even for problems unrelated to MCS because of chemical barriers such as perfumes on medical personnel, pesticides in offices, petrochemical heating systems, and so forth. Also, they often cannot tolerate the prescribed treatments. Of the 187 respondents in Phase III, twenty-eight said they avoided general dental work, twenty-five avoided medications, eighteen did not have recommended surgeries, and fifteen refused diagnostic tests. One woman said she reacted so badly to dental anesthetics (even local applications) that she chose to suffer from an abscessed tooth for two years.

Some participants reported enduring painful diagnostic medical procedures, such as bronchoscopy, cystoscopy, and colonoscopy, without the use of anesthetics. Other respondents reported using only local anesthesia for the removal of breast implants and skin tumors, and bladder and hernia repair.

Many respondents dreaded medical emergencies because they feared that the treatments administered would make them even sicker. In fact, this is exactly what happened to several. People reported that medical alert warnings clearly stated on official bracelets or necklaces were ignored; physicians administered medications and treatments to which patients had previously reported sensitivities; and reactions were not taken seriously and/or seen as psychosomatic.

Many respondents believed that they had suffered iatrogenic harm (harm caused by medical intervention). People described harm from drug effects, delay in diagnoses, treatment for incorrectly identified conditions, invasive medical tests, unnecessary surgeries, and electric shock treatments.

One woman describes becoming addicted to medications:

"In 1980, I went to a psychiatrist who put me on both tranquilizers and antidepressants. I became addicted to the tranquilizers and it took me eight years to wean myself off. . . . I still get angry when I think how they just didn't listen to me and made me feel guilty for being sick. I believe they therefore caused my physical injury and made my illness worse."

—Fifty-nine-year-old woman with MCS

Here are some other comments regarding respondents' feelings about their interactions with the medical establishment:

"I choose my eye doctor, dentist, lawyers, etc., by the odors in their offices."

"After going to doctors of environmental medicine, allergists, rheumatologists, family doctors, internists, I gave up on doctors. They can do nothing for me."

A great number of respondents' frustrations seemed to be the result of having had even life-threatening symptoms continually ignored or misinterpreted. For example, when one woman became unconscious from a reaction to hair coloring, emergency room physicians suggested that she was a drug addict. Other people with MCS had comments like these:

"For two years, between ages fifteen and seventeen, all that doctors would tell me about my problems was that 'adolescent girls have these symptoms' and they offered no help."

—Twenty-four-year-old woman with
MCS for nine years

"When no disease could be found by my gastroenterologist, he told me that he had patients a lot sicker than I am who had 'learned to live' with their symptoms."

—Woman living with MCS for eight years

"Over the years, I have seldom received treatment of any sort. Doctors did not take my complaints seriously and would send me away with the assurance that there was nothing wrong with me. So I continued getting sicker and sicker believing everyone felt as I did—only I was a weakling and a whiner for not coping like everyone else. I believed this even when I would get up in the morning and faint, when my throat would bleed for months at a time, when I had constant fevers and swollen lymph nodes for years. Why? Because *doctors* said there was *nothing* wrong with me."

—Thirty-six-year-old woman with
MCS since childhood

Some patients actually were refused treatment and sent away by physicians. One woman who had struggled with MCS for twenty-two years was told by an allergist that people's bodies just didn't do the things she described. When she reacted to the allergy testing, the allergist got angry with her and told her not to come back.

In some cases, physicians balk at seeing chemically injured patients who may become involved in lawsuits. A woman injured when a gallon of air freshener was accidentally spilled in her car said:

"When I told the first doctor what had happened to me he refused to examine me. He said he didn't want to get involved and he wouldn't charge me for the visit. I told him if he would examine my nose he would probably see physical evidence of my injury. He did this and noted that there was abnormal redness and fluid in my ears. Quickly, he said, 'But these are symptoms of a cold and I'm just going to write down that you have a cold.'"

Swearing Off Medical Treatment

For the most part, good medical care is not available to MCS patients in the conventional medical community. This has led some participants to swear off medical care entirely. One woman said, "I'm not happy about donating my body to science while I'm still alive, so I don't." Another said, "All the doctors I went to had not even heard of chemicals or pesticides hurting a person. I haven't found a doctor who even wanted to get involved. They all thought I needed a psychologist. I haven't been to a medical doctor in seven years."

Blind Faith Will Not Get You Good Treatment

Clearly, MCS patients are not receiving good care from the medical profession. Given the costs involved and the possibility of being harmed by inadequate medical care, one of the worst things the MCS patient can do is go trustingly from provider to provider, passively accepting treatments, and hoping that something will work. Here is a testimony from someone who tried to be a "good patient":

"The original otologist [ear doctor] had me tested for depression (I was not [depressed], but severely stressed.) The psychiatrist suggested a few 'talk sessions' and I readily agreed; however, he demanded I take an antidepressant (which put me to sleep at the wheel and I drove the car off the road!). He informed me he knew nothing about tinnitus or MCS, but said that if I was going to get well it would be there in his office. I laughed all the way home and didn't look back. The second otologist suggested I be put on Prozac and monitored; I began having violent headaches, nausea, and vertigo to the point where I couldn't get out of bed. The psychiatrist was supposed to be keeping careful check on me and [during his] last visit he admitted he never had a tinnitus patient and knew nothing about it. Ceasing Prozac eliminated all adverse effects. So, you can't say I'm not a cooperative patient with faith in my doctors; however, I have changed my attitude and now assume as much responsibility for my health as possible."

—Sixty-one-year-old woman with MCS for
three years, originally injured by carpet chemicals

Sometimes loved ones or primary care providers suggest that you go to a famous clinic to find out what is wrong with you "once and for all." One woman who had been sick for ten years spent her life savings doing this:

"In 1987, I got a real bad reaction (swelling in my shoulder and back, chest pains, and other symptoms). I went from doctor to doctor. One doctor did a mylegram and injected dye into my spine. I had a bad allergic reaction to the dye, but the doctor didn't understand what was going on. [She p]ut me on heart medication to stop my heart from skipping beats and other medications for swelling. [I] felt really doped up from all that. Finally, a rheumatologist sent me to the . . . Clinic. Their results showed nothing too much out of the ordinary. They could not find the cause of the dent in my head, swelling and all the other symptoms. At the end of my visit, I was upset that they could not help me. I believed it was my last hope. I used up our savings to go to the clinic. . . . Their reply was that I hyperventilate and I should come back in three years. That was *very* depressing. I have not gone to a medical doctor since."

What Works

It is possible that MCS patients have tried more remedies and treatments than any other patient group in the world. When you are left out of conventional medicine you tend to experiment. Some people have found relief with alternative treatments, including herbs, bodywork, and meditation. I collected data in 1993 on a number of treatments tried by people with MCS. This chapter deals with conventional treatments. See chapter seven for descriptions of alternative treatment options.

Alison Johnson conducted an excellent three-year study (from 1996 to 1998) on treatments for MCS by asking 351 people to rate over 160 different treatments. She distributed her findings and periodic updates in newsletters that included both quantitative data and in-depth discussions of a number of treatments. Respondents were asked to rate therapies as "effect unclear," "harmful," "didn't help," "slight help," "major help," or "enormous help." Few therapies helped more than 25 percent of the participants who tried them. Avoidance based therapies, however, were much more positive (with 95 percent of respondents rating avoidance as a "major" or "enormous" help), and some other therapies were rated fairly high as well.

Johnson's research is the largest study of treatments done to date, and although she is no longer collecting data, you can purchase her results. (See Appendix C for chapter resources and further reading.)

LeRoy, Davis, and Jason (1996) also conducted a formal study of treatments. Treatments that rated highly and had low rates of harm included chemical avoidance, creating a safe space, moving to a cleaner area, education, support groups, establishing connections with other MCS people, and meditation/relaxation.

Varying Risks

Although there is no way of knowing whether the respondents in each of these studies represent all people with chemical sensitivities and injuries, self-identified samples such as these and clinical samples from physicians' offices are the only groups that have been studied to date with respect to treatment. Both of the studies suggest that although each treatment helped some of the people who tried it, the risk of worsening was present with almost all of them.

The highest harm ratings were reported for drugs and magnet beds. (Magnet beds were rated harmful by 60 percent in the Johnson study).

Here are the harm ratings from the Johnson and LeRoy studies for several drugs.

Drug	Johnson Study *Percent Rated Harmful*	LeRoy, Davis, and Jason Study *Percent Rated Harmful*
Elavil	52	52
Prozac	56	56
Zoloft	53	56
Wellbutrin	55	67
Sinequan (doxepin)	67	59
Imipramine (Tofranil)	50	
Anafranil	75	
Tegretol	71	
MAO Inhibitors	75	
Valium	50	

The antifungal drugs did not fare too well in either of the studies. Although they were rated as helpful by a significant number of people, the harm ratings also were high.

Drug	Johnson/LeRoy % Slight Help	Johnson/LeRoy % Major/ Enormous Help	Johnson/LeRoy % Harmful
Nystatin	30/28	27/22	19/23
Nizoral	21/21	30/19	29/34
Diflucan	22/26	41/31	14/14

The removal of tooth fillings that contain mercury often is discussed as a way to improve health by reducing the body's exposure to metallic elements. Of 151 people in Johnson's study who had had their mercury amalgams removed, forty-two said that the effect had been unclear, nine rated it as harmful, and twenty-four said it was no help. Conversely thirty-five said removing their fillings was a slight help, twenty-five said major help, and sixteen said it was enormous help. Some respondents in Phase I of my research reported getting sicker from mercury amalgam removal, probably because of inhaling and swallowing mercury in the process. Although some people do seem to get better from this procedure (some even immediately), it is expensive and carries many risks, including having teeth cracked during drilling, reacting badly to anesthesia and replacement dental materials, and temporarily increasing one's mercury exposure.

How Chemically Sensitive People Improved Their Health

MSC research respondents in Phase II of my study listed the wide variety of treatments below as having helped improve their health. These items were listed most commonly:

- allergy drops/extract/injections
- sauna treatment
- homeopathy
- herbs
- proper medical treatment
- detox in general

How Is MCS Treated?

Despite routinely difficult searches for helpful physicians, the majority of participants in Phase I of my research felt that they had finally found doctors who were knowledgeable about chemical sensitivity. Although these practitioners were not all well-known experts, they took an interest in and had some knowledge about the problem. These patients saw practitioners in clinical ecology/environmental medicine (37.7 percent), general practice (11.5 percent), homeopathy (6.6 percent), chiropractic medicine (5.6 percent), occupational medicine (4.3 percent), psychiatry (2.6 percent), and immuno-toxicology (2.3 percent). An additional 29.4 percent of respondents did not answer this question. A small number of respondents found that some primary care providers also were open to learning about MCS.

> "My new primary care doctor is very interested in learning more about chemical sensitivities and welcomes the articles that I give her. She is receptive to working with me and is one of the few doctors who didn't want to send me packing out of the door because they didn't know what to do with me."
>
> —Thirty-six-year-old woman with MCS for eighteen years

Environmental Medicine

Probably the largest group of physicians to treat MCS is in environmental medicine. Although practitioners in occupational medicine have been seeing workers poisoned by chemicals for many years, treating people who react to low-level chemical exposures is the specialty of those in environmental medicine. The basic tenets of environmental medicine are summarized briefly in this chapter and in chapter one. (See Appendix C for further reading.)

In Phase I of my study, many people reported visiting practitioners of environmental medicine (referred to in the study as "clinical ecology"). Of these, 41 percent said it was of great benefit, 30 percent reported moderate benefit, 17 percent said the visit was mildly beneficial, 7 percent reported no benefit, and 5 percent reported adverse reactions.

Avoiding Chemical Exposure

According to my studies, avoiding chemical exposure is clearly the most effective intervention for MCS. Environmental medicine practitioners prescribe chemical exposure avoidance to reduce symptoms, prevent worsening of the condition, and allow the body to heal. Patients are urged to avoid all foods, molds, inhalants, and chemicals to which they react. In addition, they are encouraged to avoid chemicals that commonly cause other chemically sensitive people to become sick. Frequently, MCS reactions extend first to substances similar to your triggers, then to all different kinds of chemicals. Sensitivities also frequently extend to natural substances like food, mold, and pollens. This process is commonly referred to as the "spreading phenomenon." For example, if you become sensitive to natural gas, you are likely to become sensitive to similar hydrocarbon petrochemicals, such as propane. Similarly, if one perfume makes you sick, looking for one that doesn't is usually futile because the chemicals used are often the same or very similar. Seventy-four percent of the people in Phase I of my study labeled avoidance as having "great benefit" and not one respondent reported having adverse reactions.

Total Load

The concept of total load is important in environmental medicine because it says that the reaction you have to a pollutant on any given day depends upon the total amount of exposures your body is being forced to deal with at that point in time. The idea is that you might be more likely to have a reaction to an exposure if you are already weakened from other loads on your body, such as prior chemical exposures that day, inhalant allergies, nutritional deficiencies, reactions to ingested foods and drugs, hormonal imbalances, etc. Some have likened the total load concept to a container (the body) literally filling up or being weighted down with exposures until it can take no more. Another way of understanding total load is by using Rogers' (1986) analogy of a person with MCS setting out in a boat with a number of marked boxes that include traditional inhalant and food allergies, chemical hypersensitivity, newer mold allergies, phenol sensitivity, candida, nutrition, hormone hypersensitivity, heavy metal poisoning, stress, patient compliance (although some see this as a patient-blaming concept), and other miscellaneous factors. If the boat starts filling up with water, the number of boxes the MCS person must throw overboard depends on *where the leak in the boat is*. The lower the leak, the more boxes you have to jettison to float high enough to survive.

This may be why some people are able to get well by taking care of only one or two chemical factors (analogous to throwing only a little weight overboard), while other people must address them all. Only the very worst people have their leak located along the keel. Even if they throw overboard all twelve boxes and get rid of their entire total load, they still will continue to take in water and proceed to sink unless they are taken to a dry dock for a repair job. This dry dock is analogous to the environmental unit (Rogers 1996, 481).

Detoxification Methods

The Environmental Unit. The environmental unit is for people who are reactive to so many substances that they cannot determine their specific sensitivities, or who are so sick that they need, as Rogers says, to be taken to "dry dock." The environmental unit is a place where the environment can be completely controlled and monitored and specific sensitivities determined. The first environmental unit in the United States was established by Theron Randolph in Chicago, but it is now closed. To my knowledge, at this writing, there is no inpatient environmental unit for patients with MCS in the United States. A unit has been built in Canada, and there are a number of outpatient clinics in the United States that operate only during the day with patients staying overnight at hotels or residing with former patients who rent safe rooms.

When inpatient environmental units existed, standard procedure was to allow patients to live in a clean environment for a few days so that their reactions could be "unmasked." During this time, patients fasted on toler-ated water. Following this, patients were tested for safe waters, foods, and finally inhalants (molds, dusts, pollens), and chemicals. Progress was slow, as foods were initially eaten only one per day until several safe foods had been identified. These safe foods were then rotated. When patients finally returned home, they may have received from the clinic neutralizing drops for foods, inhalants, chemicals, and/or hormones that helped them to better tolerate some exposures. After unmasking in any unit, it is best to return home to as uncontaminated an environment as possible, which requires planning and most likely some cleaning and rearranging. (See chapter four and Appendix B.)

Creating an Oasis. To aid in avoiding chemical exposure, and because you spend one-third of your life sleeping, MCS patients are urged to create a bedroom oasis, which is a room that is as environmentally clean as possible. Eighty-six percent of the people in Phase I of my study reported getting moderate or great benefit from creating an oasis, and only two percent reported no benefit.

Serial Dilution Testing. Serial dilution is a method used in environ-mental medicine to diagnose and treat sensitivities to inhalants, such as pol-lens, dusts, and molds. This method differs from the standard "one size fits all" scratch test, in that scratch tests may examine you for a level of a sub-stance that is too low or even too high to elicit a reaction. In contrast, serial dilution testing looks not only for what substances you react to, but at what level you react. For example, you may be able to tolerate a small amount of mold, but if the dose is higher, you react negatively. Serial dilution testing looks at several levels of exposure by simultaneously injecting a series of progressively stronger solutions of an antigen under the skin. The solutions are usually diluted by a factor of five. All injections cause a 4-millimeter wheal or welt on the skin to form. An injection that causes an additional

2-millimeter increase in the wheal is called the end point. This end point concentration is used as the starting point to begin treatment for the substance to which you are sensitive. Johnson (1997) found that of the people in her study who had tried serial dilution, 6.3 percent said it was an enormous help, 31.3 percent said it was a major help, 15.6 percent said it was a slight help, 18.8 percent said it did not help, 21.9 percent said it was harmful, and 6.3 percent said the effect was unclear.

Provocation/Neutralization. Provocation/Neutralization (P/N) consists of either intradermal (just under the skin surface) or sublingual (under the tongue) testing of suspected antigens at calibrated levels similar to those for serial dilution testing. It differs from serial dilution testing in that it can be used for foods, hormones, and chemicals in addition to inhalants. Also, with P/N testing, only one dilution of one antigen can be tested at a time. If skin testing is done, physicians will assess your sensitivity by observing any reactions you may have to the substance, such as a wheal (welt) on your skin. However, to determine your sensitivity in a sublingual test, testers will rely exclusively on your own internal observations of how you are reacting to the substance. You are encouraged to watch how you feel, and to record any reactions about ten minutes or so after each test. Because only one dilution of one substance is tested at one time, P/N testing is very time-consuming and expensive. Additionally, if you are a "delayed reactor," you may need to test one substance per test period, as your reactions may not appear within the allotted observation period.

Standard allergy extracts contain the preservative phenol, and should not be used to test those with chemical sensitivities. Also, some people require the use of glycerine-free extracts due to reactivity to glycerine itself. Although antigens are available phenol-free, there is a narrower selection of test substances that are glycerine-free.

Once your antigen doses are identified through P/N methods, you will use sublingual extracts for maintenance and to help neutralize your responses to unavoidable exposures. The extracts are not a carte blanche permission for your exposure to more triggers, but they aid in avoiding constant reactions. No one knows exactly how P/N treatment works, but some people seem able to maintain more stability by using these drops. Caution: Those people whose endpoints change often have more problems because doses that once turned off a reaction may begin to trigger it.

P/N testing has been the target of much criticism from the conventional medical community. Rogers (1986) stresses that it is very tedious and exact, and requires hands-on training with an established expert for a physician to become competent in this method. Additionally, background exposures must be controlled for the testing to be accurate, e.g., if you are tested for mold in a moldy office, it can be impossible to determine your level of sensitivity accurately. Rogers is concerned that it hurts environmental medicine when P/N is experimented with inaccurately and then is deemed ineffective. In addition, it seems that some people don't even have to try it before they form a negative opinion about it. The constant criticism of P/N testing is that there are no double-blind studies that validate it and that both the development and remission of symptoms in the office may be influenced by patient and physician expectations. Rogers attempted to disprove this criticism when she did P/N testing and treatment on horses with hay fever and found it effective. However, the paper was still rejected by reviewers who insisted that P/N testing doesn't work. Doris Rapp, a leading environmental medical physician, has created videos of dramatic changes in children's behavior as they are being P/N tested for foods and other substances. Although both children and parents have testified that they have received life-saving help from P/N testing, skeptics still are not convinced.

Even individuals with an avid interest in MCS are leery about P/N techniques. Some feel that the testing itself may make patients worse. In addition, if your endpoints change often, the needed frequency of retesting is expensive and difficult. P/N testing may work best with those whose endpoints are fairly stable, and whose sensitivities are fairly limited.

Preservative-free Testing.   Johnson (1996-1998) reported MCS patients' responses to P/N testing for molds, inhalants, foods, hormones, and chemicals with and without preservatives. In all categories, she found that testing with chemicals was rated as more harmful than the preservative-free method.

Percentages of people who rated the preservative-free extracts as major or enormous help in the Johnson study included 39 percent for preservative-free inhalants, 37 percent for preservative-free molds, 23 percent for preservative-free foods, 20 percent for preservative-free chemicals, and 15 percent for preservative-free hormones. Preservative-free extracts were rated harmful as follows: chemicals, 19 percent; hormones, 18 percent; molds, 17 percent; foods, 13 percent; and inhalants, 12 percent.

LeRoy, Davis, and Jason (1996) inquired into neutralization of foods and chemicals. Neutralization to foods was tried by 188 people and found to be an enormous help for 9.7 percent, a major help for 9.7 percent, a slight help for 24.7 percent, not helpful for 27.4 percent, harmful for 11.3 percent, and unclear in effect for 17.2 percent. Neutralization to chemicals was tried by 189 people and was an enormous help for 10.6 percent, a major help for 11.6 percent, slight help for 20.1 percent, not helpful for 27 percent, harmful for 15.9 percent, and unclear in effect for 14.8 percent.

Following are the ratings of allergy injections or drops from my study.

Rated Effectiveness of Treatments
for Managing Symptoms in MCS

Treatment	Number Tried	% No Benefit	% Mild Benefit	% Moderate Benefit	% Great Benefit	% Adverse Reaction
Allergy shots (with phenol)	95	23	11	4	7	55
Allergy shots (without phenol)	95	14	20	19	33	15
Sublingual drops (with phenol)	69	14	13	14	12	46
Sublingual drops (without phenol)	98	21	17	23	24	13

Sauna Therapy. Many studies have confirmed that people retain and store toxic chemicals in their fat tissues. This means that we can experience chemical assaults not only from the external environment, but also from within. These toxins may move into the bloodstream during exercise and exposure to heat, as well as when you sleep or fast.

Sauna treatment helps to dislodge and mobilize some of the toxins stored in fat by eliminating them from the body through sweating, thus reducing your total chemical load. Using a sauna can reduce the levels of chemicals in fat tissue. Levels may continue to decline even after sauna treatments have ended. This suggests that saunas may energize the body to continue detoxifying itself.

L. Ron Hubbard, the founder of Scientology, created the forerunner of the modern sauna technique when he invented detoxification regimens to clear people's bodies of illicit drug residues, which he felt were contributing to learning and perceptual problems. The Hubbard regimen prescribes *fat mobilization* through cardiovascular exercise and nicotinic acid (vitamin B-3) and *enhanced excretion* through well ventilated heat treatment (temperature at 160 degrees instead of the usual 200 to 210 degrees in a nontherapeutic sauna). Patients are given cold pressed oils to slow intestinal reabsorption of the mobilized toxins that are secreted into the bowel, and electrolytes are monitored and replaced to counteract mineral loss. The diet emphasizes fiber and vegetables. Although the length of treatment varies, three weeks is a common time frame, with some people continuing for six weeks. The costs are several thousand dollars for the treatment and the nutrients in the medically supervised programs, and patients must be able to afford housing during the regimen.

Some people have serious reservations about sauna treatments. Cynthia Wilson, founder and director of Chemical Injury Information Network (CIIN), believes that when chemicals in your body are mobilized in the sauna, you risk further damage. Wilson says that CIIN has received numerous reports over the last seven years from people with MCS who have gone through the "quick sauna" program (lasting one to two weeks). Many of these people said they had acquired epileptic seizure activity or had had strokes while they were in the sauna. Wilson also questions whether sauna treatments provide permanent benefits or whether the effects are only temporary. When I asked Wilson whether she thought sauna treatments were helpful at all, she said that using it slowly, perhaps twenty minutes every other day, might give slow and lasting benefit with less risk.

Home saunas are available and often are more affordable and convenient. Although a home sauna may give you more control and access to the treatment, monitoring your electrolytes without supervision may be difficult unless you have a physician who can order mineral tests and can guide you in ingesting the appropriate amounts of replacement minerals.

In Phase I of my research, 40.3 percent of the people who used sauna therapy experienced great benefit, 19.4 percent had moderate benefit, 16.4 percent had mild benefit, 10.4 percent found no benefit, and 13.4 percent had adverse reactions. LeRoy, Davis, and Jason found that of 83 people with MCS who had tried sauna detoxification, 21.7 percent said it was an enormous help, 16.9 percent said it was a major help, 25.3 percent said it had been a slight help, 15. 7 percent said it did not help, 10.8 percent said the effect was unclear, and 9.6 percent said it had been harmful. (If you are interested in sauna therapy, see Appendix B for product sources.)

Additional Detoxification Methods. Practitioners of both environmental and alternative medicine may recommend other detoxification methods such as coffee enemas, liver and gallbladder flushes, and bowel cleanses.

In Phase I of my study, 40 percent of the research participants who tried coffee enemas and 35 percent of those who experimented with bowel cleanses rated them as having great benefit. Conversely, nearly 35 percent of those people who tried the gall bladder flush rated it as having no benefit at all. Many of the people (39.4 percent) who did a liver flush said it was moderately beneficial. Krohn (1996) recommends a variety of methods for natural detoxification that can be used by people with sensitivities.

There is a great deal you can do for yourself before seeing a practitioner of environmental medicine. It may be helpful to speak with people who have been treated by a particular doctor before committing yourself to a long, complicated, and expensive treatment regimen. I also suggest reading as much as possible about environmental medicine. The more you know, the better educated a consumer you will be, and the better you will choose and monitor any treatment you decide to try. (See Appendix C for further reading.)

If you decide that you want to see a practitioner of environmental medicine and are willing to pay the costs involved, which can be considerable, the American Academy of Environmental Medicine (AAEM) can provide you with a list of physicians in your area. (See Appendix C for resources.)

Experimental Therapies

There are a few therapies that are very experimental in nature (at least for MCS), but which may show promise for some people. At this point, the following therapies have very limited information available and most reports are individual case studies (as opposed to actual experiments), but some people may want to look into them. The next few sections describe such therapies.

Enzyme Potentiated Desensitization

In enzyme potentiated desensitization (EPD), low dose antigens are mixed with the enzyme beta glucuronidase (which is thought to increase the immunizing effects of the allergens), and given in a series of treatments. Edelson and Statman (1998) describe the enzyme as being extracted from abalone digestive glands. Following EPD treatment, it is thought that T-suppressor cells are produced, which then recognize and suppress reactions to subsequent exposures of the injected allergens. According to Edelson and Statman: "EPD does not abolish allergies. Instead, it increases the dose of allergen needed to provoke illness by a factor of between tens and thousands. As a result, ordinary exposures to the allergen become harmless" (p. 143).

Enzyme potentiated desensitization can be administered by two methods. With intradermal injections, the antigens, are introduced by fine needles into the forearm (shots). In the cup method, the antigens are placed in a small cup over scarified (scratched) skin on either the arm or thigh, and allowed to absorb into the skin during a twenty-four hour period. Edelson says that this slow method makes it very safe, and that the immune system will react better to antigens delivered through skin than through injections. Edelson recommends using mixtures of a wide variety of pollens, dust, dander, foods, etc., because many allergens desensitize once they are grouped together. Additionally, using a variety of allergens helps protect against the problem of developing new sensitivities. He does not, however, cite any studies that support this. Doses are given every two or three months for the first year, and the interval can be lengthened thereafter.

While undergoing EPD treatments, there are extremely strict protocols for managing diet, exposures, vitamin intake, medications, and even exercise, particularly between the day before and the week after treatment. Exposures of any kind may overload the system and, in Edelson's words, change "the 'whispered' message of EPD . . . into a 'shout' and it can reverse the effect for the allergen that is concerned" (p. 122). Even becoming overheated or using toothpaste can interfere with the treatment.

Edelson describes the need for a "very mixed" diet for food-sensitive people during the week following a treatment. He says that large quantities of individual foods will interfere with desensitization. People should therefore eat tiny amounts of food rather than normal portions and eat a large variety of food types at one time, e.g., eating a small bowl of seven or eight different grains.

Some foods and food quantities, however, may cause more trouble following EPD. Edelson states that the desensitization will not be stable early on, and that safe amounts of foods will increase in the weeks after treatment only to decrease before the next EPD dose. However, the safe quantities are said to increase progressively and eventually stabilize.

In Phase I of my study, only nine people had tried EPD. Of these, one reported it was of great benefit, five perceived moderate benefit, one reported mild benefit, two reported no benefit at all, and no one reported adverse reactions. Johnson's study (1996-1998) included forty people who had tried EPD: 17.5 percent said it was an enormous help, 20 percent a major help, 15 percent as slight help, 25 percent as not helpful, 15 percent as harmful, and 7.5 percent rated the effect as unclear.

Neurontin

Neurontin is an anticonvulsant that Dallas psychiatrist Jay Seastrunk uses to treat people with MCS. Neurontin is a synthetic amino acid. According to Seastrunk, people with MCS and chronic fatigue immunodeficiency syndrome (CFIDS) may have some localized brain injury that makes it easier for the brain to become kindled or sensitized (see chapter two) by chemicals or electrical incitants. He cites early research that found epileptic reactions may develop in humans after an extended period of time (up to fifteen years) following a traumatic injury on the opposite side of the brain from the epileptic reactions. He says:

I feel the chemical or electrical stimuli in the environment that activate these neurons become a trigger that fires previously injured or hypersensitive neurons, thereby producing a firing that can progress neuron by neuron to the furthest reaches of the brain, including the emotional area called the limbic system, or to the areas that control arousal, cognition, sensation, memory, temperature, blood pressure, pain, and motor function or any other activity that is brain mediated.

Seastrunk's research assistant Dr. Steve Krebaum (1998) said he was uncertain whether initial localized brain injuries are chemically induced or caused by some other agency. The results of brain imaging techniques, however, such as Magnetic Resonance Spectroscopy (MRS), do lead them to believe that the location of the injury determines the sensitivities in MCS.

The rationale of prescribing neurontin is to stabilize nerve cells and thus interrupt reactions in the central nervous system that are triggered by chemical exposures. Neurontin is not metabolized in the liver, rather it travels through the body unchanged, and is excreted rapidly through the kidneys. Therefore, it must be taken several times daily to maintain effective therapeutic blood levels. Seastrunk advises some patients, particularly those who "had extensive brain injury many years ago," to stay on the drug for life. However, he says 30 to 40 percent of people with MCS can stop taking the drug after two years. It is common for antidepressants to be prescribed with neurontin simultaneously, as the drug can cause depressant side effects. Seastrunk claims that 10 to 15 percent of his patients respond quickly and have little trouble with neurontin treatment, 60 to 70 percent take longer to respond, but do well, 5 percent don't do well on the program at all, and 5 to 10 percent don't comply with treatment. Seastrunk says, "Response time tends to mirror the duration of illness prior to treatment." That is, the longer someone has been ill, the longer it takes to respond to the treatment.

Thirty-six people in a study conducted by Alison Johnson (1996-1998) tried neurontin treatment. Of these, eleven reported the drug was of enormous help, nine said it was a major help, eight people said it was a slight help, and eight reported it caused harm. Johnson edited newsletters in March and September 1997 that published detailed information about neurontin with excerpts of testimonials from people who had tried it. In early neurontin trials, some people described literally "getting their life back." However, within six months, some regretted their decisions to try the drug, citing negative effects such as weight gain (even to the point of looking pregnant); edema; digestive problems, including constipation and esophageal reflux; short-term memory deficits; dizziness; acne; tremors; and more. For some, there was an improvement in emotional symptoms, although others described being "spaced out" or "numb." Interestingly, some individuals felt that neurontin masked their ability to smell dangerous chemicals, but did not prevent them from experiencing the negative effects of a harmful exposure. Still others described very difficult withdrawal symptoms when they tried to get off of the drug. One woman said, "If you are not one of the lucky ones who do better immediately, get off of (neurontin) as soon as possible." It would be wise to do further reading and/or talk with people who have tried neurontin before making a decision to experiment with this treatment. (See Appendix C for further reading.)

Antibiotic Therapy for Mycoplasma Fermentans

Drs. Garth and Nancy Nicolson (1995) discovered a microorganism called mycoplasma fermentans in their daughter's blood when she returned ill from the Gulf War and they became ill from being around her. Because the Nicolsons were both molecular pathologists they were able to identify the microorganism in their white cells through a test called a polymerase chain reaction (PCR) of the DNA. They also found that half of those tested (Gulf War and chronic fatigue immunodeficiency syndrome (CFIDS) patients) tested positive for the microorganism.

The Nicolsons recovered by taking a long course of treatment with antibiotics that are active against the mycoplasma. This treatment of four antibiotics, doxycycline (broad-spectrum tetracycline), ciprofloxacin, azithromycin, and clarithromycin, also may provide help for people with MCS who have been tested and find that they harbor the mycoplasma. Unfortunately, many people with MCS are unable to take even one antibiotic because of yeast flare-ups and other reactions to the drug.

It should be noted, the Nicolsons believe that some of the newest forms of the mycoplasma may have been engineered for germ warfare, and may be contributing to the causes of serious diseases, such as rheumatoid arthritis and AIDS, in addition to Gulf War illness, CFIDS, and MCS.

There is a very large overlap between people with MCS and those with CFIDS. Sharon Briggs a registered nurse currently collecting data for future research has been monitoring a group of twenty-three people with CFIDS who are trying the antibiotic treatment for mycoplamsa fermentans; she also is in touch with a large number of others all over the United States who are following this antibiotic protocol treatment. She says that the results have been positive; a large majority have reported that they are substantially improved and some disabled people even have gone back to work. (See Appendix C for chapter resources.)

If You Choose to Seek Professional Help

I suggest you very carefully investigate any treatment or practitioner you are considering. Medical treatment is expensive and your earning power is likely to have diminished since you developed MCS. Seeking and receiving treatment can require an enormous expenditure of time and energy (particularly if you travel to see an expert). The decision to try a treatment must balance the possibility that the treatment will be helpful against the possibility that it may fail and might actually make you worse. If paying for a treatment option will financially cripple you and emotionally devastate you if the treatment doesn't work, you need to ask yourself if you really want to empty your bank account on a bet (especially if that treatment helps only a minority of people who try it). Cynthia Wilson of the Chemical Injury Information Network (CIIN) receives at least one call per month from MCS patients who are still sick, have spent all of their money, and have been promised a cure if they can just come up with "another $1,000." Because of the frequency of false promises by some health practitioners, your delicate state of health, and very likely, your limited resources, I urge you again to do considerable research before embarking on any treatment, especially experimental potentially hazardous ones. Some of the following suggestions may help you to determine which treatments and practitioners may be right for you.

How to Investigate MCS Treatments, Costs, and Track Records

You may want to study, in detail, the particular therapies that are in accord with your personal philosophy, or that you can financially afford or feel comfortable trying. There are a number of therapies that are promoted as useful for MCS. (See chapter seven for alternative, holistic treatments.) However, no one has the money or energy to try them all. Alison Johnson's work showed that most treatments help no more than about 25 percent of the people who try them.

There is no magic bullet for MCS, although chemical avoidance helps most people reduce their symptoms substantially. I agree with Johnson, who suggests that there is something to be said for saving your money until there is an effective treatment that works for a large number of people, either from conventional or alternative medicine.

Investigate MCS Practitioners

Respondents in all of the phases of my study had a very difficult time finding accessible and effective treatment for MCS. Despite spending large amounts of money on evaluation and treatment, satisfaction with health care was low. Some respondents found some help using a variety of conventional and alternative treatments. Others tried a seemingly endless cycle of one treatment after another and succeeded only in emptying their bank accounts without experiencing much physical improvement.

Given this state of affairs, it is clear that before you make an appointment with a practitioner, you should speak with other patients who have been treated by them, even if the practitioner is well known in the field of environmental or occupational medicine. It may be possible to find out beforehand how patients are treated, a practitioner's accessibility, probable costs, and whether or not treatment was helpful or harmful. The Chemical Injury Information Network (CIIN) can provide you with a list of physicians from various fields who treat MCS patients. In addition, you may be able to get referrals from people in your local MCS support group who have tried various conventional and alternative practitioners in your area. You also can speak with people at national organizations, such as CIIN and the National Center for Environmental Health Strategies (NCEHS), who talk with hundreds of individuals with MCS each week and hear numerous stories about various practitioners.

The sad truth is that although some people's health can improve, it is rare for anyone to recover completely from MCS. This underscores the importance of chemical avoidance to prevent the worsening of your condition. MCS is a chronic condition. It is necessary to come to terms with how you will survive in the long haul, and emptying your bank account for some questionable therapy may not be your best strategy. On the other hand, some people have been helped tremendously by various treatments and practitioners.

It is important to remember that not all of your symptoms may be caused by MCS (Wilson 1999, vol. 10). When a new symptom appears, it may have a non-MCS cause, and be treatable. Wilson gives an example of a woman who attributed her terrible sinus headaches to her MCS, when actually they were caused by a deviated septum.

Before Making an Appointment

Before making an appointment with an MSC practitioner, you may want to consider the following:

- Find out what the costs will be, how much you will be expected to pay up front, and exactly for which services you will be billed. For example, will the practitioner bill you for every phone call and letter written, and if so how much will be charged? Will lab test results be forwarded to you at no extra cost or will the practitioner charge to interpret each test? For instance, if you have seven tests and you are charged ninety dollars for each interpretation (even though labs generally include a good one), your bill will increase by $630. (Your insurance company probably will not reimburse this cost.) In addition, if practitioners intend to write their own interpretations, how long will it take for you to receive the report? Some offices take months, and by the time you obtain your test results, they may be obsolete.

- *Who will do the billing and is that person accessible?* Find out who will be doing the billing, get that person's phone number, and call. If they do not answer the phone or if you do not get a call back, you have a problem.

- *Can you reach the practitioner if you need to?* Try calling the practitioner's office to see if you are able to reach a real person, even just office personnel. In some cases, speaking directly to a person, and not to a machine, is almost impossible. How difficult is it and how long does it take to obtain a quick emergency consultation with the practitioner?

- *If you are seeing an environmental medicine practitioner, find out whether the office is a safe environment.* This is particularly true if you will be paying the high costs of Provocation/Neutralization (P/N) testing. (See page 103 for more information on P/N testing.)

  You may want to ask about the heating source in the office, possible pesticide applications, the age of the building, any use of disinfectants and fragrances, new carpeting, fluorescent lighting, and any chemical use that may be a problem for you in terms of exposures. (I have seen environmental medicine practitioners' offices located in the same building as restaurants that cooked with gas, with nurses smoking in the stairwell on their breaks, where disinfectant was sprayed in the bathroom, and where outside air filled with recently cut grass was circulating through the air conditioner as patients were being tested for grass sensitivity!) All of these exposures can affect your reactions to testing. It may be that the improper control of these exposures is one reason for some of the controversy regarding P/N testing and treatment.

- *How is your insurance handled?* Does the practitioner accept your insurance and file for payment, or will you be expected to pay in advance and wait for your insurance company to reimburse you?

- *Is the practitioner a primary care physician or an MCS specialist?* Many MCS specialists expect you to have another physician as your primary care physician to take care of general medical problems and emergencies. MCS specialists tend to provide only services relating specifically to MCS.

- *Does the practitioner handle emergencies?* If you have an MCS emergency (such as a pesticide exposure, a serious work exposure, or some other problem), will you be able to obtain guidance from the doctor in a timely manner?

- *If you need to apply for disability, will the practitioner support you?*

- *Is the practitioner willing to be involved in legal disputes?* If you are involved in court litigation and you need medical evidence in your lawsuit, you need to find out—before making an appointment— whether the practitioner will help you. Not all practitioners are willing to provide written or verbal legal testimony.

- *Talk to people who have seen that practitioner.* You can place an ad in MCS-specific newsletters, such as N.E.E.D.S., asking people who have seen a particular practitioner to call you. The N.E.E.D.S. newsletter is published by the privately owned National Ecological Environmental Delivery System and will print messages from its customers in its advertising booklet free of charge.

Going to the Hospital

One of the greatest fears many MCS people have is that they will be hospitalized. They fear they will be too sick to advocate for their own safe treatment or that they will be ignored when they try to protect themselves from anesthetics, perfumes, cleaners, drugs, plastic tubing, and pesticides. Although people with MCS can never fully protect themselves while they are hospitalized, there are helpful sources for educating medical personnel and securing safe treatment for patients. Regarding education, Toni Temple (1996) has written a booklet for hospital employees, entitled *Healthier Hospitals*, in which she explains how to provide a safe medical environment for people with MCS. Her recommendations are extensive, and include structural (e.g., no carpet or vinyl blinds) and functional (e.g., no perfume) changes to minimize toxic exposures during hospital stays. Temple and others have facilitated well-received workshops for hospital employees that initiated policy changes at some hospitals. If you have the energy, you might want to provide the staff or nursing educator at your local hospital with a copy of this book and offer to organize a workshop as a follow-up. As the result of attending a workshop, for example, a community educator from a Chicago hospital created an MCS protocol that is followed whenever anyone with MCS is at that facility.

In nonemergency situations, you can write a letter to be shared with your surgeon or medical doctor before you are hospitalized. Sherry Rogers has published a sample letter in her book, *The EI Syndrome* (1986, 510–515), and suggests how you and your environmental practitioner can modify it to meet your needs.

Essential elements of Roger's letter include:

- Alert hospital personnel that you will be bringing some of your own supplies, such as bedding, food, water, etc.

- Request written orders that no one enter your room wearing perfume, aftershave, or other scents.

- Ask for a room with a window that opens into a clean area (not traffic, the parking lot, incinerator, ambulance driveway, or delivery area).

- Explain that for you local anesthetics are always preferable to general anesthetics. For example, specifically request that avoidance of carbocaine and halogenated or fluorinated hydrocarbons, which commonly are used for general anesthesia, not be used for you. (It is important to note that not all people have problems with carbocaine. In fact, some people use only carbocaine as a local anesthetic.)

- Ask that nitrous oxide be kept to a minimum.

- Although everyone is different, Rogers' letter suggests that thiopental sodium (Pentothal) or Brevital, preceded by 100 percent oxygen, be used to induce anesthesia; succinyl choline chloride (Anectine) or curare be used for paralysis; Sublimaze be used to erase memory; and Innovar, Demoral, or Nisentil be used for pain.

Several practitioners of environmental medicine believe it is not wise to rely on tests to determine your sensitivity to anesthetics because the results may not be true. You may be able to tolerate it the first time you are exposed, but not the second. That is, the first exposure may sensitize you to the anesthetic, and you might then react negatively to it during the surgery.

If you do not have an environmental medicine doctor, you can enlist your primary care physician's help in communicating your needs to your hospital ahead of time. This may not only save your life, but may give you peace of mind.

Of course, not every hospital stay is planned. To protect yourself against possible harm during emergency hospitalizations, visit your local hospital admissions coordinator and bring a letter from your doctor (if you have one) that explains your condition. Ask to have the letter kept on file. This letter should list the most important precautions to be taken if you are ever hospitalized or treated in their emergency room. (A letter on file will have greater credibility with staff than instructions from a moaning, supine person hurriedly babbling something about no perfume, gas anesthetics, or bug spray!) Note that a letter on file would not necessarily be heeded in an emergency; the best protection for a patient with special needs is to be accompanied by a strong, articulate advocate. Therefore, you might want to prepare an informed friend how to advocate for you if you must go to an emergency room or are admitted to a hospital. (See Appendix C for further reading.)

Healing Is Unique for Everyone

From the information in this chapter, you can see that the healing story for MCS is long, complicated, and incomplete. We are far from understanding exactly how the body breaks down in response to MCS and, to make matters worse, most people deny that the problem even exists. People who are attempting to heal must walk a fine and jagged line due to insufficient information about MCS and commonly encountered mistreatments. Healing is also highly personal, as no one therapy—other than chemical avoidance—seems to help everyone. In fact, one person's cure often is another's undoing. This is extremely frustrating, but it highlights the fact that only you can decide which therapies are appropriate to try. The personal nature of healing forces you to rely on your own knowledge and intuition. This isn't easy, but it certainly reinforces learning and growing.

Chapter Seven

Alternative Therapies

This chapter describes some of the holistic therapies that people with MCS have tried. The descriptions include a little about the underlying philosophy of each system and the various procedures involved with each alternative. In regard to trying new therapies, I suggest you learn about the methods ahead of time and choose those that correspond with your own philosophies of healing, or those to which you feel attracted. Since few people will have enough money to try them all, you must pick and choose wisely. Do a little reading. Making an informed choice is much safer, cheaper, and saner than going naively from one treatment option to another. More detailed information on alternative therapies can be found in Appendix C for further reading and in *Alternative Medicine: The Definitive Guide* by the Burton Goldberg Group (1994). This book is expensive, but it is a comprehensive guide to natural therapies and alternative treatments for various health conditions.

Acupuncture

A 5,000-year-old component of traditional Chinese medicine, acupuncture aims to enhance *qi* (or *chi*), which is what the Chinese call the life force circulating in all living beings. Optimum health occurs when the *qi* is balanced in its circulation along the twelve meridians or energy pathways of the human body. Each of the vital organs is associated with a meridian, and can be affected by stimulating specific areas called "acupoints," which are located along that meridian. Acupuncture treatment is administered with hair-thin, stainless steel, disposable needles that usually are not painful. The needles are inserted under the skin to stimulate the acupoints and to correct the energy flow, allowing for an improvement in health. The meridians have actually been documented by microdissection as existing separate from the blood and lymph systems (Burton Goldberg Group 1994).

The Burton Goldberg Group says that the World Health Organization lists 104 health problems that can be helped by acupuncture. Pain, particularly, is helped by acupuncture, because acupuncture stimulates the body's release of endogenous endorphins (natural opiatelike substances made in the brain) and neurotransmitters (chemicals used by nerves to transmit information). Acupuncture also has shown promise of helping people who are addicted to controlled substances; many drug treatment facilities have incorporated acupuncture into their withdrawal and rehabilitation programs. In China, acupuncture is used for anesthesia during various surgeries, including head and neck surgery. Veterinary medicine is beginning to explore acupuncture for animals. The National Institutes of Health's (1997) consensus statement on acupuncture concluded:

> Acupuncture as a therapeutic intervention is widely practiced in the United States. While there have been many studies of its potential usefulness, many of these studies provide equivocal results because of design, sample size, and other factors. The issue is further complicated by inherent difficulties in the use of appropriate controls, such as placebos and sham acupuncture groups. However, promising results have emerged. For example, showing efficacy of acupuncture in adult postoperative and chemotherapy nausea and vomiting, and in postoperative dental pain. There are other situations such as addiction, stroke rehabilitation, headache, menstrual cramps, tennis elbow, fibromyalgia, myofascial pain, osteoarthritis, low back pain, carpal tunnel syndrome, and asthma, in which acupuncture may be useful as an adjunct treatment or an acceptable alternative or be included in a comprehensive management program. Further research is likely to uncover additional areas where acupuncture interventions will be useful (p. 2).

In Phase I of my study, seventy-eight people had tried acupuncture with 24 percent finding great benefit, 8 percent moderate benefit, 27 percent had mild benefit, 29 percent experienced no benefit, and 12 percent reported adverse reactions. Acupuncture was also reported in the Johnson (1996-1998) and LeRoy, Davis, and Jason (1996) studies.

Of the 153 participants Johnson surveyed, 7.2 percent found acupuncture enormously helpful, 18.3 percent found it to be a major help, 30.1 percent said it was a slight help, 17.6 percent reported that it didn't help, 12.4 percent said it was harmful, and 14.4 percent reported that the effect was unclear. LeRoy, Davis, and Jason surveyed 132 participants. The results included 11.4 percent reporting acupuncture to be an enormous help, 14.4 percent reported it to be major help, 33.3 percent said it was a slight help, 20.5 percent reported it did not help, 6.8 percent reported acupuncture to be harmful, and 13.6 reported that the effect was unclear.

The *American Journal of Acupuncture* published a paper entitled "The Treatment of Pesticide Poisoning with Traditional Acupuncture" (Chatfield 1985) which described acupuncture treatment as substantially improving the health of three victims of pesticide poisoning. Most urban areas have acupuncture practitioners. (See Appendix C for further reading.)

Chiropractic Care

Chiropractic care is a widely used holistic treatment approach to whole-body health. It is concerned with the relationships between the spine, the musculoskeletal system, and the nervous system. More than fifteen million people each year receive chiropractic care, according to the Burton Goldberg Group (1994). Although modern chiropractic methods were established in 1895 by Daniel David Palmer, a physiology and anatomy student, spinal manipulation is thought to extend as far back as the early Egyptians. Chiropractic care is popular because of its ability to address a large number of health issues, including pain, trauma, injuries, back, and internal problems, without the use of drugs. A properly aligned spine is understood as the key to good health and is thought of as the "switchboard" for the rest of the body. Misalignments in the spine, referred to as subluxations, may exert pressure on other vertebrae or nerves, interfere with the flow of electrical impulses, or force a person into an unnatural posture that can, in turn, cause additional problems. The Burton Goldberg Group cites several studies that support the efficacy and cost-effectiveness of chiropractic care over conventional medicine for back pain and work injuries. Chiropractic care is successfully used to treat conditions of the musculoskeletal, respiratory, gastrointestinal, pulmonary, cardiovascular, and endocrine systems.

There are many types of adjustments in chiropractic practice that involve touching, stretching, and movement. All chiropractic adjustments are aimed at releasing pressure and restrictions, increasing the range of movement, and correcting misalignments. In Phase I of my study, 128 people had tried chiropractic care: 21 percent reported great benefit, 20 percent reported moderate benefit, 32 percent reported mild benefit, 23 percent found no benefit, and 4 percent reported adverse reactions. In LeRoy, Davis, and Jason's study (1996), 181 used chiropractic care: 14.4 percent reported enormous help, 18.2 percent said it was a major help, 30.4 percent said it was a slight help, 20.4 percent said it was of no help, 6.6 percent said it had been harmful, and 9.9 percent said the effect was unclear.

Applied Kinesiology

Applied Kinesiology seeks to diagnose and resolve health problems through the identification of specific muscle weaknesses. Muscle dysfunction is understood as corresponding to organ and gland dysfunction and, therefore, can be used to identify possibly weak organ systems. Postural balance, gait, and nerve function, as well as endocrine, immune, digestive, and cardiovascular functioning can all be affected by Applied Kinesiology, which aims at preventing new problems as well as at correcting existing ones.

Applied Kinesiology was invented by Detroit chiropractor George Goodheart in the 1960s, and frequently is integrated into chiropractic work. Muscles need to function properly for associated bones and joints to be adequately supported. Therefore, Applied Kinesiology is very useful for chiropractors. Because specific muscles are associated with specific organs (e.g., the deltoid muscles are specifically associated with the lungs), they are used to monitor the functioning of those organs. Certain nutrients (e.g., vitamins, minerals, glandulars) that may help a patient to heal, for example, can be tested immediately for effectiveness by placing them on the patient's tongue and checking to see whether the associated muscle becomes stronger or weaker. Applied Kinesiology is often used in sports medicine and has been an aid to some world-famous athletes.

In Phase I of my study, of the seventy-six people who tried kinesiology, 34 percent described great benefit, 22 percent moderate benefit, 25 percent mild benefit, 18 percent described no benefit, and no one reported harm.

Johnson's study (1996-1998) included 124 people who used Applied Kinesiology. Of these, 9.7 percent said that it was of enormous help, 28.2 percent said it was a major help, 22.6 percent said it was a slight help, 17.7 percent said it didn't help, 2.4 percent said that it had been harmful, and 19.4 percent said the effect was unclear. These two preliminary studies indicate that Applied Kinesiology may help—to some degree—more than half of the patients who try it.

Contact Reflex Analysis

Contact Reflex Analysis extends the theory and application of Applied Kinesiology to allow for greater detail and more complex diagnoses. It is a method of determining root causes and preventing health problems. It works by testing any of the approximately seventy-five reflex areas on the skin that correspond to organs, glands, and bones. As practitioners probe reflex sites with their fingertips, they use muscles as circuit indicators, to determine whether body circuits are functioning correctly.

Muscles weaken considerably when the practitioner locates a reflex site that has had its energy flow interrupted. Contact Reflex Analysis can locate subclinical problems, i.e., physiological problems in their early stages that have not yet manifested as organ disease. The system was developed during the past thirty years by a chiropractor named D. A. Versendaal (1998) and others in the industry.

Contact Reflex Analysis is taught to health professionals in continuing education courses and at conferences. Versendaal has hired a researcher to document the usefulness of Contact Reflex Analysis so it can be taught in a more formal education environment.

Bodywork

Bodywork therapies share the goal of improving the functioning of both body and mind, often using movement, touch, or energetic therapeutic interventions. Some, such as Rolfing, massage, and Hellerwork, focus on working with body tissue to restructure the body. Feldenkrais and the Alexander Technique work more with movement to correct postural problems that may affect various systems, including the brain and nervous system. Energy therapies, such as polarity therapy and therapeutic touch, strive to improve health through balancing the body's energy patterns. The participants from my research studies rated each of the seven body therapies. The results are presented at the end of this section, on page 125.

Massage

Most people are somewhat familiar with massage, which is an umbrella term for a collection of bodywork methods that manipulate muscle tissue for therapeutic goals. The Burton Goldberg Group (1994) cites studies that show massage is beneficial in treating injury-induced trauma, stress, headaches, muscle problems (such as spasm or pain), and temporomandibular joint (TMJ) problems. Massage can help the body to eliminate toxins, reduce pain, increase blood flow, relax, and recover from scarring. Furthermore, massage may help prevent the development of additional health problems, by reducing or releasing tension and prolonged constriction from the body.

Rolfing (Structural Integration)

Ida Rolf, a biochemist, invented the Rolfing technique. When an osteopath treated her for an injury, she became convinced of the importance of good body structure for both physical and psychological functioning. Rolfing seeks to align the body properly to improve functioning and health.

Often, people unknowingly have minor and, sometimes, major misalignments in their posture that interfere with their movements and clear mental functioning. The work involves the manipulation of the fascia, an elastic membrane that surrounds all muscle tissue. The fascia is important because it covers all muscles that influence posture and if the fascia is constricted, it may restrict muscle and joint movement. Deep pressure is used to work on the fascia, one body segment at a time, with the aim of creating less restricted and more balanced movement. Sometimes people have emotional responses to Rolfing, because emotional trauma can stay lodged in muscle tissue for long periods of time. The Burton Goldberg Group (1994) cites studies that show Rolfing induces smoother movement, reduces stress, and even enhances neurological functioning. Other systems of bodywork evolved out of Rolfing, including Aston Patterning and Hellerwork. (For a discussion of these systems, see the Burton Goldberg Group 1994.)

The Alexander Technique

The Alexander Technique was invented by a Shakespearean actor who used the study of his own posture to cure himself of losing his voice. The technique uses touch, movement, and awareness of one's own habitual misuse of bodily position to correct harmful habits that can lead to disease. The Alexander Technique is practiced by more than 2,500 people worldwide, including people in drama, dance, speech, and athletics (Burton Goldberg Group 1994).

Sessions involve receiving gentle instructions for postural change as well as hands-on help from the practitioner to prevent continual repetition of harmful patterns.

Feldenkrais

A physicist who healed himself from a sports injury without having to undergo surgery invented Feldenkrais. Similar to the Alexander Technique, Feldenkrais seeks to interrupt negative movement patterns to allow the body to move in a freer manner. Self-image and breath are both seen as important influences on the function and movement of the body. Feldenkrais does not *teach* people how to move, but rather has each person *discover*, through experimentation and the release of old patterns, the healthiest way of moving for themselves. Because of its ability to help people move with more ease, Feldenkrais is used to treat injury, stress, and illnesses that have caused restricted movement.

Trager

Trager is a movement reeducation technique that uses touch, including rocking, pulling, and rotational movements, to loosen stiff muscles and joints. Trager was developed by Milton Trager in 1927 and, similar to Feldenkrais, aims to release old tension patterns in the body. Trager uses mentastics, which are dancelike movements that help the body learn to move more effortlessly. Its goal is to modify the feedback that the nervous system receives from body tissue to improve the person's sense of well-being. Trager is used for injuries, diseases that affect neuromuscular function, such as multiple sclerosis, and for athletes. The Burton Goldberg Group (1994) says that more than 7,000 people have received Trager training.

Polarity Therapy

Polarity therapy revolves around releasing blockages and restoring proper energy flow to the body in an electromagnetic sense. It was developed by Randolph Stone, a chiropractor, osteopath, and naturopath, who was interested in electromagnetic energy and the body. Polarity therapy uses a variety of techniques, such as pressure point contact/manipulation, breathing, reflexology, and exercise. The Burton Goldberg Group (1994) says that polarity therapy can effect positive changes in well-being, physical health, energy levels, and self-understanding. It is taught to practitioners worldwide.

Reflexology

Reflexology is a holistic healing technique that uses gentle massage of reflex points in the feet that correspond to various organs and systems throughout the body. The feet are thought to be a microcosm of the body; pressure exerted on specific points affects the corresponding body parts. In *The Art of Reflexology*, Dougans and Ellis (1992) say that the goal of reflexology is to trigger the body's return to homeostasis, i.e, restore balance through tension reduction and relaxation. It is an energy technique because, as Dougans and Ellis say, six main meridians, which connect with major bodily organs, travel to the feet. Massage at these meridians can remove blockages and allow the *chi* (energy) to circulate freely. Reflexology is essentially electrical in nature, with the human body likened to a battery that conducts electrical energy. Although this technique is medically unproven, practitioners report very positive effects. The Burton Goldberg Group (1994) says that there are almost 25,000 certified reflexology practitioners worldwide, and that it is the primary form of alternative treatment in Denmark.

Reiki

According to Janet Strubbe Wittenberg (1996), a certified Reiki master, Reiki is an energy therapy where the practitioner becomes the channel for energy that affects the patient, opens the chakras, and energizes the body.

Proponents of Eastern philosophies believe that the chakras are seven energy centers that reside along the spine and in the head. An imbalance in a chakra may mean an imbalance on the physical level that might be associated with a blockage or illness. The practitioner lays hands on the patient's body allowing energy to flow through where needed. The energy flow may create actual sensations in the patient, such as electricity, warmth, or tingling. Reiki's goal is to increase physical and mental energy. Reiki advocates say that this treatment method can also be done as distance healing, where the patient and the practitioner are not physically in the same location. In *Essential Reiki*, Diane Stein (1995) says that the practitioner's body has received Reiki "attunements," which open and clear their energy channels. Practitioners are then connected to the universal *chi* and can channel increased life energy to themselves and others. Attunements are given one-on-one from a teacher and open the student's latent abilities. The hallmark of a Reiki practitioner is said to be heat emanating from their hands when they are placed on patients for healing purposes.

Therapeutic Touch

Therapeutic Touch, or T Touch, was developed in 1972 by Dolores Krieger and Dora Kunz, and combines several modalities including visualization, energy field/aura repair, and laying on of hands. Often, no physical contact is needed and the session consists of the practitioner determining blockages in the patient's energy field or aura through the use of rotational hand movements two to six inches away from the patient's body. Both practitioner and patient are centered (calm) and quiet; the practitioner aims to correct problems, such as obstructions, and reestablish a free energy flow. The Burton Goldberg Group (1994) cites studies that have shown T Touch to alter enzyme activity, accelerate wound healing, relieve pain (including headaches) and stress, ease asthma, and reduce fever. It is taught in colleges, in many countries, and is a component of many Lamaze pregnancy classes. T Touch also is used by veterinarians on animals.

Herbal Medicine

Herbal medicine is a system of natural healing that has been practiced for thousands of years. Historically, women were the herbalists in their cultures, but throughout the nineteenth and twentieth centuries, the use of medicinal herbs diminished in Western culture, partly as a result of women not being allowed to practice medicine. In fact, many women who were burned at the stake as witches in Europe and Colonial America actually were herbalists (Ehrenreich and English 1973). With the rise of allopathic medicine in the nineteenth century there was considerable resistance from physicians to

Effectiveness of Body Therapies in Phase I

Name of Technique	Number Of People Who Tried The Technique	No Benefit	Mild Benefit	Moderate Benefit	Great Benefit	Adverse Reaction
Alexander Technique	8	13%	75%	0	13%	0
Massage	115	12%	32%	23%	31%	1%
Polarity Balancing	39	28%	31%	8%	33%	0
Reflexology	59	19%	27%	24%	31%	0
Reiki	23	26%	39%	26%	9%	0
Rolfing	10	20%	33%	10%	20%	20%
Trager	8	13%	50%	25%	13%	0

herbal cures. Although in most areas of the United States herbal medicine is no longer considered mainstream, it is not difficult to find practicing modern-day herbalists. For those areas where herbal medicine is not easily accessible, information can be obtained through books, tapes, newsletters, and correspondence courses.

There are at least two different perspectives within the field of herbal medicine. Some herbalists say that only whole plants should be used for medicinal purposes; others believe that the active ingredients should be extracted from the plant and guaranteed as present in particular strengths in specific formulas. The first perspective is more in line with traditional herbalism and holistic medicine, while the latter is more closely imitative of modern pharmaceuticals. Because the holistic approach is integral to traditional medical practices in most rural cultures, the World Health Organization has urged integrating this system with allopathic medicine inasmuch as herbal medicine is already the people's health care, and thus well accepted.

With the rise of holistic health practices in the developed nations there also has been an increase in the practice of herbal medicine. Consequently, now is an excellent time to find good information on native plants that may be useful for treating MCS. For a fraction of the cost of some of the experimental MCS therapies, you might learn useful knowledge that will put you more in charge of your own health. Although herbs may not cure MCS, they may offer safe, inexpensive relief from some symptoms and allow some people to strengthen specific body systems that have been ravaged by chemical injuries. Herbs each have particular actions they perform in the body based in part on their constituents, e.g., some are astringents, which staunch bleeding.

Some of the most common MCS symptoms, such as headaches, joint pain, digestive problems, anxiety, and others, are easily addressed by herbal medicine. Nevertheless, you should exercise caution when you begin to experiment with herbs. Because people with MCS have very sensitive reactions to all kinds of substances, they should be extremely careful using herbs, particularly if serious food reactions are at issue. One precaution might be to try a minute amount of an herb before taking a full dose. Additionally, be sure that your herbs are organically grown so that you will avoid reactions to herbicides and pesticides. Another general caution with regard to herbs is that some are toxic; toxic herbs can easily be confused with safe ones when collecting in the wild. Also, many herbs have contraindications. That is, they may cause harm under certain conditions. For example, there are a number of herbs that should not be used during pregnancy because they may relax the uterine muscles too much (e.g., sage), or even stimulate a miscarriage (rue and black cohosh). So be careful, a little learning can be dangerous. If you do decide to use herbs as medicines, you might start by consulting a skilled herbalist while you study and slowly begin experimenting with safer herbs on your own. There are some very safe herbs for self-use with which you could confidently begin your study and experimentation. Some of the safer herbs with no contraindications include: chamomile, dandelion, burdock, and thyme. Each herb has a number of different actions, however, and you should be sure that none of the actions work against what you are trying to achieve.

The wonderful thing about herbs is that they can be used to strengthen, integrate, cleanse, and nourish your body in a holistic way. They do not have to be expensive as you can grow them yourself, if you have a safe organic area, and then dry them or use them fresh. There are several ways of storing and using herbs, with some techniques keeping the herbs closest to their natural state. Herbs can be prepared fresh or dried as teas. They can also be preserved in tinctures of grain alcohol, in glycerine, or even water. Some people think that alcohol is better at extracting the medicinal components from the plants. Herbal tinctures come in small dark bottles with droppers. These tinctures can be taken directly under the tongue, mixed with a little water for drinking, or dissolved in hot water to dissipate the alcohol before it is drunk. The most processed method for storing a plant is pill form. Although some companies guarantee the potency of their pills, the dried, powdered capsuled product is a long way from its original state. Many herbs are so bitter or foul tasting, however, that tinctures and pills are the best way to use them. (If you have ever tasted wormwood, valerian, or feverfew, you know what I mean.)

There are several ways that you can begin to learn about herbs. One is to learn the properties of a few very safe plants in which you are particularly interested and then to use them to strengthen your system. This is somewhat the approach of Susun Weed (1989), who lauds the healing properties of common plants, such as nettles and dandelions.

Another approach is to learn to categorize herbs by their "actions," which define their various medicinal effects. I had been reading about herbs for twenty years and couldn't keep them straight until I learned what their "actions" were. There are many wonderful books on herbal medicine and reading some will greatly increase your knowledge. (See Appendix C for further reading.)

There are various methods of preparing herbs for use. As a rule, you make infusions from leaves and flowers. This means that you pour boiling water over the dried or fresh herbs and allow them to steep. Roots and barks, however, are harder, and therefore must be boiled directly in the water to extract medicinal components. Herbs should be steeped or boiled for about twenty minutes and strained before use. Although the amounts of the herb used for preparation vary, often a teaspoon to a tablespoon is used per pint of water for roots and barks, and slightly more for leaf and flower infusions.

For people who need scientific proof of herb efficacy, evidence has accumulated for many plants to the point where even conventional medicine is investigating and using them. It must be remembered that many pharmaceuticals are extracted from natural products; e.g., digitalis, which is a powerful cardiac stimulant and diuretic, is made from of the common herb foxglove.

Plant uses that currently are supported by strong research include:

- Gingko for Alzheimer's disease and other dementias

- Echinacea for infections

- Bilberry for capillary circulation to the eyes

- Chamomile for digestive upset, inflammation, and as a gentle sleep aid

- Dandelion for increased digestive health and as a diuretic

- Feverfew for migraine headaches

- Garlic for lower cholesterol and blood pressure, and as an antimicrobial

- Milk thistle for liver damage from chemicals

- Passionflower for nervousness or hyperexcitement

- St.-John's-wort for depression

Aromatherapy

Aromatherapy involves the inhalation or external use (on the skin) of concentrated plant oils to treat both emotional and physical problems. Because the olfactory system (which governs your sense of smell) has many neural connections to the limbic system (which controls emotions and motivation), it makes sense that plant oils can affect a person's emotions and sense of well-being. Deanne Jenney (1997) says, "Aromatherapy uses scents to influence moods and pain and to treat and cure minor ailments. The essential oils work to encourage health and bring the body into balance."

Essential oils primarily have the same properties (or at least the major constituent) as the plants from which they were distilled: they can be antimicrobial, relaxing, invigorating, and relieve pain. The Burton Goldberg Group (1994) points out that it is not the essential oils' aroma that has the medicinal effect, but the pharmacological properties of the oils, which penetrate body tissues due to their small molecular size. Although they are referred to as essential oils, they are not really oily. Instead, they are concentrated liquids that evaporate in the air and are not water soluble. Essential oils should be stored in dark, sealed bottles away from any light and air. Oils can be delivered to the body either through olfaction (the process of smelling), which brings the healing elements of the oils to the brain, lungs, and blood, or through skin contact (massage), which allows them to enter the bloodstream and vital organs. A few oils can be used internally through the digestive system, but it must be kept in mind that they are very concentrated.

The historical use of aromatherapy goes back to the Egyptians and, through Ayurvedic medicine, the Hebrews, Greeks, and Romans. Jenney says that the French perfume industry probably began as a result of the aromatherapy the Crusaders experienced in their travels. Oils are extracted from fresh (or sometimes dried) plants through steam distillation, cold pressing (for citrus), or the use of vegetable oil, alcohol, or solvent for very delicate plants. Jenney says that to extract oils from delicate plants, like rose and jasmine, they are coated with a chemical solvent. Most essential oils are diluted with carrier oils, such as vegetable oils, which require refrigeration.

The Burton Goldberg Group (1994) cites aromatherapy as effective for bacterial respiratory infections, immune deficiencies, skin disorders, cystitis, herpes, arthritis, and stress management. Studies show that certain calming oils can alter brain waves and induce calm and well-being. Some examples of extracted oils include the well-known tea tree oil, which is used as an antiseptic; thyme oil, which is used to prevent or treat infection; and chamomile oil, which is used to relax and relieve stress.

With the already sensitive olfactory system in MCS, you might ask whether aromatherapy is something to avoid, or whether nonchemically extracted oils would actually make positive use of your sensitive olfactory system. Since no studies to date have specifically investigated aromatherapy use for MCS, the question remains unanswered.

If you do decide to experiment with essential oils, be sure that they are truly pure, nonchemically extracted, and meant for medicinal use rather than fragrance. Prices will vary from oil to oil because of variations in the harvesting and other factors. The Burton Goldberg Group points out that good oils are usually expensive. It can sometimes take 1,000 pounds of a plant to produce one pound of oil. If you find a product line that has a uniform price for each of their oils, this is probably a bad sign, and may indicate oil adulteration. (See Appendix C for further reading and resources.)

Homeopathy

Homeopathy relies on remedies that, according to the homeopathic "law of similars," actually can *cause* symptoms in a healthy person.

Homeopathic remedies begin as dilutions of natural plant, mineral, or animal substances. Remedies are activated through "succussion" (shaking), and then rediluted and succussed again several times until, at very high levels of dilution, only an "imprint" of the substance is left; no actual molecules of the remedy source remain. The more diluted the remedy, the more powerful it can be. Studies have shown that homeopathic remedies release specific electromagnetic signals (Burton Goldberg Group 1994).

According to the Burton Goldberg Group, approximately 3,000 providers practice homeopathy in the United States compared with 5,000 in France, 6,000 in Germany, and 25,000 in India. The Royal Family of England has been treated by homeopaths for centuries. The World Health Organization has urged the global use of homeopathy along with conventional medicine in attempt to meet world health care needs.

Samuel Hahnemann founded homeopathy in the late eighteenth century when the use of leeches, bloodletting, and cathartics was standard medical practice. His work was based on the principle that "like cures like," a principle well known to Hippocrates, Paracelsus, and to Ayurvedic, as well as modern allopathic medicine.

For example, radiation can cause tumors, but it can heal tumors as well. Hahnemann tested homeopathic remedies for six years before writing about and practicing with them. He was greatly persecuted for differing from the medical establishment (some things never change) and, at one point, his work was publicly burned. His original testing, which founded classical homeopathy, was based on "type" or constitutional remedies. Therefore, homeopathy does not treat the disease per se, but the person who acquired the disease because of emotional, physical, or spiritual imbalances. This means that each temperament and type of person corresponds to one specific homeopathic remedy. Symptoms are seen as the body's attempt to heal rather than as inconveniences to eliminate. In classical homeopathy, the task of the practitioner is to understand and assess a patient's health and/or condition through use of many pieces of information about the person; and then to figure out the correct remedy, which will move the patient toward a better state of health.

Homeopathic remedies are used not only at the constitutional level, but the symptom level as well. For example, in recent years, some companies have made a variety of remedies that include newer allergens in addition to the classical substances used by Hahnemann. These include allergens that neutralize inhalant allergies to grass, pollen, and weeds; irritant substances, such as poison ivy and poison oak; and mixtures to help the body clear pesticides from its systems. It may be possible, either through homeopathic practitioners or self-study, for you to find some remedies that will help you. In chemical injury, the body has been so seriously altered, that it seems it would be very difficult to identify a type remedy. However, some people with MCS have reported receiving considerable help with this method. In Phase I of my study, 126 participants tried homeopathy: 20 percent reported great benefit, 22 percent moderate benefit, 26 percent mild benefit, 23 percent reported no benefit, and 9 percent reported adverse reactions. LeRoy, Davis, and Jason (1996) found that of 187 people who tried homeopathy in their study, 11.2 percent reported enormous help, 24.6 percent major help,

25.1 percent reported slight help, 16.0 percent reported no help, 12.8 percent reported the effect was unclear, and 10.2 percent reported harmful effects.

Flower Essences

The original thirty-eight Bach flower essences were established by Nelson Bach, a renowned London physician. In 1930, Bach gave up his medical practice to devote himself to finding safe remedies that would help people overcome illness and that could be used by anyone for self-healing. The Bach essences are all made from flowers, trees, and bushes, and are safe for use alone or with other methods. The essences are created by imparting the "life force" of a plant to a water-based remedy. These remedies then interact with body systems on vibrational energy levels, much like homeopathy. Flower essences are said to work on the emotional and soul levels, allowing the body to heal by restoring balance to the mind.

The Bach remedies are based on the most common negative states of mind. For example, there are five remedies that address five kinds of fear. The remedies can be used as type remedies when they correspond to the basic essence of a person's personality, or on a symptom level for relief of a situational upset. The most well-known remedy is called Rescue Remedy. It is a combination of five remedies that restore emotional balance in times of great upset, fear, or trauma. It contains star-of-bethlehem for shock, rock rose for terror and panic, impatiens for mental stress and tension, cherry plum for desperation, and clematis for the out-of-the-body feeling that may signal fainting or loss of consciousness. A large number of additional remedies have been developed by the Flower Essence Society, which is a "worldwide organization of professional health practitioners and interested laypersons who are devoted to the development of flower essence therapy" (Kaminski and Katz 1996, ix). Some people have more trust in the original thirty-eight remedies developed by Bach, while others are open to the later developments, which offer more options.

The Burton Goldberg Group (1994) cites a number of well-known practitioners, including George Goodheart, the founder of Applied Kinesiology, who use flower essences as adjunct therapies for more lasting benefits, or even in lieu of allopathic drugs. (See Appendix C for further reading.)

PART III

PSYCHOLOGICAL AND PERSONAL GROWTH

Chapter Eight

Coming to Terms with Chronic Illness and Disability

Part of coping with MCS is coming to terms with having a chronic illness. *Chronic* means that you may experience ups and downs, and that the condition is long-term. This does not mean that you can't be helped. It doesn't even imply that some people won't get better. But for many, if not most people, MCS is a chronic disability; this must be accepted. Some degree of acceptance will relieve you of the desperation felt by those who search frantically for a cure, empty their bank accounts, and perhaps harm themselves in the process.

If you are like many people with MCS, you probably became very excited at the first suggestion that something might help you *no matter how much it cost*. You were willing to try anything, in the belief that in the long run it would be worth it because even if you went into debt for your treatment, you would be made well and could justify the cost with your newly regained health. The possibility of the treatment not working or even making you worse was not factored into your equation.

Desperation can make you susceptible to every high-cost vitamin or mineral food supplement and newfangled therapy that comes along. With each failed high-cost attempt to get well, you may have become more depressed and frustrated, and you now may feel that the roller-coaster ride is no longer worth it. I know one woman with MCS who used to joke to practitioners that she was saving her money for jewelry rather than giving it to them. She got a lot of pleasure from the jewelry and she is still kicking.

Another woman has the following advice about seeking a cure:

- Stop trying to find a cure.

- Accept the illness and do your best to find as many ways as possible to keep yourself comfortable, busy, stress-free, and well nourished with good food.

- Find ways to relax and socialize.

- Do something to help others with MCS.

- Don't feel sorry for yourself. Everyone has health problems; this is yours.

- Make the best of it because you can't change it; those who pressure themselves to find a cure sometimes just make it worse.

- Educate those who want to learn and stop trying to convince those who don't.

Consider the possibility that if you are to get well, it may not be a high-cost therapy that will help you. And, "never say never" in regard to getting well: I once talked with a woman who had MCS who said she had been greatly helped by a faith healer. (See chapter ten for a discussion on spirituality.)

Sociological Effects of Chronic Illness

A perspective on the sociological effects of chronic illness can help you to stay calm while you choose which treatments to try, begin to understand your difficulties, and realize that you are not alone. Even if you are one of the lucky ones who does not have MCS for the long-term, understanding something about the sociological effects of illness in general will help to prepare you for encounters with providers in the medical profession. It also will help you with those people who are influenced by popular conceptions about chronic and poorly understood health conditions.

The helping professions have not always been kind in their assessments of people with difficult health problems. For example, those with chronic pain frequently are perceived as complainers, or as using pain for "secondary gain"; some psychologists try to prove that women with breast cancer have unhealthy ways of handling anger; and many psychology textbooks still say that asthma is triggered solely by stress and psychological factors.

Attitudes about MCS Patients

Brodsky, Green, and Ograd (1989) describe women who have MCS as having a "decompensative psychological illness that results in a change in intrafamily dynamics." They are described as feeling relief from not having to deal with the overwhelming demands of home, family, and job; and from having others take care of them. Their burdens have been lifted and they become the burden themselves. This is not very different from how providers describe people with other health problems. Consider these statements about a woman with head and back pain cited in the journal *Women and Aging*:

> At its simplest, the pain was a powerful means for expressing her disaffection with her life situation in general and the marital relationship in particular. At a more complex level, pain served the purpose of correcting what family theorists have described as "hierarchical incongruity." This concept is predicated on the assumption that while a symptomatic partner in a marriage assumes a dependent position, the symptom also empowers that individual, which in turn corrects the power imbalance in the marriage. In short, pain enables the person in the one below position to gain the upper hand (Roy 1994, 80).

In none of the cases cited in the article was the pain described as valid or the experience of the sufferer honored. Chronic pain and MCS may share the characteristics of chronicity and lack of response to standard medical cures. Both syndromes frustrate physicians, and patients themselves come to be seen as problems. In some other conditions as well, the patient bears the brunt of our culture's difficulty with poorly understood systemic health problems. Goodheart and Lansing (1997) say:

> There are many myths about the causes and cures for unpredictable diseases, such as multiple sclerosis, rheumatoid arthritis, chronic fatigue syndrome, postviral syndrome, and post-Lyme syndrome. These diseases are not readily tolerated in our technological solution-focused society because of the aura of uncertainty that surrounds them. People with ambiguous diseases are often viewed as being depressed or psychosomatic, malingering, or using their symptoms for psychological secondary gain. Of course, any disease or symptom may be used for conscious or unconscious manipulation, but ambiguous diseases present an easier target for hostility or dismissal (p. 29).

These authors then tell of a woman who was experiencing weakness, pain, and difficulty walking. Physicians attributed the problems to psychological causes. Believing this assessment, the woman didn't make accommodations for herself, even when it meant crawling around her house in order to be mobile. She was determined not to "give in" to her pain. Finally, a better trained physician diagnosed her as having postpolio syndrome. This kind of faulty diagnosis is common in MCS and those who have it struggle to continue trying to live with full functioning because they are culturally required to live as though they were "well." Consider the following words from an MCS patient:

"I was ill equipped to face illness, to accept and abide by these new requirements of my body. Then, as my illness wore on, I struggled against the limitations it imposed, because of an inherent habit of pushing limits and overcoming obstacles to fulfill my responsibilities without complaint."

Families in Denial

Commonly, families withhold "permission" for the person with MCS to have a "nonlegitimate" illness or disability. For example, in Phase II of my research, people were actually forbidden to talk about their MCS. Many respondents described relatives walking out of the room if they discussed their sensitivities. This happens on a more subtle level with cancer and other illnesses, although there is often a show of support in the critical stages. But when a family member is forbidden to talk about their health concerns, the situation is abusive and dysfunctional, and would not and should not arise if good care was being provided. Goodheart and Lansing (1997) say:

> Ideally, when a person has a chronic physical illness, an assessment of the family should include gathering information about the disease and the ordeal the family will be up against; the point in the family life cycle at which the disease occurs; the family structure; the family history and beliefs about the illness; and the ways in which a family relates to the treatment setting. This assessment should enable the therapist to anticipate problems and enable the individual and the family to adapt effectively to chronic illness. Perhaps someday such a goal will be attainable. In reality, early assessment of the family rarely happens (p. 154-155).

The authors are correct that an early assessment rarely happens, especially in this day of managed care. For MCS patients, it almost never happens. But with the education of psychotherapists, it could. The goal of doing early assessments would be to support family members as they adjust to living with a loved one with a chronic illness. It is distressing to families to suddenly have members' roles disrupted by disability, yet compassionate support from professionals could help tremendously.

Compassionate Models

Because of the culture's negative attitudes toward the chronically ill and, until recently, the lack of available psychological services, there was very little published material available. (See Appendix C for further reading.) Strauss (1984) wrote compassionately of illness from a sociological perspective, but the psychological community has been slow to address individual and family issues relating to chronic illness.

Jenny Altschuler (1997), however, in *Working with Chronic Illness*, recognized the bind inherent in having "illness in a world defined by health." In reference to "delegitimized" illnesses, she says:

> [A]ll ill people have to integrate at least two descriptions of themselves, that of being a person in their own right and being ill. However, some ... have to integrate a third description: experiencing themselves as unwell, but not being regarded as legitimately ill. This [third description] profoundly affects how they are treated by both family members and professionals (p. 4).

Altschuler's work applies to all people with health problems. Understanding how everyone in the family is affected by an ill family member, including children with ill parents, can help to normalize some of the trauma of MCS as part of a dynamic process that occurs with all serious health problems. Although the specific demands of each condition differ, people with MCS are not alone in facing delegitimization, loss, and extreme hardship due to illness.

It is informative to have friendships with people who have other chronic illnesses. Although their illnesses may be more socially acceptable than MCS, and they may receive better health care, they still suffer the same difficulties with maintaining an income, having enough energy to complete tasks, paying medical expenses, and trying new treatments that don't work. For example, my friend with Parkinson's disease can dine in restaurants, but if his medications fail, his body may freeze and he will have to be carried out by others. (I once helped to drag him out of a bookstore under the gaze of numerous staring patrons.) Similarly, my friend with Crohn's disease doesn't have to cope with avoiding all petrochemicals, pesticides, and fragrances—as do people with MCS—but no one would envy the periodic emergency trips she must take to the hospital for yet another bowel resection. My point is that although there are many unique aspects of MCS, people who suffer from it have much in common with people who have other injuries, disabilities, and illnesses. This knowledge may help you to "normalize" some of your suffering.

Goodheart and Lansing (1997) offer a multi-faceted model for understanding people's various responses to chronic illness. The authors cite two writers, Holland and Rowland, who name "five Ds" that create problems in adapting to chronic illness. All can occur at any stage in adapting to an illness and all express the concerns of people with MCS. The "five Ds" include:

- Distance in intimate relationships

- Dependency issues

- Disability and the obstacles it poses to achievement

- Disfigurement and the fear and anxiety of Death

Goodheart and Lansing believe developing and adjusting to a chronic illness entails first a disorganization and then a reorganization of self, which includes accepting the illness and its limitations, lifestyle changes, and more. The authors describe a six-stage process:

1. In the first stage, "Initial Response," you recognize that something is wrong. Symptoms at this point may be explained away or ignored until it becomes apparent that the problem is persistent.

2. During the second stage, "Awareness of Chronicity," you may become anxious or fearful or enter denial. Once the message sinks in that the problem is chronic, more anxiety and a grief reaction are likely to occur. Many conditions wax and wane for a long time before diagnosis is possible. So, the second stage can be a time of ambiguity and seemingly endless waiting when clear answers are not forthcoming.

3. The third stage is "Disorganization." Goodheart and Lansing describe this stage as the beginning of the disorganization process; you may experience disturbances in work, education, family roles, and general quality of life. Anger is a natural result of the frustration at this stage and social isolation begins:

   The patient's negative internal messages go hand in hand with the messages from the outside world. The responses of other people have an extraordinary impact at this vulnerable psychological crossroads in their inner life experience. Patients' losses are growing. They face the internal loss of a familiar sense of self, function, and identity, and they may be faced with the external loss of support or contact with important other people at work, in the social milieu, or even among family members.

   Although some give up, most continue to try to retain some stable sense of self:

   Most people struggle courageously to reorganize themselves internally, without conscious awareness of the process or assistance that would help them to navigate the disorganizing transition period (p. 38).

4. In Goodheart and Lansing's fourth stage, the "Intensified Wish for a Cure," the patient expands the search for help through conventional and alternative avenues, religious quests, and other means. The desire is for a return to "normal," to extrude the illness once and for all. Self-blame may enter the picture as the search for the cause of the illness continues. Magical thinking in a variety of forms may result when the wish for a cure goes unsatisfied:

> [Patients] may believe that the illness is a punishment for misdeeds or poor habits or may imagine that the problem lies in not trying hard enough because of laziness or lack of moral fiber, grit, and determination. At the other extreme, patients may blame themselves for working too hard, having Type A personalities, or overdoing exercise. A tendency to minimize one's role in illness or to maximize it to the point of believing one can control the illness may be incorporated into the individual's magical thinking process (p. 39).

5. At some point, the person recognizes that the illness cannot be undone or erased and enters the fifth stage, "The Acknowledgement of Helplessness." Here, they are now free to mourn/grieve for what will never be the same. Simultaneously, the adaptation process can now truly begin as people turn their energy toward finding strategies and coping mechanisms for dealing with the illness. In this stage, they also begin the process of restructuring their life around the illness-imposed limitations. (See chapter ten for an overview of what respondents in Phase III of my research said about the adjustment process and about how MCS has affected their sense of identity.)

> Patients respond differently to disease, disorganization, and helplessness, depending on their capacity for creative adaptation in their lives, the severity of the illness, and the support available in their environment. They are challenged to find coping strategies as the disease process changes and as they are changed by it. Coping strategies are successful only to the extent that they are congruent with patients' normative personality style and level of functioning (40-41).

The point about coping strategies being congruent with your personality and functioning level is very important. Everyone has to cope in their own way. One woman I know with mild/moderate MCS has a very highly visible and responsible profession. Because she is assertive and not afraid of others' opinions, she is able to persuade psychologists, attorneys, judges, and many others not to wear perfume in her presence. She warns them to leave their scents and scented clothing home, so that if she becomes irritable it can be for a good reason! Not everyone is this comfortable with asking for cooperation, but this is a woman who actually thinks it's funny when other people publicly criticize her. Would that we could all be so effective and confident!

6. Goodheart and Lansing sum up stage six, "Adaptation to Illness," as the time when people reorganize around the illness:

> Despite serious obstacles, many patients are able to develop a restructuring of their lives and internal sense of stability. They are able to reorganize in a healthy way. A few are so brittle they do not adapt; instead, they collapse psychologically. Some have an encapsulated neurotic adaptation with a limited range of possibilities; they become subsumed into the patient role or are viewed as society's discards or cranks. *Some are transformed, like the phoenix rising from the ashes, and show significant gains as they reorganize their lives* (p. 41) [emphasis mine].

The challenge is to become this phoenix; there are plenty of phoenixes in the MCS community. (See chapter fourteen for examples of people who have made valuable contributions in spite of their illness or disability.) There is a strength that comes from acceptance, meaningful work, and taking personal responsibility for your life. This strength is evident in these people who are role models for others with poorly understood illnesses and disabilities. It is a process—sometimes a long and painful one—but once someone accepts that they may not fully recover, they are free to explore what that means. When you understand that our society has not done a good job of dealing with any chronic illness, let alone MCS, it helps you to realize how strong you are to have coped as well as you already have. Sometimes you just have to stay in survival mode and not feel guilty about it. One woman understood this when she had the following encounter with a mental health provider:

> "He wanted me to function from more of my creative side instead of from my desperate survival mode. I thought that would be nice, but I didn't think talking to him was going to solve my pressing medical problems. I guess he didn't realize how much creativity it takes to survive with this illness either. Or how much courage, stamina, and planning it took to go see him, just in case he might be able to help me. He was nice but he didn't have a clue!"

Acceptance also challenges you to decide on what level you want to approach your chronic illness. The woman I met who had been helped by a faith healer had approached her illness on an energy level. This does not mean that she believes that MCS is a psychological problem, as she doesn't. But working on a level beyond the physical, for her, offered a way to intervene in a physical problem that appeared to be intractable.

I believe we are never truly stuck. There was a door into the predicament and, although it may seem to have disappeared, there is another door out. It is not the same for everyone; everyone has to find their own door. Remember, though, it does not necessarily have to cost you your whole bank account to turn the key. The paradoxical position of accepting and coping with the fact that your illness may be chronic, while being open to healing from a number of sources (that will do you more good than harm), may be the healthiest approach to living and still thriving with MCS.

Chapter Nine

Share This Chapter with Your Therapist

If You Weren't Crazy Before You Got MCS, "You Are Now"

Multiple chemical sensitivity is an extremely difficult condition with which to cope. It is understandable if you are feeling distressed. The condition demands the impossible, while threatening to take away your resources in the process. The first step toward facing the psychological challenges of MCS is to give yourself credit for the coping you *already* have done. Consider the following: What have you done well? What changes have you made that have improved your health or prevented it from deteriorating further? What very difficult challenges have you faced with creativity and strength? If you credit yourself for what you already have done, it will be easier to move forward and to face more challenges.

People without MCS don't realize that there is nothing specific about you that caused you to get MCS, and you are not inherently different from people without MCS. Just as pregnant women are really no different from non-pregnant women in that they are simply in a different condition, multiple chemical sensitivity is a condition that can affect anyone. Before you developed sensitivities you were basically just like other people. The need for some people to distance themselves from individuals with disabilities and illnesses and from accident victims, is perhaps a way for them to pretend that these circumstances can't or won't happen to them.

Some people also subscribe to the "just world" phenomenon, which is the illusion that bad things happen only to those who deserve them. This belief provides an artificial escape from potential danger, for if you are just "good," then you will be spared. People often use this theory to distance themselves from rape victims or to blame them, i.e., if the rape victim had only locked her car doors, then the rape wouldn't have happened. Of course, this is not even close to the truth since many victims are raped in their homes by people who know them, including dates and spouses. Somehow, however, the "just world" phenomenon perpetuates an illusion that is less painful than the truth.

Given the difficulties that MCS can cause, this chapter is designed to help you think about how you might be reacting psychologically to the extreme limitations caused by MCS and to decide whether or not to see a therapist. The last quarter of this chapter is written specifically for therapists working with MCS patients.

Psychological Baggage

Although MCS is not a psychological illness, it does not preclude the possibility that you have some unrelated psychological baggage with which to deal. We all do. As long as your other personal issues—whatever they may be—remain unresolved, they will interact with your MCS-imposed limitations and create further discomfort for you. Taking care of any issues that are unrelated to MCS can lighten your psychic load and free up more energy for coping constructively with the MCS. Just as importantly, learning how MCS interacts with and affects your psychological vulnerabilities will help you to cope more successfully.

Assertiveness

Have you typically been a shy and sensitive person who now needs to perform the thankless and assertive job of asking for special accommodations to survive? If your modus operandi has generally been a passive style, i.e., to give of yourself, do what is asked, and never complain, it may be extremely difficult to come to a point where you are comfortably able to state your needs assertively. Whether it is because of personal habit, style, discomfort with being the center of attention, or the belief that you don't deserve "special treatment," the task of negotiating your social life will be more difficult without at least a little work in the psychological arena.

A therapist can help you work on being more comfortable with assertive behaviors. There are a number of good self-help books that could help you with this as well. Another option is to practice on your own using what George Kelly, one of the major personality theorists, called fixed role therapy. In fixed role therapy, the therapist writes a sketch of a person who embodies the qualities that the client wants to develop. So, in this case, you would write a page-long description of a person with good assertiveness skills. In this sketch, you should describe the ideal person's thoughts as well as behaviors. For example, you might write something such as, "Sally finds it easy to explain her needs, as she realizes that her health depends on it. Negative feedback from others is not upsetting to her because she knows that it is common for people who are different to be treated negatively." After clarifying the written sketch, the client then role-plays being the ideal person with the therapist. Next, the client pretends to be this person for approximately two weeks, and has several therapy visits during this time to discuss how the process is going. You could experiment with doing this on your own and see how it feels to try a different behavioral approach in one area of your life. If you do try it, carry your sketch with you, refer to it often, and be aware of how it feels to try a new behavior.

Another tactic of changing assertiveness behaviors might be to identify with an animal you can relate to that is assertive and that you admire (but be careful who you choose to tell that you are doing this, as some people may demean you in the process). For example, you might be a lion who is protective of itself, its home, and its young. Or, you might be a scrappy badger who doesn't hesitate to use its bite if threatened. Being assertive means facing your biggest fears—one of which could be rejection. Most often, however, people will respect you for standing up for yourself, and you are likely to have at least *some* advocates in the process.

Self-Esteem and Self-Worth

Self-esteem and self-worth issues may surface if you are treated badly by others in response to your accommodation requests. Individuals with poor self-esteem, or with past abuse issues may find this behavior extremely painful; while people with more of a "thick skin" will be less devastated by others' behavior. Learning how to "stay tough," regardless of input from others, will help you to stay on track and to get your needs met. Abuse issues can be tackled with the help of a competent therapist or through the use of self-help books and/or support groups. It is interesting to learn how "thick-skinned" people think about others' feedback. They often have great ways of keeping it in its proper perspective, seeing it for what it is, and going forward. For example, when I get negative feedback on a journal article, I am usually devastated. My friend Arnie, on the other hand, assumes that he got a bad reviewer. (See chapter ten for more on self-worth and identity.)

Overachievement

How about being an overachiever? Have you ever proven your worth by achieving, creating, doing, going, and otherwise perhaps overdoing? If your dynamic is that of the overachiever, conditions such as MCS or chronic fatigue immune deficiency syndrome, which cut your productivity, will be extremely painful because they will block your usual way of coping. If you draw your self-esteem from achieving important goals, and your achievement is cut in half (or lost entirely), either you have to do without half (or all) of your self-esteem or adjust the way in which you measure it.

Many people measure their achievements by the contributions they make in their professional careers. You can attempt to adjust your career so that it interferes less with your health by working more at home, working different hours, or working in a different area. If your job is less than ideal, you may have to rethink it entirely, i.e., you may have to find a job that is not damaging to your health, and/or move toward a profession that is compatible with environmental health. Everyone with MCS has something to offer; and your productivity does not have to go completely downhill forever.

Procrastination

On the other hand, if you are a procrastinator and have trouble getting things done, the health problems you have may provide an endless source of good reasons to continue procrastinating. You might have to resort to "to do" lists and schedules, with rewards built in for reaching milestones in your progress. A realistic, daily "to do" list can be a rewarding help. Make a list of tasks you would like to accomplish; as you complete each task, check it off. When everything is checked off the list, you are finished. (It is not fair to add more tasks for that day.) Any reward system that you can build into this exercise will help. Behavioral therapists recommend that their clients make a reinforcer list, which is a list of items or activities that are personally rewarding. The items on this list must be available and possible to achieve, i.e., if you can't travel, your reward can't be a trip to Florida. Some suggestions include spending time with friends, buying or borrowing a book you have been wanting, taking a bath, reading a magazine (without perfume inserts), or setting aside a specific amount of money toward something you have been wanting to purchase. Whatever it is you choose, be sure to reward yourself for what you accomplish.

Personality Style

Individual personality styles may dictate the type of emotional pain people with MCS experience. For example, extroverts may have a more difficult time with isolation than will introverts; but introverts may find it difficult to explain their needs and protect themselves in relationships. Isolated extroverts can experience tremendous emotional pain from the lack of stimulation. Although it can be very difficult, it is crucial for extroverts to find resourceful and creative ways to have contact with others. My favorite example of this is from a woman in my study who arranged horse trail rides in the mountains "because life ain't no spectator sport."

MCS can drag you so far down that you forget that there may be some things that you *can* do. Search for them and try to keep yourself from becoming completely isolated. Most people will not be riding horses in the mountains, and many of your activities may technically qualify as "spectating." Enjoying and sharing sights with other people, however, is still living, and may keep you at least vicariously connected to the outer world. (See chapter eleven for more on social support.)

MCS-Specific Issues

If the effects of MCS could be summed up in three words, those words might be loss, loss, and more loss. It is traumatic to lose access to almost everything you have ever wanted, worked for, and thought you would have. Of course, not everyone with MCS loses everything. In fact, you will see in chapter ten that some people even feel they have gained something from having MCS. But, there is no denying that loss is a common theme in people's descriptions of the life changes that occur post-MCS. Some of the losses people experienced were described in detail in chapter three.

Other psychological issues that might result from having MCS are included in this chapter. The following descriptions are normal responses to living with a poorly understood and limiting condition. They are described here to "normalize" them as much as possible and to help sensitize therapists to what their clients might be feeling.

Psychological/emotional reactions to MCS can be divided into direct and secondary reactions. Direct reactions are those that people experience as a direct effect of chemical exposure, e.g., crying and depression after an exposure to natural gas. Secondary reactions come from having to cope with the direct reactions as well as with the long-term reality of living with MCS. It is important to understand both types of reactions.

Direct Reactions

Usually, direct reactions are experienced within a very short period of time after being exposed to a chemical, food, or other incitant. The timing can vary for each person. Some people seem to react almost immediately, while others have more delayed reactions. For the delayed reactors, it is more difficult to sort out exactly what caused the problem. Direct reactions can manifest as depression, anxiety, panic attacks, irritability, restlessness, confusion, anger, and other responses.

> "There were pesticides being sprayed on a field near my home. I was outside doing yard work and all of the sudden I started to shake and became extremely angry. Angrier than I have ever been. I seem to have lost control. I wanted to put my fist through the wall, anything to release the pressure. I started screaming and throwing things. It was awful. I never felt so out of control. I find this happens when I'm exposed to pesticides."
>
> —Thirty-four-year-old woman with MCS
> for five years

Alison Johnson (1996) found that feeling irritable and angry and, to a lesser extent, even violent, were not uncommon reactions to pesticides, perfume, foods, and petrochemicals. Depression and panic attacks also were listed as reactions to a number of exposures. Johnson asked 239 participants about psychological reactions to ten substances, including pesticides, perfume, natural gas, foods, mold, pollen, dust mites, PMS, diesel, and tobacco smoke. The following percentages of participants experienced reactions to at least one of the incitants, while many participants encountered numerous emotions simultaneously: 73 percent became irritable, 60 percent felt angry, 29 percent felt violent, 26 percent became paranoid, 62 percent were depressed, 41 percent felt anxiety/panic, and 29 percent felt suicidal.

Sometimes reactions depend upon the timing of the variables, such as hormonal cycles:

> "Each exposure can cause different results depending on how I feel that day, how long I'm exposed, and where I am in my menstrual cycle. After ovulation, I become increasingly more sensitive. I'm most vulnerable a day or two before my period. I schedule appointments and activities according to my cycle."
>
> —Thirty six-year-old woman with MCS

Direct reactions also may go beyond simple emotional reactions to mimic serious cognitive deficits, such as those seen in delirium or schizophrenia, although these seem to be less common. A respondent who worked at a chemical lab described this:

"I felt out of touch with reality during the ten years I worked in the chemical laboratory. It felt like my brain was floating—it didn't feel a part of me. I drove extremely slowly. . . . I did not feel in control unless I drove very slowly. I drove through red lights. I knew they were red, but I couldn't react. I talked slow (still do). Walked slowly. Couldn't follow instructions, trembled unbelievably. Couldn't remember things I needed to remember. I slept anytime I sat down. I was definitely out of touch with reality."

—Fifty-two-year-old woman with MCS
for eighteen years

It is important to be able to identify as many direct reactions as possible, as this will help you to sort out your true emotions from the reactions your brain is having to harmful substances. Although cumbersome, keeping a log of activities and reactions may help with this. Psychological reactions that are environmentally triggered may appear as the result of intermittent exposures, or may be chronic if you live or work in a toxic building. Gas-sensitive people who live with gas heating or cooking appliances may have headaches, depression, and irritability that remit somewhat while they are at work or out of the house for extended periods of time. This is a clue that the exposure is in the home. It is very important to identify or rule out environmental causes for psychological reactions before you attempt to counsel yourself or someone else about the problem.

Direct reactions often feel out of control. The challenge is to not allow the stresses of a reaction to cause you to behave contrary to your personal ethics. It is important to emphasize that we are still responsible for controlling our behavior. MCS is not an excuse for violence, acting out, or perpetrating harm on others. Of course, this is a gray area because with cerebral reactions you may not be in full control. However, that is all the more reason to take responsibility by practicing chemical avoidance, for having a strategy to remove yourself when you do get exposed, and to remember that you are vulnerable during a reaction and need to take special care in your behavior. This includes being careful when you are driving, interacting with others, verbalizing, and making decisions. It can be a great help if a close family member or friend can recognize when you start becoming confused and help to remove you from an exposure. However, not everyone has someone to do this, and the bottom line is that it is not someone else's job to control us.

Secondary Reactions and Effects

Secondary reactions and effects to MCS are the psychological and life consequences of coping with the long-term effects of a debilitating illness/disability, and may include some of the following:

Loss

Multiple chemical sensitivity may rob a person of a job, friends, education, access to community resources, and even attractive clothing, cosmetics, and home decor. Losses may be deep and require grief work and great flexibility for the person to thrive in spite of such drastic loss.

Isolation

The physical isolation that results from being unable to tolerate many public environments, and the mental isolation that comes from having a condition that no one understands can be either severe or catastrophic stressors, especially when they are added to the stress of illness and financial loss. Ignorance and maltreatment from others can further strain and isolate the person with MCS.

Fear

Living with MCS requires constant vigilance, especially if reactions are debilitating or life-threatening. People can come to fear places that were once a source of entertainment and fun. Malls, movies, parties, and other outings can no longer be approached light-heartedly if you must be ready to vacate when you encounter perfume or smoke. In addition to the daily stress of such unpredictability, you may find yourself fearing for the future, since your sensitivities to chemicals tend to include more and more chemicals. You may fear you will lose even more with respect to your livelihood, home, and physical and mental abilities.

Anger and Frustration

Anger and frustration are normal reactions to loss, misunderstanding, and bodily harm from exposures, discrimination, and misdiagnosis. You will need a way to process this anger if you are to avoid having it control you.

Obsessive-Compulsive Behaviors

Avoidance of environmental triggers can result in behaviors that resemble obsessive-compulsive characteristics, especially to people who do not understand how important avoidance is for those managing MCS. Precautionary MCS measures may appear rigid and lacking in spontaneity. For example, watching for someone to light a cigarette, phoning ahead to check on the potential pesticide contamination of a building, avoiding a large numbers of foods, airing out mail to reduce the risk of fragrance exposure, and washing new clothes in vinegar and baking soda many times before wearing them may seem odd to some people. If your character is judged on these types of behaviors, you may mistakenly be accused of having obsessive-compulsive disorder.

Self-Blame

People with MCS may wonder how they got sick and whether they could have done anything to avoid it. Also, those who continue to deteriorate also may distress themselves with questions like, "Why didn't I get a water purifier sooner?" or "Why did I continue to live in that house with oil heat?" The medical paradigms that blame illness on emotions or assert that "everyone gets what they deserve" or that we "create our own worlds" continue to inappropriately fuel this fire.

Lack of Choice Regarding Emotional Reactions

Most people have at least some choice about which emotions they will express in public. People with MCS, however, may be caught off guard by chemical sensitivity reactions that might be cerebral and could be triggered at any moment without warning. These reactions can cause you to demonstrate chemically induced irritability, tears, or nervousness in situations where there may be negative consequences for these types of behaviors, e.g., work.

Lack of Privacy Regarding Health

People who have health problems that do not interfere with their work can choose how much of their health information they will make public. For example, if you had an ovarian cyst, you would not necessarily have to tell your boss. However, if your health requires that you make environmental accommodations in the workplace, privacy does not exist. Furthermore, it doesn't help when journalists, such as John Stossel of *20/20*, add public humiliation to the mix by espousing multiple chemical sensitivity as a psychological disorder (1997).

Loss of Choice Regarding Lifestyle

MCS often dictates so much about the specific conditions that are required merely for survival, that people have very little choice regarding their preferred lifestyles. For example, one outgoing MCS woman has been forced to endure isolation, which does not suit her or her style, and thus is a source of even further stress. Having once enjoyed working with inner city, underserved populations, she now must be content to work in a carefully chosen, clean, rural environment, if she works at all. In this way she is prevented from making her chosen professional contribution. It is important to note, however, that this does *not* mean that she will make *no* contribution. Another woman with MCS said this:

> "This illness has changed my sense of choice. I think that choice is extremely important. Prior to [having this] illness, if I worried over or was unsatisfied with a situation [such as a job], I always felt

there were many choices and I'd be able to change any situation that was difficult or dissatisfying. Presently, I am only able to work out of my home environment, and I am unhappy with my limitations."

Negative Attitudes Toward Authorities/Conventional Medicine

People with MCS have had to self-educate and advocate for themselves to survive. Having received little or no help, or even mistreatment from conventional physicians, they may come to expect rejection and a low quality of care. Hence, by the time they get to therapy they may inaccurately appear to be angry, oppositional, or paranoid to the potential helpers who do not connect these behaviors with the client's history of receiving inadequate medical and psychological care.

Confused Attributions

A person with MCS may become anxious or depressed as a result of a chemical exposure, but may not be aware of what the exposure was. Because there is no shortage of stress in our society, the person may blame the upset on a psychological stressor, which, although present, did not cause the reaction. The person is thus co-opted or tricked into mistakenly questioning their psychological coping ability. This is extremely important to come to terms with if that person is not to alienate friends and co-workers by blaming social and/or work situations for upsets that are actually caused by chemical exposures.

The Loss of a Stable, Continuous Identity

Anselm Strauss (1984) discusses the loss of a continuous sense of identity that occurs when someone is chronically ill. With any chronic illness, the person's sense of self and well-being may fluctuate depending on the current physical state. Because chemical exposures cause people with MCS to have emotional reactions that feel so different from their usual state of mind, they may experience a discontinuous sense of identity. That is to say, when not reacting to chemical exposure, someone with MCS cannot imagine being so ill. On the other hand, when they do have a chemical reaction, they cannot remember feeling well, or feelings concerned with growth and direction. Therefore, the sense of personal identity comes to be punctuated by periods of limbo, during which a person with MCS suffers and waits for exposure effects to wear off.

These "down periods," when a person with MCS is recovering from a harmful exposure, also are disruptive to relationships. Regardless of an MCS person's ability to be accessible—or not—during a down period, other people's lives continue during the recovery process, and repeatedly having to catch up socially can be difficult. (See chapter eleven for a discussion of relationships.)

The Role of the Psychologist

Mental health professionals perform a variety of roles in relation to MCS, such as assessments (including neuropsychological), rehabilitation counseling, insurance-related screening for disability, advocacy, or therapy. There is a great need, however, for educated therapists to provide support to those who are coping with the devastating losses reported by chemically sensitive people.

I receive periodic telephone calls from women with chemical sensitivities who ask for referrals to therapists in their areas who will understand their condition. (I have even received calls from homeless women who still regard therapy as a priority.) By the time I receive one of these phone calls, the life disruption is likely to be severe, and without some sort of supportive intervention, the person may be at risk for committing suicide. Unfortunately, psychological intervention for people with MCS often has been anything but supportive. In fact, contact with mental health practitioners for respondents in Phase II of my study was felt to be particularly troublesome. A total of 549 mental health providers were contacted by respondents who sought psychological help. Of these, only 17 percent of the practitioners were educated about chemical sensitivity, and 36 percent were in some way helpful. People reported having felt harmed by mental health providers in various ways, including having their symptoms of chemical sensitivity ignored or deemphasized (63.6 percent), receiving psychiatric labels (54.5 percent), being given psychoactive medications (44.3 percent), having psychiatric hospitalization suggested (17.6 percent), and/or being admitted to psychiatric hospitals for symptoms of chemical sensitivity (14.9 percent).

One respondent reported that she sought out psychiatric help to deal with the effects of the illness on her life, but that her reports were discounted. Instead, the practitioner suggested MCS was solely caused by problems in her relationship with her mother.

The Role of Evaluator

The most negative treatment from providers occurred when the provider was in the role of "evaluator." One woman with MCS describes her experience dealing with a less than helpful psychiatrist:

> "'Severe hypochondriac'—the psychiatrist from social security administration wrote this on his report. It was humiliating and frustrating because he just did not understand the illness and really

didn't care. I have discovered that women (seems to be especially if you are single) seem not to be taken seriously. I have been told by so many medical doctors, who didn't know what was wrong with me in the early years or didn't understand the illness, to get a job (I was so sick that I had to leave my great job) and to get married!"

—Forty-year-old woman with MCS for
thirteen years

Inappropriate psychological labeling was particularly upsetting for respondents. Some respondents were labeled by mental health providers, but others were given mental health labels by physicians and other professionals. Over half of the respondents from Phase I of my study received mental illness labels, including depression, psychosomatic illness, schizophrenia, panic disorder, neurosis, posttraumatic stress disorder, mania, delusional disorder, and "it's all in your head."

In many cases, people were psychologically labeled simply because they claimed to be affected by chemicals, regardless of whether they had psychological symptoms. For example, some respondents were described as having "olfactory delusions" because they were able to smell chemicals that others were not. In some cases, the evaluators took it a step further and labeled people as "schizophrenic," due to olfactory delusions. Respondents described experiencing erosion of self-confidence, ostracism, anger, and extreme trauma as a result of this kind of treatment by health providers. As an extreme example:

"That doctor has not given me one psychological test, yet he says I have a delusional disorder. He granted my disability on psychiatric terms. He even told me in an interview that I should be placed in a mental institution. I am outraged at the incompetence of our medical doctors."

—Fifty-three-year-old woman with MCS
for nine years

Gender-bias in mental and physical health diagnosis is not uncommon. Many of the problems receiving short shrift from the medical profession are those that afflict women. The history of women's health reads like a comic book of error and mishap.

Unfortunately, this is the heritage of the health system in America, especially with women being doctors for only a relatively short period of time (Lawrence and Weinhouse 1994). It is not surprising that women's health complaints may still be ignored and attributed to psychological variables, as in this instance:

"The label I received was the 'It's in your head' kind. I tried to talk to my doctor about some of my symptoms and concerns, and he gave me the name of a psychiatrist. Later, when my ex-husband complained of the same symptoms, this same doctor sent him to an allergy specialist."

—Sixty-one-year-old woman with MCS
for thirty-six years

Unfortunately, if therapists rely on professional journals for help with treating people with MCS, they will find little useful writing on helping or coping with this disease. In fact, there are a number of researchers committed to proving that MCS *is* a psychological illness. To this end, they have conducted and published "studies" that, in some cases, have managed to show that people with MCS demonstrate some psychiatric symptoms. These symptoms have then been used to make the case that MCS is a psychiatric illness. However, simply demonstrating that people have *some* symptoms is not enough to classify MCS as a psychiatric illness. To truly make the case that people with MCS are psychiatrically disturbed, all of the following conditions would have to be satisfied:

1. Any physical causes for the psychiatric symptoms would have to be ruled out.

2. The psychiatric symptoms would have to have caused the MCS.

3. The group with MCS would have to have more psychiatric symptoms than people *with other chronic physical illnesses.*

There are no studies that have demonstrated these conditions. In fact, researchers rarely have the understanding that MCS patients should even be compared to others with chronic illnesses.

Problems with Psychological Research and Diagnosis

Some of the problems with the research and clinical work that conceptualize MCS as a psychological condition are discussed below.

Experimenter Bias

Even before some studies begin, there may be the problem that "experimenter bias" will affect their accuracy. *Experimenter bias* means the person conducting the study has an interest in proving a particular conclusion. That is, if your mental stability was being questioned and a researcher interviewed you with a preconceived notion of your psychological state, the outcome would not necessarily be accurate. It is as if the biased researcher says, "I think you are mentally unbalanced; let me interview you and prove it." Then, based on the interview that follows, the researcher concludes that indeed you are mentally ill. Experimenter bias can affect both the selection and examination procedures of studies and does not result in valid work.

Inadequate Medical Screening

Often "traditional" medical tests will not indicate chemical damage even when it is present. To date, we have not found a consistently reliable test that will identify MCS damage. Even cholinesterase tests, which should accurately show when someone has had an organophosphate or carbamate pesticide exposure, do not always show low levels of acetylcholinesterase (AcE). People with MCS do show physical indicators of the damage caused by chemical exposure, but often only during in-depth testing that examines the body systems likely to be affected. Examples of these in-depth tests include immune profiles, SPECT scans, close examination of the nasal mucosa, and red blood cell (rather than plasma) measures of nutrients.

Not Listening to What Patients Say

When researchers have their own agendas, they rarely listen to what MCS patients are reporting. For example, Simon, Katon, and Sparks (1990) believe that "psychological vulnerability strongly influences chemical sensitivity." To support their theory, they note the case where a large number of plastic workers reported MCS-like illnesses following the introduction into their workplace of new plastics materials containing phenol, formaldehyde, and methyl ethyl ketone. Although the researchers said plastics workers who developed MCS had more prior depression and anxiety and had more reported psychological symptoms than those who did not develop MCS, the largest predictor of who developed MCS was the preexistence of *medically unexplained physical symptoms*.

Despite the fact that many of the complaints were neurological (including headaches, fatigue, dizziness, nausea, dyspnea, and cognitive disturbances), the authors summarize that "no medical diagnosis or immunological abnormalities were found to account for the vast majority of the workers' systemic symptoms." Given that the testing was done soon after exposure, and that immune tests do not measure neurological damage, it seems that the "panel of specialists" did not listen to the workers. That is, rather than listen to workers and tailor the testing to the complaints (i.e., use neurological exams), the "panel of experts" chose to use inappropriate evaluation methods (immune tests).

No One Is Listening to Gulf War Veterans

Gulf War veterans cannot get officials to take their claims of chemical exposure seriously. In fact, not only is the government not listening to what the veterans have to say, but they also deny any possibility of chemical warfare or damage at all. For example, even though numerous Gulf War veterans and their partners complain of caustic sperm, the official response to them is, "There is no reason to test the sperm." Almost humorously, Sylvia Copeland, chief of the CIA Persian Gulf War Illnesses Task Force, explained that the CIA did not speak with anyone who was in the Gulf as part of their investigation, but reviewed only "intelligence" information. When questioned as to what was "intelligence," she replied that it was anything written on paper by the staff "from foreign sources." In other words, the CIA made sure that they did not find out anything that they did not already know. Representative Christopher Shays (R-Connecticut), chair of the Subcommittee on Gulf War Veterans Illness, replied, "That doesn't seem very intelligent." He summed up the importance of the CIA input into the hearings as follows: "Your statements here are almost meaningless then, because you're telling me that you can only check with foreign sources. But when we have our own troops who claim they're exposed to chemicals, you're not allowed to talk to them" (House Government Reform and Oversight Subcommittee 1996).

Fitting New Problems into Old Categories

Often MCS patients are called somaticizers and hypochondriacs. In my view, these labels represent nothing other than a smug and condescending attitude. It is important to remember that many diseases formerly thought to be the creations of somaticizers were appropriately identified as soon as suitable medical technology was invented. For example, it is now formally recognized that temporomandibular joint (TMJ) can cause headaches, digestive problems, neck and back pain, and a host of other symptoms. Chronic fatigue, formerly seen as psychologically caused, is now recognized as a physical condition by the Centers for Disease Control. In fact, a host of immunological abnormalities has been found in chronic fatigue patients when sophisticated testing is used for blood work. Another disease formerly thought to be of psychological origin is multiple sclerosis (MS). Now proven to affect the brain and/or spinal cord and to cause partial or complete paralysis, MS may first manifest as psychiatric-like symptoms for as long as the first ten years (Klonoff and Landrine 1997).

Unfortunately, Gulf War veterans with physiological problems also have been labeled as psychologically disturbed. Dr. Frances Murphy, neurologist and Director of the Veterans Affairs Environmental Agents Service and of the Persian Gulf Referral Service, testified in Congressional hearings to this effect. She said that 187,000 gulf veterans have been seen in ambulatory care clinics complaining of fatigue, skin rash, headache, muscle and joint pain, memory loss, shortness of breath, diarrhea and other gastrointestinal complaints, sleep disturbance, and other complaints that had become "very familiar" to VA physicians. Regardless, Murphy also said that the Gulf War veterans did not have a "pattern of unexplained illness," rather that "a large number [of Gulf War Veterans]" had "well-established physical and psychiatric conditions." It seems that the veterans' diagnoses were shunted into other preexisting categories, such as anxiety disorders, rather than the physicians examining, in detail, the pattern of symptoms actually experienced by Gulf War veterans. Patients with MCS are treated likewise. The forcing of MCS symptoms to fit into accepted psychological diagnostic categories is described by these two women:

"The first experience [I had] at the U. of WA was frustrating. I thought the interview/consultation was straightforward. [However,] the evaluation statement [included] symptoms I have never had and did not report, such as sweaty hands, rapid heartbeat. . . . These seem to [have been] added [only] to support the [man's] theory about MCS being "posttraumatic" or anxiety induced. I am well aware of situations in which I feel anxious, but anxiety about chemicals does not participate in my illness."

—A woman with MCS for six years

"I was asked if I would be willing to have a psychiatric evaluation when I applied for social security disability. His assessment was 'a very long history of what appears to be severe panic disorder with agoraphobia.' He felt that attributing my 'migraine headaches and breathing difficulties to various irritants reached an almost delusional proportion.' At first I felt quite angry at his assessment, but then realized this is quite typical of the narrow-mindedness the medical profession in general has taken. Note: The psychiatrist recommended the use of Xanax and Prozac. I said 'No thanks.' He says I have very poor insight into my illness and I have difficulty seeing it as a 'psychiatric disorder.' He thinks it's likely I would respond well to medication treatment. This doctor was quite dramatic. While I was sitting in his office, he pulled his wallet out of his pants and slammed it on his desk and said he was willing to 'bet this on it,' referring to his drug treatment program for me. I felt that little gesture was really 'professional.'"

—Forty-five-year-old woman with MCS

Inappropriate Labeling

Some researchers completely discount the physiological problems of MCS and instead inappropriately label MCS people as having psychological disorders. For example, Rosenberg, Freedman, Schmaling, et al. (1990) believe people with MCS have personality disorders. They say that some MCS patients are dramatic and hysterical, and thereby explain their symptoms with emotion and flare. The authors label other MCS people as obsessively detailed and fastidious. They say these patients bring in lists of symptoms and a timeline of how they got sick, and describe their illness with less emotion. The authors say that these people appear "to be primarily ideational (obsessive/paranoid) character." The MCS patient, therefore, regardless of personal style, is doomed no matter how they present their illness, as there always is a label to be applied to delegitimize their experience.

Patient Experience Is Not Considered During Test Interpretation

People's individual responses to items on psychological tests often are not interpreted within the context of the patient's life experiences. For example, some items on the Psychosocial Adjustment to Illness Scale (PAIS) (Derogatis 1986) on the Health Care Orientation subscale ask about a person's attitude toward medical care. In Phase I of my research, people with MCS did not have much good to say about the medical treatment they received. Normally, this is interpreted on the PAIS as having a cynical attitude toward providers. The problem with this interpretation, however, is that the evaluators assume that adequate health care exists for the patient's condition, and that providers have given the patient appropriate information. Because most physicians are unfamiliar with, or do not believe in MCS, results from the Health Care Orientation scale need to be interpreted in context of these realities. The patients' recognition that they have been poorly cared for is probably a sign of good reality testing rather than a sign of a cynical attitude.

Contamination of Depression Inventories with Somatic Items

Most measures of depression, such as the Beck Depression Inventory, contain items that ask about physical symptoms. These types of tests, however, assume that the physical symptoms are caused by the depression. If these same measures are used with people with physical illnesses, they receive elevated scores on depression for having physical symptoms. There-fore, these scores are not valid measures of mood disorders. To avoid this problem, some researchers use the Geriatric Depression Scale or some other measure that is not contaminated with somatic items. But many researchers don't. Research using inappropriate testing methods to evaluate as depressed people who have MCS or other physical illnesses is invalid because it fails to control for physical illness.

Using Control Groups from the General Population

A number of studies have compared those with MCS with a control group matched by age and income, but not physical illness. These studies show that people with MCS are more upset than those without physical ill-nesses, but nothing more. To prove people with MCS had psychopathology, you would have to compare them with a control group of people with other chronic physical illnesses. (Of course, since these experimenters do not believe that MCS is a physical illness, in their minds this would *not* be a suit-able control group.)

Ignoring Studies that Support Physical Explanations

Researchers sometimes choose to ignore studies that clearly support a physical explanation for MCS. For example, some studies test for and incor-porate both the physical and psychological issues involved with the disease. My two favorites are these:

In an early study (Bertschler, Butler, Lawlis, et al. 1985) found that people with MCS appeared healthier on psychological testing after receiving treatment for their sensitivities with environmental medical tech-niques, including avoidance, neutralization, and nutritional supplements. That is, patients had better mental health simply by reducing their sensitivities.

Similarly, Bell, Peterson, and Schwartz (1995) tried to separate physio-logical from psychological indicators by examining self-reported illness caused by odors in a nonclinical population (people who were not MCS patients). They found that people who had cacosmia (an exaggerated sense of smell) were more likely to have close family members with *physical* as opposed to *psychological* illnesses. Physical illnesses that run in the family could result from shared heredity or a shared toxic environment (or both). (See chapter two for the causal theories of MCS.)

Attitudes and Beliefs about MCS

We are a culture that wants desperately to believe that a positive attitude will make everything all right. To that end, we have every kind of mind over matter training that you can imagine. Love, positive attitude, and optimism are all supposed to mitigate the effects of serious disease. Those with positive attitudes are supposed to recover faster from cancer. Books prescribe affirmations that correspond with illnesses. My favorite is Louise Hay's affirmation for constipation, which is: "I willingly release the old and welcome the new." This is not to put down the work of Louise Hay, as there are people with AIDS who credit her work with keeping them alive. This attitude can be tricky, however, when you are nose deep in a neurotoxic exposure. Because neurotoxins alter brain chemistry, simply trying to maintain a positive attitude will not be enough to stay healthy. In one instance, a woman with MCS was determined to use affirmations to help her avoid having a reaction to diesel fuel. She was faced with having to drive several hundred miles without air-conditioning in the summer, and decided to say affirmations aloud the entire twelve hours. When she arrived at her destination, she did indeed have a somewhat smaller systemic reaction than normal (because she was breathing through her mouth the whole time). But her throat was raw from breathing diesel fumes through her mouth and saying affirmations for twelve hours.

It's hard to fight biochemistry, as described by this participant:

"I used to experiment with laying on of hands, mental suggestions, Science of Mind, etc. I really believed people could become well with a change of consciousness. I was wrong, and I sincerely regret some of my advice. . . . I realize I have no control over the illness. I thought my mind could handle it. I cannot prevent the reactions when I'm in the chemicals. I've tried all my training and nothing works."

—A woman with MCS for twenty years

Janice Strubbe Wittenberg (1996) says that studies show that 50 to 75 percent of all problems that manifest as pain or illness are "emotional, social, or familial in origin." How could this ever be proven? Evaluators may think that problems are from family of origin, for example, but then we must again examine the possibility of evaluator bias. There is, in fact, evidence for evaluators missing serious illnesses. In one study (Fishbain and Goldberg 1991), for example, 62.5 percent of people with the label of "conversion disorder" later developed organic brain disorders compared to 5.3 percent of those with the labels of "anxiety" or "depression." A conversion disorder diagnosis is given when a person appears to have lost the function of a body part, such as an arm, but no medical reason can be found for the dysfunction.

I am not against affirmations, positive thinking, and other mental and emotional interventions. In fact, I support them if they are used wisely. But when Wittenberg says, "Things can hurt you if you think they can. This means it is possible to decide against reactivity and extreme fatigue," I have to disagree. Most people with MCS didn't think chemicals could hurt them until long after the damage was done. Theories of positive thinking should not be used to punish people who are sick by implying that they thought their way into the illness. A 63-year-old woman with MCS says, "I've been told I didn't have to have a swollen tongue and hiatal hernia if I didn't *want* to. Do these perpetrators believe it's interesting and loads of fun to have tubes stuck down one's throat?"

If positive thinking techniques can be combined with wise management and chemical avoidance, then you have a great package for coping. (See chapter twelve for more about coping.)

Summary for the Client: How To Make Psychology Work for You

Although there are some theories to be wary of when considering psychotherapy, there is no denying that if you find the right therapist, you may have great success with better coping and dealing with MCS. The following seven points are a checklist of how you might use psychology to your benefit.

1. Work with a supportive therapist to sort out non-MCS, family-of-origin psychological issues.

2. Determine how having MCS might complicate the non-MCS, psychological issues you discover in therapy. Learn how these issues might complicate your coping with MCS.

3. A therapist can help you to directly cope with MCS. For example, developing skills that will help you ask for the accommodations you need and figuring out how best to do it; learning time and energy management skills; dealing with losses, anger, mistreatment, fear, and frustration; and deciding how much effort you want to put into maintaining particular relationships.

4. You have the right to interview and choose a therapist. Many therapists offer either a free or reduced fee consultation in which you can meet and decide whether to work together. You are hiring the therapist; you can interview them in this session to see how you feel about the therapist's ideas and general approach. Before you go to your first meeting, however, be sure to inquire about the office environment and ask about any special accommodations you may need. For instance, you may want to ask some of the following questions:

Questions to Ask Potential Therapists

• "What do you know about chemical sensitivities and injuries?"

• "Can you accommodate my special requests?" For example, you may ask if the office is fragrance-free or if pesticides or petrochemical heating is present. Is the therapist willing to see you outside of their office if their environment is not safe?

• "How would you work with someone with this problem?"

• "What is your orientation?" Although today most therapists are eclectic or integrative (meaning they use a mixture of techniques), some subscribe closely to one theory that more or less guides most of their work. For example, if a therapist tells you that they are psychoanalytic, you most likely will hear a lot about your hidden defenses and your attraction for your opposite sex parent. If the therapist is "client-centered," this means that they subscribe to the theories of Carl Rogers. These therapists are likely to listen to you and reflect back to you your feelings as they understand them. Note that there are many different types of orientations to which a potential therapist may subscribe.

5. Do not work with a therapist who doesn't believe in MCS. If you had diabetes, would you go to someone who didn't believe in diabetes and planned to lead you to believe you could eat more and more sugar? Many anti-MCS articles have advised therapists to get to know their clients and build trust by never directly challenging their beliefs. Then slowly, the therapists try to get the clients to change their belief that chemicals are making them ill.

6. Carefully research any therapy suggested to you. For example, most people with MCS who reported their experiences with antidepressants did not do well on them. This does not mean that you wouldn't respond well to certain drugs; but before taking them, you at least need to know as much as you can about them and what the experiences of others have been. (See chapter six for further information on antidepressants.)

7. Share this chapter with your therapist. The more they know about the problem, the more effectively you can be helped.

Making psychology work for you—as opposed to against you—is dependent on other topics, such as social support and identity. (See chapters ten and eleven for more information on these topics.)

Good coping involves psychology, spirituality, support, understanding chronic illness, getting enough decent medical help to prevent decline, cleaning up your home to prevent further exposure, and understanding the political situation in relation to MCS. It is a large package and every piece is important. By looking at it one piece at a time, perhaps you can negotiate your way through the maze of surviving—and even thriving—in spite of difficult odds.

Therapist Summary: Suggestions for Treating Clients with MCS

This is a brief introduction to therapy considerations for counseling people with chemical sensitivities/injuries. You can learn more by listening to people who tread the path of the impossible—living in the modern world while it is poisoning them. Goodheart and Lansing (1997) say that the treatment tasks for the person with chronic illness and their therapist are fourfold:

1. Facing the assault on self and identity

2. Working through the reorganization or reshaping of self

3. Reconsolidating the new self and achieving stability of self despite an unstable body

4. Providing follow-up structure/process to maintain progress made

More succinctly, Goodheart and Lansing say: "The adaptive goal of psychotherapy for these patients (the desired outcome) is the stability of self and identity in the face of the body's instability and uncertain course." The person with MCS needs to be helped to retain positive qualities that they had prior to developing MCS, and to develop new ones in response to coping successfully with their health.

Do Not Jump to Conclusions About a Personality Profile

Psychologists are fond of finding personality profiles for everything. For example, when sick building syndrome (SBS) came to the public's attention researchers searched for a personality profile that would make some more susceptible to SBS than others. The profile was never found. In fact, Scandinavian studies have found that SBS is influenced by the following variables: gender, preexisting asthma or rhinitis, a history of atopy (which is a type of allergy), job category, photocopying, VDT use, and handling carbonless paper (cited in Ashford, Heinzow, Lutjen, et al. 1995). To best assist your MCS client, it would be beneficial to everyone involved if you did not rely exclusively on information from extraneous personality profiles.

If You Can't Be a Positive Support, Refer the Client to Someone Who Can

Just as "neutrality" is often interpreted negatively by other oppressed groups (e.g., gays/lesbians), not taking a stand will be interpreted negatively by the MCS client. Although some researchers/writers suggest gaining the MCS patient's confidence before slowly trying to get them to change their belief that chemicals are making them sick, your patients will see through this. You will waste their time—and yours—and you may be ethically responsible for making them sicker if they experience exposures at your suggestion. If you cannot be supportive, refer your client to an associate who can.

Beware of Treatment Recommendations That Ignore the Clients' Complaints

There are many treatment recommendations available that ignore the MCS client's experience and complaints. For example, Black (1996) suggests, "Treatment of coexisting psychiatric disorders, including depression and panic disorder, will help to reduce symptoms of illness and disability." What if the symptoms, however, are caused by chemicals to begin with, as MCS clients assert? Black continues, "Patients with 'reactions' (e. g., panic attacks) to chemical exposures, for instance, may be able to tolerate exposure to disagreeable odors once the panic attacks are blocked." In this instance, Black is ignoring the evidence that solvents can cause panic attacks (Dager, Holland, Cowley, et al. 1987). Black further says, "On the other hand, patients with somatization disorders can be monitored for the emergence of new symptoms, which can then be placed into context. This will help to reduce unnecessary testing and other medical procedures that may contribute to the patient's disability" (p. 354). By "placed in to context" I assume that Black means ignored, since the person is assumed to somaticize their psychological discomfort. Similarly, "reduce unnecessary testing" can be taken to mean that these new symptoms are not to be investigated and thus the possibility of overlooking end-organ disease development is great. Given that patients of Heuser, Wojdani, and Heuser (1992) and of Levin and Byers (1992) have developed autoimmune disorders, the ethics of this approach are questionable at best, and they are complicit in using psychology to silence those harmed by contamination at worst. Practitioners can and should be held liable for ignoring indicators of potential disease.

Suggestions for Supportive Interactions with MCS Clients

It is not difficult to become familiar with the major characteristics of MCS. There is a growing body of MCS-related literature, and well-educated clients will provide therapists with much useful information. Although it is not the client's responsibility to educate their therapist, many clients are happy to find someone who wants to understand the problem. Having a strong, relevant understanding of MCS combined with strong clinical skills will allow for people previously neglected by mental health professionals to receive an important source of support.

Utilize the Skills You Already Have

People who have other disabilities and chronic illnesses share many of the same problems of chemically sensitive people. Although each chronic illness is unique, any special knowledge, training, or experience you have in any area of disability/chronic illness will increase your sensitivity and will be helpful in understanding this population. Therapists will see that people with MCS share the financial and work difficulties of those with a variety of conditions. Similarly, disappointment with medical providers is common in those whose conditions are poorly understood, or can be maintained, but not cured. Isolation, too, is common for anyone of limited energy or mobility.

What distinguishes MCS from other illnesses is probably a unique constellation of variables, including the lack of access to safe buildings, financial and job resources, and medical information or treatment; the personal isolation; poorly understood physical suffering; and the inability to tolerate items that most people not only take for granted, but are practically the basis of our entire material culture.

Understand Toxicology

Even if you will not be doing testing and evaluation of MCS patients, it is important to understand something about the effects toxicants have on people's bodies, particularly the nervous system. The field of neurobehavioral toxicology explores the effects of toxins on the brain and behavior. (See Appendix E for a list of suggested readings in toxicology; and Appendix C for further reading and resources.) Arnold (1997) explains the importance of being able to provide resources on toxic injury to physicians, as they may not be well informed about likely neurological effects.

If you will be providing testing and evaluation of people who have had toxic exposures, you may need more training, particularly in the area of neuropsychology, as well as knowledge about the appropriate measures for toxic injury. It would also be beneficial for you to understand the overlap between toxic injury and other conditions on test results, and to be current in your knowledge of neuropsychological testing and toxic tort, which is court litigation regarding toxin-related injuries.

Sensitivity Levels Determine Lifestyle

There will be great differences in the necessary lifestyle modifications between those with mild sensitivities and those whose sensitivities have become severe. Many people without sensitivities are able to understand mild or isolated reactions, but draw a blank when confronted with someone who is virtually unable to tolerate any exposures. Some people with MCS are unable even to be near other individuals who will secondarily expose them to odors that they have picked up on their clothing or hair.

Some Reactions Will Mimic "Psychiatric" Symptoms

Chemical sensitivity/injury may create severe stress, anxiety, and depression both as primary reactions to exposures and as secondary reactions to loss and disintegration of previous lifestyle. Critics have used the presence of neurological reactions as grist for suggesting that chemical sensitivity is a psychiatric disorder. However, petrochemical exposures can cause depression (Randolph and Moss 1982), anxiety, and even panic attacks (Dager, Holland, Cowley, et al. 1987). In fact, many people with MCS report having developed phobias after the onset of the chemical sensitivity, but no research has directly addressed this.

At the same time, any preexisting or unrelated mental health needs should not be ignored. Certainly, other concerns do not disappear just because a person has developed sensitivities. Deciphering when the issue at hand is specifically MCS-relevant can be a shared task with the client, and will require a good working knowledge of MCS-related issues as well as a sensitivity to the dynamics operating for specific clients in specific contexts.

Be Flexible

Some clients will need modifications in the office setting. Small modifications might include removing air fresheners, potpourri, perfumes, and other odors from the office. Some clients will be unable to go to the office at all, even with these modifications (perhaps due to the heating system, pesticides, or perfumes used by other clients). It would be best to see these individuals in their homes. Additionally, with these clients, cancellations are more likely to be the result of erratic energy levels and illness due to unavoidable exposures than to resistance or lack of follow-through. Furthermore, financial difficulties may prevent many people with MCS from obtaining therapy unless some flexible monetary arrangements can be made.

Help Your Client Mourn and Come to Terms
with Any Losses

Each client will have endured some losses caused by their health condition. You may want to inquire how your client thinks their life would be different without MCS. According to respondents from Phase I of my study, common losses include educational opportunities, professional success, financial stability, relationships, and nurturing possibilities, including motherhood.

Help the Client Plan

In between exposures, clients may require assistance in making plans for themselves as to what they will do once they are aware that they have suffered a debilitating exposure. Because some exposures entail mental confusion as well as physical illness, clients may do well to plan, in advance, what they will do during or immediately after a debilitating exposure. Some of a client's special needs during such times may include needing to ask for physical assistance, getting away from the offending chemical, taking a particular remedy that mitigates ill effects, taking special care to control irritability brought on by the exposure, etc.

Monitor the Client's Level of Support

Everyone has varying levels of support and conflict in their relationships with other people. Therefore, MCS clients may need some assistance negotiating their close relationships with other people who invariably will demonstrate various levels of belief in and support for those with MCS. Therapists with training in family counseling may be in unique positions to help in this way, but should guard against conceptualizing the sensitivities as "symptoms of family dysfunction" rather than as valid problems in their own right.

Clients Struggle with the Issue of "Lost Time"

Each harmful exposure or long period of debility may mean "down time" or time in which the client is unavailable to others or unable to accomplish much in terms of effortful work. Of course, the inability to work will be a problem for those who are employed, and may lead to friction with co-workers and bosses, as well as to financial problems. The inability to be available to others is likely to take a toll on both intimate and casual relationships. For example, Barshay (1993) has written of her experience with chronic fatigue and MCS. She says, "I do not have the energy to make new friends or even to keep up with women I already know; for an extra telephone call in my day will often bring on an exacerbation of symptoms." Even when the client is feeling good, conditions such as MS, MCS, and other illnesses with a variable course, create the unpredictability of not knowing how one will feel on a particular day. This makes it very difficult for anyone to make social plans. In addition, when in long periods of illness, if friendships are not nurtured, the person with MCS may come out of the experience looking forward to seeing friends again only to discover that they are unavailable. People who have gone on with their lives in the client's absence may not understand the prolonged hiatus, and may have trouble resuming the previous level of intimacy.

Help Clients Validate Their Own Knowledge

Even clients who are considerably educated about their condition can forget that *they* are the experts in regard to how chemicals and the illness/ sensitivity process affects them. For some, avoidance may even be a matter of life and death. Yet, people with this condition are in the position of having to be assertive about something that few people understand or respect.

Help the Client Plan for a Future That May Include Disability

Although some people with MCS recover to some extent, and a small number report recovering completely, many do not. Considerable fear may be associated with an unknown course of illness. The client may need help making plans to confront work problems, financial difficulties, and perhaps more physical disability. Another aspect of long-term planning includes helping the client let go of earlier goals that are now unattainable. Since chemical sensitivities dictate what environments are feasible, there will be roles that must necessarily be abandoned or never attained.

Resist Pressuring the Client

Although your intentions may be pure, you should resist pressuring a client into trying specific cures or treatments. Esten and Willmott (1993) have written of some therapists' need to "cure" clients of having a disability: "With all good intentions the therapist tells the client of diets, snake venom treatments, special exercise programs, and vitamin regimes that will rid them of the problem." This is not to say that there are no helpful interventions for MCS. On the contrary, many participants in Phase I of my study reported obtaining help from a variety of treatments. However, it is the client who must make the decision to try yet another type of therapy. These decisions must be viewed in the context of knowing that the client has probably already spent considerable money, time, and energy trying various treatments. One exception to this is simple avoidance. If you have clients who refuse even to try to protect themselves by avoiding continual exposures, then you will not be able to help these clients until they stop denying the problem and decide to deal with it.

Help the Client Come to Terms with Constant Challenges to Identity

If the condition progresses, each increase in the level of sensitivity poses new challenges for the chemically sensitive person. If new sensitivities develop, further life restrictions may ensue. Clients with MCS are in the position of having their contextual background shrink with increasing limitations until much of what is identified as "self" is no longer available. One respondent dealt with this by actually giving herself a new name, as she felt that her old self was "dead" now that she was forced to live an entirely new and isolated lifestyle. Although this upset family members, for her it represented a tangible way of naming her experience and moving forward. Other clients may struggle with the need to be ever vigilant regarding exposures. Still others may need to mourn the loss of a spontaneous lifestyle. Clients with MCS, perhaps much as those with MS, need to confront, integrate, and mourn each new loss or change in themselves if functioning slowly diminishes. Friedman (1993) has discussed the tremendous personal shock of becoming quadriplegic in an instant as a result of a car accident. Conditions like MCS, in contrast, *may* have the "advantage" of spreading slowly over time, thus giving a therapist the opportunity to offer support as one stable element in the degeneration process.

Support the Client's Move to the Political Arena

If possible, and if clients wish it, helping them to connect with advocacy organizations may urge them on to a new level of growth. Many MCS sufferers have made serious contributions to public education and legislative advocacy in relation to MCS and the environment. For many clients, this will happen naturally as they learn of legislative and educational projects. Others may need to be made aware of the major organizations that have been formed to deal with MCS-related issues. Therapists should be familiar with these organizations to provide resources and remain current on political and legal discussions in the area. Many health providers with an interest in the area join a number of these organizations for self-education and to procure resources. (See Appendix D for organizations to join.)

Be Willing to Go to Bat for Your Client

Therapists may be asked by clients to provide them with letters and various communications that will aid in procuring resources. Because cultural biases often dictate that MCS patients will have to see psychiatrists when pursuing worker's compensation or disability benefits, a letter from a sympathetic mental health professional who knows the client may help dilute damaging information from an industry-based psychiatrist.

Be Willing to Help in Practical Matters

Clients with MCS face the task of searching for safe housing, organic foods, chemical-free furnishings and clothing, etc. Information of this sort may be needed by clients who have just recently recognized their sensitivities, while clients with longer-term experience will be educating the therapist.

Understand the Importance of the Environment

Don't compartmentalize clients or what you learn while seeing them. For some chemically sensitive people, their condition is their call to education and activism in regard to the environment. This quest often leads to a bottom line understanding that environmental degradation is so pervasive that people's biological systems are breaking down under the strain. Considerable anger results from the fact that other people do not seem to take this seriously. What follows may be a commitment to activism. Probably the most validation/respect a therapist can show for the MCS client is to become educated about environmental issues and commit to a style of life that has minimal negative impact on others' health. People with MCS have discussed the irony of going to chemically contaminated offices with perfumed providers in order to "heal." Therapists who truly understand MCS are necessarily placing themselves on the path of the environmentalist. If you learn from your client that wearing perfume makes chemically sensitive people ill and denies them access to every place you wear it, can you then—in good conscience—go home and put on perfume to wear during your evening out?

Basically, the person with MCS needs to build a new foundation of self that includes the MCS without purging positive unique self-qualities. Since so much of self is relational, this can be extremely difficult in isolation, and part of therapy may be helping the client to brainstorm possibilities for social interaction. (See chapter ten for more information on social support.)

Chapter Ten

Against the Odds

Identity, Loss, and Possibilities for Growth

Having a chronic illness or disability is bound to have some negative reper-cussions on a person's sense of self; however, having a condition that is dele-gitimized and demands some degree of isolation, such as MCS does, creates even more challenges. In Phase III of my study, participants were asked how their sense of identity had changed as a result of having MCS. This chapter describes some of their responses. You may find that you have experienced some of these feelings, or you may have entirely different perspectives on how MCS can affect someone's sense of identity.

Hijacked: My Life Is on Hold Until I Get Well

Some people with MCS were deeply involved with buying equipment, visit-ing physicians, and pursuing the "cure." Simultaneously, these individuals had a sense of, "This is not *really* me. This awful thing happened to me and it has eclipsed everything I know about myself." People with chronic illness, especially people with MCS, desperately wanted their old selves and their old lives back. There was a sense of feeling tired, empty, and strange—so much so that it was difficult to have anything to say to other people. The following quote from a woman with MCS captures the essence of people who felt their lives were "hijacked":

> "I don't feel like I have a sense of self anymore. Sometimes I really hate myself. (I hate what I have become due to this illness). Deep down, I am the same person (feelings, wants, etc.)—but I am so overwhelmed by having to live in isolation and feel so empty and lonely that I also feel the old me is gone forever. I miss people. There is no way to deal with this except to take one day at a time. I talk to a few people on the phone, but am unable to see anyone (except very occasionally one or two people like myself)."

Possessed: How Did I Become So Irritable?

People with MCS described experiencing unwelcome negative emotions that either were primary reactions to chemicals or secondary reactions to the trauma of having MCS. Both were extremely frustrating and unwelcome. These reactions were also contrary to their self-image in terms of what people had wanted to become, before they became ill. Feeling angry or irritable were two primary complaints, as one thirty-eight-year-old woman who has had MCS for three years described: "I have a squirrel in the yard who will come and take food from my hand. I am also the type of person who never gets upset when my kids spill something accidentally. During my sickest time, I would actually aim for squirrels and birds while driving in the car."

One person described the discomfort of having to focus on self-care. She says, "I feel very 'needy' and I was *never* . . . that way before." Likewise, a woman who has had MCS for more than seventeen years explained, "I never thought of myself before. It was always my family or some friend who needed some special attention. Now I must always consider, 'How will this affect me?' So I feel that I have become self-centered, but it is necessary to survive with any happiness."

Two women who have MCS and are quoted below describe other unwelcome, long-term secondary changes:

> "I am a lot more cynical, I do not trust anyone anymore. My sister said she used to think I was the nicest person she knew after [so and so]. She said it appears that I still try sometimes, but I am just not as nice as I used to be."

"I have [a master's degree] and sometimes I can't even write a paragraph! My whole sense of security and who I am has changed. My husband says I have lost my adventuresome spirit. I am paranoid about exposure to pesticides. Food allergies radically alter my personality."

Paradoxically, although primary reactions to chemicals often include intrusive anger or irritability, some people experienced a "blunting of emotions" as a long-term phenomenon. These people felt "robbed" of aspects of their essential selves.

"[M]y ability to feel on an emotional level has changed significantly. I am *intellectually* emotional rather than really feeling, and I feel *flat* most of the time when I'm not having reactions. When I'm having reactions, anger, confusion, and frustration are most prominent, and often much out of proportion to the event [to which I am reacting]."

—Fifty-two-year-old woman with MCS
for twenty years

"MCS has deeply affected my ability to enjoy life. It has strangled my fun, loving, kind, true self. I find I can now be very jealous, mean-spirited and depressed very easily."

—Forty-six-year-old woman with MCS
for one year

One woman, after suffering two acute incidents of prolonged exposure (both skin and respiratory) to a pesticide, described losing her entire personality, energy, and ambition for six months. It took two years to recover her full "affective" or emotional life.

Many study participants expressed anger at the unfairness of having so little control over their behavior, despite having spent years developing their personal growth.

Driven Incognito: I Won't Let Anyone Know

Some people with MCS hid their sensitivities and pretended to be well in order to "pass" for normal. For example, they kept toxic appointments at hairdressers, they failed to speak up about exposures that were affecting them negatively, and generally they hid their condition to avoid other people's censure.

People hid their reactions and sensitivities to deflect negative feedback from others, to maintain some semblance of a "normal" life, and for the benefit of others. Unfortunately, the same people who hid their sensitivities described enduring excruciating pain (e.g., headaches) privately while continuing to function. One woman, for example, explained that you should never let your pain interfere with your relation to someone else and, for this reason, she always cheerfully "did" for her family even if she was suffering:

> "I believe with all my heart, you should never put your pain onto someone else. As sick as I am, I'm a pleasant person. It keeps our marriage working and happy. No matter how I feel, I still do my housework. I still cook. . . . I can tolerate a great deal of pain. This is the way I survive."
>
> —Fifty-eight-year-old woman with MCS for thirteen years

Robbed: This Is Not the Life I Planned

No children, when asked what they would like to be when they grow up, reply, "I'd like to be a sick person." The realization that MCS will greatly alter your previous perceptions of career, home life, hobbies, travel, athletics, and retirement plans can be traumatically shocking. MCS can mean having to redo all of your goals and plans in midstream. (It can be somewhat like finding out halfway across a lake that you are not going to make it to the other side.) The anger, loss, fear, and confusion that are generated can be overwhelming.

> "I feel I have lost my sense of identity. My life is so sheltered and alone compared to the way it was before the MCS. I have very limited contact with people. I feel I am unable to express myself. I have had to learn to live basically at home in my safe environment in order to survive. Sometimes I feel I have lost contact with the rest of the world and what is going on around me. It has caused me a lot of emotional stress. Luckily, I have a very loving and understanding husband who allows me to let out my angers and emotions and listens to me and tries to understand what I'm going through. This is my way of dealing with things, and I am determined I am going to get better.
>
> —Thirty-four- year-old woman with MCS for five years

> "Working near or with smokers, perfume users, in moldy dusty areas, and the refusal of everyone involved to understand or moderate behavior has determined my life course. [People's behavior

regarding my sensitivities is] very unsatisfactory to me and has left me destitute financially: Limping along, struggling from exposure to exposure, from job to job, has created an insurmountable obstacle to my accomplishing what I wished to carry out."

—Sixty-two-year-old woman who has
been chemically sensitive since childhood

The pervasive loss that is caused by long-term illness can be an insidious trauma (Root 1992); yet sufferers of delegitimized illnesses receive very little recognition or support. It is no wonder that people who are chronically ill sometimes become involved in addictive behavior. One man, for example, became a heavy user of alcohol and marijuana after he was involved with a chemical accident that destroyed his health and left him confused, unable to concentrate, and plagued by nightmares. In another case, a woman with MCS became addicted to overeating:

"I feel trapped at home and extremely bored—as a result, I have seemingly developed a compulsion to overeat. I'm sure it's to fill the gigantic void I feel in my life. I also beat up on myself a lot and I am extremely unhappy. Through it all, though, I always wear a smile and am cheerful around others, while on the inside, I have a great big ache."

—Fifty-one-year-old woman with MCS
for three years

Dislodged: I Don't Know Who I Am

Along with feeling "robbed" of their identity and sense of self, people with MCS described being severely "dislodged" from all of their familiar roles. Another way of describing this is that they experienced a loss of self-positioning. That is, we all play multiple roles in our lives that cause us to relate to ourselves and others in social, professional, parenting, romantic, sexual, and other roles and relationships. These roles and relationships, however, may disappear when health no longer is robust enough to fulfill them. For example, a teacher who was poisoned by an oil heating system says, "My career is now destroyed because my health has been ruined. I don't feel life has much purpose and wish I could just die and get it over with." A forty-seven-year-old woman who has had MCS for fourteen years says, "I feel worthless. I was a school psychologist who was consulted by students, teachers and principals all day every day. I am now isolated and desperately miss the stimulation and mental gymnastics [I used to experience at work]."

One woman with MCS since adolescence pointed out that her life was greatly affected by continually having to wear a mask in public that protected her from inhaling unsafe chemicals. She says, "Having to wear a mask, covering my face, takes away identity. People stare [at me], children are even afraid."

One role that American culture particularly values is mental acuity. For some people, however, even this diminished once they become chemically sensitive. For example, a forty-seven-year-old woman with MCS for five years says, "For me, I was always proud and secure in my intelligence. This illness has taken away one of my most prized possessions. My mind was part of my identity."

Even material possessions, such as clothing, furniture, and houses, are important elements of identity in Western culture. Having to give up makeup, fashion, and/or a beautiful home were stressors for many individuals. Generally, however, many people moved beyond these values:

> "Having lost my home . . . and all the pretty things and antiques, I find that life and happiness is not in possessions, but within each individual. If I dwell on this loss I am unhappy, but if I dwell on how to make tomorrow better, well, I am happy."

> —Sixty-nine-year-old woman with MCS
> for over seventeen years

Sometimes, physical circumstances were so seriously challenging that they posed further trauma. A fifty-three-year-old woman with MCS for more than fourteen years says, "I sat in my car for a *year*! I would sleep at another [chemically sensitive person's] house at night and use my car in the daytime so that I would not inconvenience them too much. I also had to sleep in my car for a month."

The sexual roles and relationships of MCS people were also affected by their illness due to their declining energy levels and other physical problems. Unfortunately, having tension in this area often can cause further stress in a person's one, close, ongoing relationship. As a rule, all roles that demanded attention and energy were affected by MCS.

Deserted: No One Cares About Me Anymore

People with MCS struggled with what it meant to lose connections to people they knew from work, social circles, and even their families. Friends often deserted them. Even children, spouses, in-laws, and parents were not immune from potentially writing off those with MCS as hypochondriacs. Desertions by loved ones caused people to face the void of isolation and, often, suffer from the lack of something or someone to hang on to.

> "I am no longer the same person I was before. My life used to be full of friends, family, children, flowers, and I loved my job. Since the carpet was installed, my life has been one nightmare after

another: I was treated like a crazy person, I became terribly thin, the more I tried to get help, the more I was labeled as crazy. My friends pulled away from me, I changed jobs four times, and now [I] try to work out of my house. I feel like my life has no meaning, no future, no one has offered me hope, my phone never rings, the people I cared about most have stopped coming to see me. I even look different. I can no longer have my hair or nails done, my weight has gotten out of hand, my clothes don't fit. I cry a lot alone. There is no one to listen, no one to care and, worst of all, nothing anyone could do anyway."

—Forty-one-year-old woman with MCS for five years

Some people became most desperate and "hit bottom" when they were forced to face the fact that people who they once thought would stand by them did not.

"I feel like people laugh at me and they don't believe me. I'm made fun of by co-workers. [I was] refused a promotion because of my health and was told so by my supervisor. I have [a] poor memory. I just mainly stay at home since I'm on sick leave from work."

—Forty-two-year-old woman with MCS for fifteen years

"It's had a devastating effect on my life. My dreams have been shattered. Life has merely become a matter of survival, as if I'm in a prison camp. My self-esteem has been damaged due to hostility and ridicule from co-workers and management. I was formerly optimistic and confident in my ability to overcome obstacles. Years of poor health and increasing, persistent obstacles have made me sad and bitter. . . . The future is bleak. As my health worsens and money continues to dwindle, I fear that I will end up with only one option."

—Thirty-six-year-old man with MCS for six years

Goaded: MCS Is Forcing Me to Grow

In Phase I of my study, we had the nerve to ask whether people had experienced any significant personal growth as a result of having MCS. Some respondents were not amused and responded with statements, such as, "Hell no, why should I, stupid?" and "No. MCS is a royal pain in the tuchas." And, "This question annoys me."

Some respondents were humorous, including, "I (*have*) thirty-pound fluctuations in my weight three to four months at a time." And, "I had a small *growth* on my arm." Some participants, however, were able to meet the challenges and imposed isolation of MCS, and made it work for them. People read, listened to tapes, and/or developed their spirituality:

> "The isolation has taught me to be very creative. The unpredictability of both illnesses has taught me to enjoy today, and do the best I can each day. I've learned to focus on what I *can* do and not on what I *cannot* do. I've developed my spirituality and have decided God's goals for me are different than the ones I had for myself."

> —Fifty-five-year-old woman with MCS
> since childhood

Sometimes, you can experience personal growth that occurs as a result of having MCS, whether you seek it or not. For instance, one chemically sensitive person says, "I now know more than I ever wanted to know about housing construction, food growing and processing, skunk behavior, clothing manufacturing, how to use aluminum foil tape, variations in water heaters, the life and habits of mold, etc." Other respondents say:

> "Of course! Since I have been 'evicted' from society, I spend most of my time reading—half are books and articles about chemical poisonings and sick buildings—at least now I know I'm not crazy! The other [half of the] time I spend reading spiritual literature, thinking, meditating, and writing—the spiritual interests I never had enough time to have in my life before. I am trying to use this to my advantage to change my life."

> —Forty-one-year-old woman with MCS
> for twenty-one years

> "I've become humbler and appreciate beauty more in nature, music and art. My disability gave me more opportunity to read (in the sauna), to take longer vacations in Europe (where they have electric trains with no smoking cars), and I tried hiking in the Alps because I thought it might help my MCS, which it did. At the same time, I discovered a marvelous activity and some unspoiled mountain villages without motorized traffic. I've also had more time for vacation photography."

> —Fifty-nine-year-old woman with MCS
> for twelve years

> "If I had continued to have a comfy life, I don't know if I would have embarked on this path. My illness was something that

certainly pushed me in that direction—I was desperate for answers. Now I've learned so much about positive thought and God's love, etc. . . . this exploration of mine has not caused me to wake up one morning symptom-free, but it has given me the strength, grace, and tenacity to cope with all of it day by day."

—Twenty-four-year-old woman with
MCS for one year

Having a chronic illness can foster personal growth in ways that include everything from specific personality changes, such as becoming more assertive due to having to advocate for oneself, to life-transforming discoveries of spirituality. Common themes reported from respondents included appreciating who your real friends are, getting priorities straight, taking more time to live in the moment and savoring the "little things," valuing supportive family members, learning new skills that are MCS-compatible, and living a healthier lifestyle in general. "Living in the present" and "acceptance" were related themes that many respondents said they experienced. For example, one woman with MCS says:

"Perspective is really everything. You can still use time wisely in many ways: I have worked with acceptance of where this disease may lead, but refuse to wallow in worry and fear. Instead, I simply try to live each day so that I don't regret any aspect of it tomorrow. And, I try to keep things in perspective by asking myself 'If you knew you had two weeks or two months (etc.) to live, how much would this matter? What changes would you make and what things would you do that you've postponed?'"

Reconnected: Defining New Relationships

Most people went through some version of Goodheart and Lansing's (1997) disorganization and reorganization process of coping with MCS (see chapter eight), although some seemed to get stuck in the disorganization component. Many people, however, began to rebuild fulfilling connections with others who have and do not have MCS. Sometimes, support groups were the initial connections. Family members who at first had trouble understanding, sometimes came around and were supportive. Other times, people made new friends by getting involved with MCS activist work (see chapter fourteen).

One important element of growing, meeting your needs, making wise treatment decisions, etc. is finding your "pack" (Estes 1992). When Estes talks of "finding your pack" in her book, *Women Who Run with the Wolves*, she is referring to finding your rightful group of people with whom you can express your essential self. The isolation caused by breaking old, no longer healthy connections leads to the process of eventually finding where and with whom you do belong.

Fortunately, there are those who apparently have the sense to see you as deserving respect and affection (despite the fact that you're not quite what's expected). These people may be family, friends, or new acquaintances (with or without MCS) who have enough maturity not to write you off for having a disability that requires specific considerations. Many multiple chemical sensitivity activists, support group leaders, and members have formed healthy connections with others, both in and outside of the MCS community (see chapter fourteen).

Integrated: Feeling Like a Person Again

Through acceptance, support, patience, time, and (for some) spirituality, some people emerge through the maze of chemical injury with a sense of self—even a more expanded self—intact. For some it took a long time. For others, it occurred surprisingly quickly. People learned to construct a self and a life that included (perhaps was even driven by, but was not obliterated or smothered by) MCS. This process included learning new skills, healing, and understanding the early pain, accepting that you may not be a material success or that you may fall short of realizing the goals you established before you became ill.

Commonly, people developed great pride in their accomplishments, successful coping skills, ability to educate others, and the strength required to survive the trauma of a life-rearranging condition. In the early stages of MCS, people rarely predicted feeling this positive about such a debilitating disease. For example, one woman remembers a phone conversation she had when she first learned she had MCS. The woman with whom she was talking said to her with surprise, "Oh, you still want to get rid of this illness?" With some consternation, the respondent said, "Yes, of course, don't you?" To which the woman replied, "Oh, no. I wouldn't trade everything this illness has taught me," and proceeded to list the high points of having MCS. It would be eleven years before the receiver of this message would be able to see things in a similar light.

Many people described their lives as "integrated," not only *despite* having MCS, but commonly *because* they have MCS. For example, one woman who has MCS says, "I have been physically damaged, but I have rebuilt myself as a result. I am more conscious [of] what I eat/drink, and how the body is a wonderful entity." Other individuals agree:

> "As a challenge MCS is hard to beat! I can't begin to list all the ways I've grown but here's a sample: Reconnect with the earth— air, water, animals, flowers, and beauty. Tremendous deepening of faith and learning to deeply value all aspects of my life. Learning to

release fears of loss, death. Dismantled (more or less) type A behavior. Learned to live in today. To set boundaries and deprogram codependency (you can't mind other's business on a teaspoon of energy). Made some wonderful friends in other MCS folks. Learned to feel my feelings and to love myself as I am rather than for what I do (former workaholic). The suffering has been mind-boggling, but the learning has been miraculous. A much healthier and real relationship with spouse and children and friends. 'Tis a gift to be simple.'"

—A woman with MCS for many years

One woman made MCS sound like something everyone should want to have as she itemized her MCS-induced areas of personal growth:

"Tremendous spiritual growth, self-awareness, more of an ability to love and take care of myself. The ability to listen to my body, intuition and higher self. The realization that doctors don't have all the answers and that I am my best source when questioning a decision or treatment. Seeing that everyone has some kind of challenge to work through, be it physical, emotional, mental, or spiritual. Choosing my friends more wisely and dealing with family and people in general in a new and different light. Learned about higher purpose and serving humanity and the planet."

—Thirty-six-year-old woman with MCS
for fifteen years

Coming to Terms with MCS

Much like other illnesses or losses, coming to terms with MCS can be a long process marked by stages of denial, anger and, finally, perhaps, at least partial acceptance. This long-term process is nicely illustrated by the experience of the following thirty-seven-year-old woman who has had MCS for twelve years. She says:

"My identity was totally lost at first. I used to tell people I had, after developing MCS, entered the twilight zone. Life was unreal all of a sudden and felt surreal. I was not able to do things that were normal, like wear my clothes (which had chemical detergents) or walk in a building (that was new or gas heated or just painted). The good news, though, is that now I realize I'm not the problem, the synthetic chemicals are. I'm just a product of nature in an over-industrialized man-made world. I'm not saying it's easy. I'm just saying I can see the problem and it makes sense to me that the human body can only withstand so much in this age of synthetics. Now, regarding my sense of self. I'm still working on that one. Talk about low self-esteem. At first, I felt like I was just existing and totally dependent on others for help.

"Fortunately, I have a family that supports me financially, which lots of people don't. But emotionally, I've had to learn how to deal with sitting around because I can't go places. Next, I have to deal with a parent who supports me financially, [and] though I'm so grateful, I feel like a burden. Then . . . I perceive others thinking what a burden I am, and so on. But over the years, I know deep down [that] those who know me realize I'm doing the best I can. I want to do for other people, but I'm so needy they still do for me. I hate it. Shall we go into the worthless feelings? It'll all lead into how I deal with this or try to express myself. Well, I've tried self-help groups and talking with people, and that helps a lot. But bottom line, I have to deal with *me*. I spend lots of time alone as I can't pick up and go places all day long like I used to. The only thing I know to do is try to get a grip on life by learning about spirituality. I liken MCS to someone who has hit a rock bottom in their life with an addiction. What's left at the bottom? To me, it's been the nudge that has pushed me to see life differently with a relationship between myself and a higher plane . . . which, in turn, redefines how I should see life, rather than the way I expected it [to be]. I'm working on this. I just keep my mind open to new ways of seeing life."

Enraptured: Connecting to My Spiritual Self

Some people went beyond forced growth or even acceptance/integration and described a spiritual connection that sustained them, and made MCS bearable. One forty-year-old-woman who has had severe MCS for ten years says, "The loneliness and despair that I felt when I was not in control of my body or environment has been replaced by an awareness that I can depend on God for help and can come through things." Others with MCS also describe how spirituality and/or religion has helped them to live more successfully:

"The most important thing I have found is being assured my God is always by my side. If I ever feel lonely, angry, etc., . . . I ask Him to rename it, He always responds. He is a constant companion to me and will be to anyone else. He has made my life so different and so much more pleasant. He has not removed my burden, but He has certainly helped me bear it."

—Sixty-nine-year-old woman with MCS
for seventeen years

"My most ingenious practice is not mine, but God's. He granted me a healing experience that began the healing process in my body. Without it, I would still be pretty much incapacitated. Even though I'm not completely well yet, I'm 100 percent improved over three years ago."

—Forty-one-year-old woman with MCS
since adolescence

"*Tremendous* personal growth! I have spent a great deal more time working on my inner self rather than my outer self. I have found a perseverance that I never realized that I had. My faith in God has become much stronger, and I've changed my lifestyle to involve myself in those things that I now feel are really important."

—Thirty-three-year-old woman with MCS
for one year

Most, but not necessarily all, of the people who made it to a place of self-forgiveness, thankfulness for good relationships, and a sense of new purpose wrote about a new spiritual life. They were not referring to a "God cured me and now I can use chemicals" mentality; they were writing of the humbling experience of surrendering to divine love and intervention that then initiates healing and growth. Respondents continuously described coping with the impossible—with divine support—through all of their difficulties, forgiving themselves and others, redefining their purpose and, in the end, being thankful for MCS because it put them on a path of personal growth.

For many, living with and coping with MCS required some form of faith. That is, MCS asks the impossible, and they need something extraordinary to support them in their healing. Many found this support through a spiritual commitment, which often took the sting out of their worst fears. After all, it has been said that even death no longer has power over you, if you have faith in a Higher Power. Coping with MCS is so difficult that prayer seemed to provide the daily guidance that people needed to face continuing daily challenges.

Many people mentioned prayer as their most important practice when facing MCS. But some of the emotional numbing that can occur in MCS can make building a spiritual connection even more difficult. Prayer, to be effective, requires an open spirit. Passionate emotion can help people open spiritually. You can take your emotional upsets, for example, and use them by praying passionately for help. Things don't have to be serene for you to open this door. If you are constricted in what you can feel, however, the challenge may be greater.

You may want to pursue inspirational reading from your own religious or philosophical perspective. There are some very helpful books from the Christian, Jewish, Eastern mystical, and many other traditions. (See Appendix C for further reading and resources.)

Where Does This Leave You?

Although this chapter addresses the pain of loss of self in MCS, I hope that it also offers encouragement with the knowledge that many people moved beyond their losses to rebuild themselves, despite tremendous obstacles. If your MCS is mild, then hopefully you will not experience the level of isolation and loss that some people have had to face. If you have a more serious problem, perhaps knowing that many with MCS have achieved tremendous growth in spite of their problems will provide you with some encouragement. You may want to assess where you are now in terms of your sense of identity. Ask yourself the following questions:

- What have you given up?

- What parts of your self are no longer expressed because of your losses?

- Have you experienced any personal growth despite the MCS?

- Do you feel totally confined or can you identify ways that you have actually grown from the experience?

- Would you want to give up everything you have learned since developing MCS?

- If you have grown, how can you continue to support that growth?

If you have not grown, can you do something to set yourself on a path of personal or spiritual growth.

There must be something you have developed as a result of having MCS that you may not have gained otherwise. Make a list of these variables. Ask yourself what skills you now have that you did not have before. Does anyone else need them? This woman found someone who did. She says, "I have become the PTA environmental health liaison at my daughter's school and that role has proved to be a tremendous help. It challenges me and I am constantly acquiring new information and networking with new contacts."

Most people with MCS eventually become tremendous resources. There is definitely someone who needs your unique knowledge. Make a list of ten people who you think may benefit from hearing what you know and see who is open to receiving it. Even if only one person listens, you will have educated someone. (See Appendix C for further reading.)

Sometimes accepting yourself just as you are is the first step toward change. For some reason, it seems that experiencing surrender is necessary before change can occur. That is, try to:

- Accept that you have MCS

- Accept that it may be lifelong

- Accept that there may be some reason that you just can't see for you having MCS

- Accept that whatever that reason is, it will be revealed to you

- Accept that you are still a worthwhile person even with MCS

Everyone lives in danger all of the time. Having a condition such as MCS just makes the danger more poignant and makes you more aware of it. Fully accepting this existential approach may lead you to a greater acceptance of the reality of death. Once that happens, there is nothing left to fear. You can begin to face your condition with true strength. One woman describes it like this:

"There was a long time when I was afraid that MCS was going to kill me. I worried and worried, convinced that even my friends with cancer felt better than I did, and that there must be some terrible thing in me that was really serious. I remember the day that I said, 'Well, then I will die.' It was total acceptance of that possibility. I see now that I needed to do that to take away some of the illness's power over me. It is fourteen years since then and I haven't died yet. In fact, I see that I have a contribution to make, and as long as I'm still kicking, I'm going to make it! As long as I am able, I'm going to say my piece."

—Forty-year-old woman with MCS for
more than twenty years

The sad fact is that not everyone makes it to a point of considering personal growth. Sadly, there are suicides in the MCS community. However, some of those who have been close to suicide have eventually turned their situations around such that they are no longer in despair. There is no simple formula for getting to the point of acceptance. At minimum, it requires enough physical improvement to at least be able to think straight and have some positive experiences. For each person, however, there is a way. Each person's way may differ, but all ways seem to share the components of surviving "trial by fire," enduring forced self-reliance, furthering education about toxins and health, and forging a spiritual connection.

Some people with MCS have managed to make tremendous contributions that help other people with the condition as well as the public in general. They are inspirations to others, and examples of what is possible even with a severely limiting disability.

For instance, Cindy Duehring (who unfortunately died in 1999) was a marvelous example of the kind of contribution that can be made, despite extensive MCS-caused limitations. She won the Right Livelihood award, known as the Alternative Nobel Prize, from the Swedish parliament for using her illness in the service of humankind. Hopefully, hearing the testimonies of individuals who have experienced personal growth will motivate you to use the next four chapters to help you move in a more positive direction.

Chapter Eleven

Mobilizing Social Support

A variety of chronic illnesses has been studied for the effects of social support—or the lack of it—on the patient. Low amounts of social support are directly linked to increased symptoms and higher death rates in the chronically ill, even after finances, health behaviors, physical activity, obesity, and preventive health care utilization have been taken into account. Greater amounts of social support are associated with improved cardiovascular, endocrine, and immune function (Uchino, Cacioppo, and Kiecolt-Glaser 1996) and strongly relate to psychological well-being. Interestingly, the amount of social support that people *perceive* they have may be more important than the support they actually receive (Barrera 1986). However, it is not known exactly how perceived support exerts this influence on health (Shumaker and Hill 1991; Thoits 1995).

Many studies show that patients with chronic illnesses have a difficult time maintaining social support. This may be due to the fact that pain, functional difficulties, and spending time in bed all limit social contact. Some researchers have explained the reduction in social support for the chronically ill with the "stigma hypothesis" (Peters-Golden 1982); others explain the lack of social support with the "social activity hypothesis" (Bloom and Kessler 1994). The stigma hypothesis holds that the healthy will avoid and stigmatize those with illnesses and disabilities. The social activity hypothesis holds that as illness progresses, people are less able to participate in social interactions.

In support of the stigma hypothesis, Peters-Golden (1982) found that women with breast cancer reported receiving inadequate support, particularly compared to the support that well people expected to receive if they became ill. Furthermore, a substantial number of Peters-Golden's healthy respondents said that they avoided people with cancer, and that they viewed people who discuss their illness as being maladjusted. Twelve years later, Bloom and Kessler (1994) concluded that the stigma no longer applied to breast cancer, but that people do lose social interaction opportunities as a result of both role change (with the ensuing loss of portions of identity) and reduced ability to participate.

Because of reduced energy, discretionary activities disappear as the ill person struggles with survival issues, such as work. Increased time must be spent resting to compensate for energy used in work or other necessary activities (known as "down time" to those with MCS), and the social activities that may provide supportive exchanges cannot occur.

> "Most of all I miss the ability to give to others. . . . I want to talk to these people about something other than my problems and my illnesses, but it is very difficult. All of my time and all of my energy seem to be consumed with coping with my circumstances. There is little energy to be involved in other activities that are not related to my health problems and that could be shared with non-MCS people."
>
> —Forty-one-year-old woman with MCS
> for six years

In the case of MCS, both stigma and restraints on social activity seem to operate to limit opportunities for social support. People with chemical sensitivity may be at risk for problematic interactions with others due both to their requests for chemical-free environments and the poorly understood nature of MCS. If healthy people are likely to stigmatize people with physical conditions, such as cancer, they are even more likely to avoid those with a condition that is often seen as psychological. Thus, people with MCS may be avoided or become the targets of negative attitudes from others. Furthermore, social activity itself is diminished by the need to avoid chemical exposures, thus reducing the person's opportunity for social interaction.

Levels and Sources of Social Support

In Phase I of my study, I used the Personal Resource Questionnaire 85 (PRQ85) (Weinert 1987) to ask people with MCS about their level of perceived support, their support needs, and to whom they turn to for meeting these needs. (See Appendix A for more details.) Perceived support is the support someone believes would be forthcoming if needed. Received support is the support that one actually has received.

Perceived Support

Gender, health status, and fatigue strongly influenced people's perceived levels of social support. For example, according to respondents in Phase I of my study, women perceived higher levels of social support than did men. Also, if a person's health improved, they perceived higher levels of support than if their health condition worsened. People who were fatigued perceived lower levels of social support. Severity and length of illness did not affect perceived levels of social support.

Receiving Support

People with MCS receive support from various sources, including support groups, partner relationships, family members, friends, professionals, spiritual advisors, and neighbors.

Support Groups

A little more than half of the Phase I participants (53 percent of women and 63 percent of men) had some contact with a support group on a weekly (22 percent) or monthly (15 percent) basis. Unfortunately, the difficulties associated with accessing chemically unsafe public and private buildings limited many respondents to phone contact with other support group members. Interestingly, I found that having contact with a support group did not affect a person's perceived level of social support. Those with high levels of contact (monthly or greater) had a tendency to perceive higher support, but the effect was not strong enough to be called "significant." Similarly, severity of condition was weakly associated with high support group contact.

Partner Relationships

Other support available to Phase I participants occurred in partner relationships. Sixty-one percent of the participants said that they were in romantic relationships and had higher perceived support than those not in relationships. People who rated their partners as being very supportive perceived higher levels of social support than did those who rated their partners as being less supportive. About half of participants said their partners were very supportive, one-third said somewhat supportive.

Just over three-quarters of those in romantic relationships said that their partners believed "fairly strongly" or "very strongly" that chemicals caused their symptoms. However, some reported that their partners believed "not at all" (3.4 percent), "very little" (2.9 percent), or "somewhat" (16.4 percent) that their illness was caused by chemicals.

Thirty-one percent of participants experienced a romantic breakup since becoming chemically injured. Almost three-quarters of these people believed that their illness contributed to ending their relationships. Only 26 percent said that the illness contributed "not at all" or "very little" to the breakup. This is not so different from what Alison Johnson (1996) found when she asked 243 people with MCS: "Has your condition been a significant factor in a divorce?" Only 15.2 percent said yes, 68.3 percent said no, and 16.5 percent were unsure. Although the rumors are that most people with MCS are "abandoned," you can see from these two studies, this is not always the case.

People with MCS find it particularly stressful to be disbelieved when they assert that chemicals make them ill. Consequently, perceived social support scores are positively related to having a supportive partner who believes that chemicals are making the person with MCS ill. Not surprisingly, people who suffer romantic breakups after becoming sensitive to chemicals and who believe that MCS is the cause of the breakup report lower levels of support.

Family Members

Support from family members is crucial for people with any kind of illness or disability. For MCS patients, this support can mean the difference between successful coping and tremendous suffering. Many respondents who felt well-adjusted credited their families with providing the compassion and understanding that allowed them to maintain a high quality of life. Partners, in-laws, and children who accommodated to the MCS person's needs were literally lifesavers.

Many people with MCS, however, felt painfully isolated from families, especially in instances where family members were asked to be chemical-free. Many Phase II respondents did not receive positive support from their family members. Unsupportive behaviors included:

- Refusing to understand the nature of MCS sensitivities

- Wearing perfume

- Disbelieving that MCS was a true physical illness

- Refusing to discuss the chemical sensitivity

- Excluding the respondent from family get-togethers

- Calling the respondent a malingerer or a hypochondriac

- Being verbally abusive

- Refusing to visit

- Making the respondent the target of humor

- Cutting off communications entirely

- Deliberately exposing the respondent to chemicals

Although these are some very abusive behaviors on the part of families, more prevalent were testimonies of loving support from spouses, immediate family, and a few close friends:

"I have my own pulma-aid machine that makes breathing easier. Otherwise, [I rely on] the moral support of my husband, family, and friends. They don't laugh at me and are very understanding. They bathe special for me and visit a lot. We have all adjusted to socializing at our house. We have weekly to bimonthly dinners, [play] card games or watch videos. When you aren't isolated from life, it really helps.

—Thirty-eight-year old woman with MCS
for fifteen years

Loving family support was even able to help some people move beyond merely coping with MCS. Some individuals used the support of their family to help them be role models for how best to live with a chronic illness, such as MCS:

"I want to help other persons who have not had the good fortune to have a loving wonderful husband who sticks by you through thick and thin [and] wonderful children who know their mother isn't crazy. I've learned to put people and things in perspective by learning to say 'That's their problem if they don't understand.'"

—Fifty-nine-year-old woman with MCS
since childhood

Sexual Relationships

Sexuality is a concern for many people who have lost their sexual vibrancy. Nothing has been written about this in the medical literature, but many people with MCS report sexual problems:

"For me the greatest loss is the ability to share affection with my wife.... I am impotent and can't even have relationships with [members of the] opposite sex. Of course, my sense of self is compromised. [I'm] not sure, [but] I may kill myself eventually. I have

noticed though, that I am able to express and develop my spirituality since I have been unable to work and socialize.

> —Fifty-year-old man with MCS for
> twenty-three years

One woman responded to the question, "Is there any goal or activity
you have wanted to pursue but haven't been able to pursue?" with "A full
and rich sex life with my husband, like before I felt so sick."

In Phase I of my study, respondents answered these questions about
sexuality from the Psychosocial Adjustment to Illness Scale (Derogatis 1986).
Here are the percentages of people who reported particular sexual problems:

Problems in a general relationship as a result of illness:

No change in our relationship.	30.8%
A little less close since my illness.	15.1%
Definitely less close since my illness.	7.9%
Serious problems or a break in our relationship since my illness.	19.3%
Did not answer question.	26.9%

Loss of interest in sexual activities as a result of illness:

Absolutely no sexual interest since illness.	8.9%
Marked loss of sexual interest.	35.7%
Slight loss of sexual interest.	22.0%
No loss of sexual interest.	18.7%
Did not answer question.	14.8%

Decrease in the frequency of sexual activities as a result of illness:

No decrease in sexual activities.	10.2%
Slight decrease in sexual activities.	20.0%
Marked decrease in sexual activities	33.4%
Sexual activities have stopped.	19.0%
Did not answer question.	17.4%

Change in the pleasure or satisfaction from sex:

Sexual pleasure and satisfaction have stopped.	10.2%

Marked loss of sexual pleasure or satisfaction.   21.0%

Slight loss of sexual pleasure or satisfaction   23.0%

No change in sexual satisfaction.   24.9%

Did not answer question.   21.0%

Interference in the person's ability to perform sexual activities even though still interested in sex:

No change in ability to have sex.   33.4%

Slight problems with sexual performance.   28.5%

Constant sexual performance problems.   11.8%

Totally unable to perform sexually.   5.2%

Did not answer question.   21.0%

Intefererence with sexual relationship causes arguments:

Constant arguments.   3.0%

Frequent arguments.   8.2%

Some arguments.   24.3%

No arguments.   35.7%

Did not answer question.   28.9%

You can see that for some people, sexual and intimate relationships were affected, but that the experience was by no means universal. Sexual functioning is difficult when you are feeling unwell and when stressors have mounted. In addition, we know very little about any endocrinological factors involved in sexual functioning for those with MCS because the area has not been studied.

Dating

Chemically sensitive people without spouses sometimes attempt dating, but describe obstacles that frequently prevent an intimate relationship from getting off the ground. Some people refuse offers because they feel it is unfair to the potential dating partner to even attempt a relationship. Others tried and failed because there was so little they could do together.

"I would like to be in an intimate relationship. I recently started dating, but it is very difficult because of my reactions when I'm out.

I want to so much, but don't also have the energy. Most people want to date healthy people.

> —Thirty-eight-year-old woman with MCS
> for fifteen years

It is true that MCS is not exactly conducive to personal ads. Consider this imaginary ad. Who do you think would respond to it?

> Woman with chronic illness who cannot go to restaurants, theaters, movies, parties, or any public building that has been sprayed for insects or where others are wearing fragrance is seeking potential dating partner who does not smell for chemical-free outings and to share boring food. Sex for me is a thing of the past, and I'm often in pain. I can't use makeup or get my hair done, but I'm beautiful on the inside.

Or this one:

> Man who cannot work, but with good heart, seeks woman who does not wear fragrances, or dry-cleaned or fabric-softened clothes. Must be content not to go out much in public including restaurants, theater, or parties. I'm on social security. House attractively lined with aluminum foil to seal out chemicals.

There is also the possibility that you will find a person who doesn't mind dating someone who is ill, but whose motivations may not be the most loving or healthy:

> "[It's] very hard to attract a 'healthy mentally' man to me. Most men who would be interested in me have some kind of mental health problem, i.e., too co-dependent on my being sick so they feel needed!

> —Thirty-five-year-old woman with MCS
> for three years

By now, you've got the idea that dating is extremely difficult for those with MCS. Surprisingly, however, some people not only dated, but also found meaningful relationships. Some even married in spite of having MCS.

Parenting

Because parenting is such a consuming responsibility, it can be extremely difficult to perform when you have MCS. Multiple chemical sensitivity demands so much coping energy and rearranges your life without your consent. For some people, the constraints of MCS prevent them from ever becoming parents.

"The effects of the chemicals on my body left me so exhausted, I was experiencing so much confusion and difficulty making decisions, I couldn't imagine the complexity of the addition of a child."

—Woman with MCS for six years

If this were the case in any other illness, there would be many books written about it by now. Motherhood is such a mandate in our culture that large numbers of women deciding not to have children for health reasons should draw a lot of attention. But it doesn't. Even the feminist journal in which I published my article "Multiple Chemical Sensitivity/Environmental Illness, and Life Disruption" suggested that the part about not having children be cut.

Unfortunately, MCS prevents some who do have children from being all they want to be in those relationships. Parents with MCS may not be able to attend school conferences, sporting events, plays, and other activities that involve their children. In some cases, the difficult symptoms and mood changes further interfere with parenting responsibilities. One woman with MCS said, "Over twelve years of constant headaches three or four days a week [that were] severe enough for vomiting left me a poorer mom than I would like to have been. Also the irritability was (and is) at times a problem. However, my children always knew they were loved, and [they] have good self-images."

Successful Strategies

An illness in a family member is a call to responsibility. In MCS, the illness usually precedes any knowledge about the condition. That is, you may feel sick before you have any idea what is causing your illness. You may almost feel caught in a time warp and will understandably turn to significant others for self-validation. It is crucial that they be there for you. Goodheart and Lansing (1997) say:

> Patients' negative internal messages go hand in hand with the messages from the outside world. The responses of other people have an extraordinary impact at this vulnerable psychological crossroads in their inner life experience. Patients' losses are growing. They face the internal loss of a familiar sense of self, function, and identity, and they may be faced with the external loss of support or contact with important other people at work, in the social milieu, or even among family members (p. 38).

Family members have a responsibility to one another, and just as you would be expected to support a family member who developed cancer, your loved ones need to support you in this "invisible illness." In some sense, family members need to hear that "not believing" in MCS is no excuse. That is, wedding vows do not include the caveat "unless she gets MCS." Relationships that are already strained or of poor quality will be hit the hardest when MCS is present, and they are likely to disintegrate under the pressure. If your relationship has an Achilles heel, MCS will find it.

On the other hand, I have never been told by anyone with MCS that their previously supportive and kindly spouse suddenly became abusive because they developed MCS. Usually, if a spouse becomes abusive or a relationship becomes unhealthy, there were indications of it before the MCS developed. For instance, when I ask what the relationship was like before, I often hear something like, "Well, he did drink."

At some point you may have to decide that an abusive relationship is not worth it. Although it can be terrifying to go it alone when you are so vulnerable and needing help, some people's behavior can be more harmful than helpful. One woman, for instance, who has had MCS for five years, says her husband "unjustifiably calls me names, ignores me, orders me to not talk (anytime), [and offers] no affection, no sympathy, no help."

Dealing with Friends and Children

Many people in my study talked of the difficulty of having their children's friends be fragrance-free. Some adolescents even stopped inviting people to their homes as they were embarrassed by their parents' demands. I think this is copping out. The chemical-free atmosphere of the home must be preserved for the safety of the MCS parent, just as wheel-chair ramps are required when a family member is in a wheelchair.

It takes a lot of effort to educate and "clean up" a friend for visiting, but it is worth it. You can make little kits of safe soap, shampoo, and conditioner for friends' use when they visit. Discourage their use of chemical fabric softeners (there are safer ones now) and mothballs. Perhaps they can keep a change of clothes in a plastic bag to use when they visit you. Once someone is educated, then you can go on to other things, such as having real interactions. People need to be educated and to know that simple things like fabric softener are so impregnated with toxins that they make a large number of people sick.

It is not acceptable for adolescents to give up on parents with MCS any more than it would be to give up on a parent with any other type of physical challenge. You are still the parent in your household, and as such, should hold some authority. Family systems should not become so skewed and out of balance that the parents no longer have their children's respect.

You may feel that you are an inadequate parent because of your inability to attend your child's school events and other functions. However, you can still be a parent where it counts. Even if you don't attend every activity, you can listen, care, advise, and support your children. Parents with disabilities can be respectable, nurturing, and available, and it is up to you and your spouse or partner (if you have one) to arrange life in your family so that this occurs.

There are many things that you can do as a family. Learn to be creative in your planning. Maybe instead of going to a street fair and breathing perfume and propane, you can go on a picnic and eat organic food and take a small walk. With planning and adjusting you can still share some activities. If you can be relieved of some of the activities that make you ill or exhausted, you may have more energy left for more important and meaningful parenting tasks. When grown, your child will not remember every PTA meeting that you missed, but rather the overall picture that is largely composed of the quality of the relationship you provided.

Quality relationships preserve appropriate parental authority. When family therapists look at families in distress, they look at power, boundaries, communication, and roles. All of these are relevant to the MCS family. Parents should always have sufficient authority in the family to effect change, and provide a safe and loving environment for their children. If a parent has become disrespected and disempowered by the family, then that power needs to be restored to that parent. The inability to breathe perfume is not a character flaw and should not set you up to be the family scapegoat. Do not accept this reassignment of authority.

Furthermore, boundaries between people in healthy families should be strong enough so that each person has his or her own identity and room to grow. However, boundaries should not be so rigid that people can't communicate and share. If the boundaries are too rigid, there is no intimacy. If the boundaries are too permeable, then the family is said to be enmeshed. An enmeshed family blurs the identities of its members and does not allow each person an adequate amount of personal space or privacy.

Do you think that MCS has affected the boundaries in your family? For example, children do not belong in the parents' discussions about experiences of sex or conflict. With an ill parent, this boundary may tend to dissolve while the children are taking care of the parent, or the well spouse or partner comes to rely more on the children. For healthy family functioning, however, the couple's relationship should be preserved complete with an appropriate parental boundary.

Roles also are an important piece of a family's identity. Has MCS changed the roles in your family? Some practical aspects of the parental role are bound to change when you have limitations, but the cognitive (mental) aspects of the parenting role should be maintained. Who plays what role in the family? Initial therapy sessions with a family reveal so much about how members relate, such as who speaks for whom, who relates to whom, who gets listened to, and many other functions. Ideally, each person in the family is able to communicate directly with every other member without translation by a third member, each person is listened to, people speak for themselves, and no coalitions form that exclude any family members.

Recognize the Stress Family Members Face

Although healthy relationships do not usually suddenly disintegrate due to MCS, even healthy and supportive family members might experience extreme stress in response to the losses and demands of MCS. The losses inherent in the condition fall not only on the person with MCS, but on their significant others and children as well. Activities, finances, housing, future plans, and customary ways of spending time together are all disrupted. Even small things, such as decorating the home, can be sources of conflict in relationships:

> "In my case ... MCS can contribute a great deal of stress to [the] 'romantic' relationship, as you put it, especially if the two people are married or living together. It is a challenge to provide for one's physical needs as well as balancing the other person's need for freedom in using the house according to his needs and wishes (to feel it's his 'nest' too). A mattress, a piece of furniture, computer, synthesizer, or a redecorating or repair job may cause major problems. Objecting to what seems like a reasonable, mundane request leads to extra conflicts, extra negotiation unless both people are very mature and 'evolved.'"

> —Fifty-six-year old woman with MCS for
> six years

The well partner has the pressure of performing the duties that the other can't, as well as coping with reduced income, communicating with in-laws who may not understand, and having to care for the MCS person when they are debilitated. To make matters worse, the well partner has to "explain" repeatedly to others why the significant other can't fill up the car, drive to the mall, help out a neighbor, etc. The well partner's own interests and activities get put on hold, while trying to make things better for the MCS patient. But what happens when this task lasts fifteen years? Where is the personal development of the well partner? It seems that some are able to cope and grow in spite of the terrible stresses. In response to the question, "Have you experienced any personal growth as a result of having MCS?" one woman wrote:

> "No, but my husband has. He discovered he had the strength to stand by me and support me, even though doctors opposed my opinion of my illness. He would say, 'I know my wife, and she's the last person who would want to be sick, or who would fake illness.' I couldn't have asked for more constant support, even through some very rough times. We had plenty of ups and downs,

but he always came through for me. This in turn has deepened my love for him, and made us a stronger team."

—Sixty-year-old woman with MCS for four years

But the well partner should not be expected to put all personal aspirations on hold. Altschuler (1997) talks of the need to remain current with the needs of the well family members including adolescents and young children. Although time may feel as if it's "on hold" for the ill family member, others in the family are progressing through life's stages and have important needs that must be met. Taking some time to address this specifically instead of allowing all resources to be swallowed by crises would be helpful to all family members, and can be done in therapy or by the family independently. But it needs to be done.

Try Not to Let MCS Cut Off All Positive Activities

Your family probably used to have fun together and engage in outings before MCS threatened to limit all of your access to enjoyable leisure activities. There may still be some things that you can do with your significant others that you haven't tried. You can use the following exercise to create an Anti-Isolation Activity Grid to brainstorm activities to share with both family and friends.

Anti-Isolation Activity Grid

To begin you need an 8½ x 11 sheet of paper bisected in half with a vertical line. Then do the same with a horizontal line so that you have the paper divided into four quadrants. You will use this paper to make an activity grid. Have the vertical line measure how rewarding an activity is. The higher up on the line, the more rewarding the activity. The horizontal line measures how ill you get from activities with the farthest point on the right being the most ill. Now, write in activities according to how rewarding they are and how sick they make you. Think of potential activities as well as those you already engage in. Those that are fun, but make you very sick, should be in the top-right corner. Those that make you sick and are no fun in the bottom-right corner. The lower left will be for activities that are no fun but which do not make you sick (e.g., washing dishes). The corner you are interested in is the upper left, as the higher up the activity the more rewarding it is. The farther left on the paper, the less sick it makes you. There should be at least some activities listed there that you might be able to pursue. Try hard not to limit yourself to the lower-left quadrant.

Many people tell me that they go only to the health food store and to the doctor. This is sure to be a depressing existence. Is there anything in the upper-left quadrant that you can do that you haven't tried? Don't let yourself say that MCS has taken everything in the world away from you. When someone loses her or his sight, they gain a recognition and appreciation for other abilities and senses that previously were used in more limited ways. Find out what you still have that is unaffected and develop it. Think of any qualities that you still have that mean something to you and use them to enhance your life. Your activities in the upper-left quadrant should reflect the gifts you still have.

Use the grid to find activities to share with loved ones and friends. Have your significant other do the activity grid with the same two schema that you used. That is, the vertical axis is how rewarding an activity is to them. The horizontal axis will be how ill an activity makes you, the MCS partner. Then look at the grids together. Those activities that are in the upper-left quadrants of both should be the things you do together. Those in the partner's upper-right will be those that they do alone. These will be activities that are well liked by your partner, but make you ill. In the lower-right quadrant, place the activities that are not very rewarding to your partner, but which make you ill. Perhaps pumping gas and cutting the grass would go here. These are the activities that the partner may have to do for the household. If the partner truly hates one of these tasks, this may be a perfect chore for which to hire an adolescent neighbor. Some of the activities in the lower-left grids of both people (unenjoyable to both spouses, but don't make anyone ill) might have to be picked up by you to avoid overwhelming the well partner.

Friends

Many people say they find out who their "real friends" are when they develop MCS. As some old friends fall away, others help and becme closer. In addition, people meet new people with MCS who often become close friends and confidants, even if only in phone relationships. You may have to accept that you are not able to have the quantity of relationships and activities that you had before having MCS. But this doesn't mean that you have to do without all quality relationships. It does mean that maintaining your relationships may be trickier and require some creative work on your part. Some of the following suggestions may help.

Be Clear in Stating Your Needs

It is hard to overestimate the importance of being clear and direct in regard to your needs. One respondent visited her in-laws' home, arriving

Anti-Isolation Activity Grid Example

HIGHLY REWARDING

animals

street fairs

writing   reading

bookstore   hiking

coffee house

gardening   work

travel

music

theater

DO NOT GET SICK   GET VERY SICK

movies

housecleaning

pumping gas

NOT REWARDING AT ALL

only to find windows open with pollution entering from other homes, scented candles burning, and heavily perfumed guests. Now she will not go back to this home. To avoid similar situations, your needs can be spelled out ahead of time by asking lots of questions and making statements about what you can and cannot tolerate: "Will windows be open? Will guests be wearing perfume? I cannot attend if they do. I am also sensitive to scented candles, animals, etc." You will have to spell out every detail, as people are generally uninformed about their environment. One woman began volunteering at the animal shelter walking dogs, after explaining that she would not be able to walk any dog that had been recently bathed or sprayed for fleas. When she saw a commercial product in the kitchen and asked about its use, she was told that they were using it to kill their weeds, but not to worry because "that's an herbicide, not a pesticide."

Similarly, it is best not to wait until a crisis is present to communicate your needs. As this woman found out, in crises, without prior preparation, people naturally expect you to pitch in as they do:

> "I was seen as lazy and irresponsible in a family crisis when my mother got sick. Agreed, I hadn't told my family much about my condition beforehand, but that was because when I broached the subject I got negative responses. (At that time I didn't know as much about it as well.) If I had it to do over, I would have forged ahead earlier, and not waited for a family crisis to bring it out into the open."
>
> —Fifty-six-year-old woman with MCS for six years

Everyone has their own idea of what a friend is. Having MCS may limit your being able to qualify as a friend in someone else's estimation. One woman, when going through an extremely difficult time following pesticide poisoning, was missing many get-togethers with her work friends. One such friend informed her that if she wasn't there, those friendships could disappear. There was no understanding on this person's part that the woman with MCS was virtually unable to go anywhere beyond work. However, this same person also has fragrance-free parties to allow the woman with MCS to attend. It also did not occur to members of this group to visit her at her home or ask if she needed help. Their definition of a friend was someone who came to the get-togethers. Yet these people respected the needs of the others in the group when they had traditional health problems such as minor surgeries, etc. People may have only pockets of awareness regarding MCS, as it is very difficult to conceptualize MCS when you don't have it. The same person who informed this woman that she could lose her relationships, often thought of her when she was on vacation. The person would think, "My friend with MCS couldn't even safely come here." That was one of her pieces of being aware of MCS.

Heroic Efforts May Be Needed

Some respondents reported going to extreme efforts to ensure social interactions. One person described creating a new "family" outside of biological relatives. One woman who had an extremely positive attitude in spite of severe limitations—she had lived in her horse trailer for a year—only felt safe socializing outdoors and so organized trail rides in the mountains. This woman overcame her limitations and maintained a social group through some creative planning. Her life has gradually improved ever since.

There must be something that you can do, even if it is only to walk in the park (beware of pesticides), meet at your home with a book group, walk dogs, or play cards. Finding that something may be difficult, and there may be periods when every outlet seems to disappear. But creative individuals with MCS have written newsletters, had phone pals, educated the community, and otherwise found outlets. Although the job of connecting with other people is made more difficult by being unable to work, it is also true that you have more time. A little of this time can be spent figuring out possibilities for social interactions.

Is there anything in the upper-left quadrant of your activity grid that could include other people if you organized it? Do you have a friend with whom you could walk in the park, plant a garden, start a book club, etc.? (How about planting a woman's mid-life garden with organic herbs that help with menopause?) Find something that you can do that can be shared and find others who would enjoy it too.

You Have the Right to Be Treated Respectfully

Even if people don't understand your condition, this does not give them the right to mistreat you. After all, even if MCS were a psychological ailment (which it is not), you still do not deserve to be abused for having it. Unfortunately, you will receive your share of mistreatment due to ignorance and misunderstanding. No one escapes this.

While reading Jack Berkson's *A Canary's Tale* (1996) about his bout with MCS, I started to think, "Well he is being treated okay so far. Perhaps it is because he is a known and respected ex-state legislator and an attorney. He also is a man and may command more respect from those who have sexist ideas about women." But then Jack had to go to the hospital and was harassed miserably by an aide wearing aftershave. Even Jack couldn't escape abuse from ignorant health care workers. (By the way, this is a very serious, yet funny book about one man's coping with MCS.)

Some friends will support you during bad times. Find them and accept their help. Your worth is not determined by the opinions of abusive others. The more sensitive you are to others' opinions, the more difficult it will be for you. But, as this woman pointed out, some people will criticize you regardless of what the issue is.

> "I haven't changed. Though what I can do for others has changed. I did go through a period of hurt and [wondered] why when many of my longtime friends dropped me. I have found new friends and people who respect me much more. I have found that having MCS and my struggle for survival has earned me that respect and compassion from others.... I have also found a small percentage of people who will criticize you, but if it isn't MCS it would be something else."
>
> —Sixty-nine-year-old woman with MCS
> for seventeen years

Try to Be Happy for Those Who Have "Normal" Lives

It's hard to listen to accounts of parties, vacations, and other outings and experiences of those who have what we call "normal" lives. Hearing of other people enjoying what you have lost may inspire envy, sadness, longing, depression, or even resentment. You will probably need to learn how to avoid allowing negative emotions to take over every time someone describes having a nice time out in the world. Your negative responses probably will improve as you find better ways of being active in ways that mean something to you. Others may not spend their energies the way you would, and they may not recycle everything they use, but then neither did you before you got MCS. They haven't had MCS as a teacher, and are doing the best they can. (They might even learn something from you in regard to health and environment in the long haul.) To be a friend to them, however, you must be able to be happy for their ability to enjoy their lives and communicate this to them. Becoming consumed by resentment will only make everything more painful and cause you to feel more isolated.

Determine Who You Can Educate

Just because some people don't understand MCS doesn't mean that they can't. You might want to consider who might come around with a well-thought-out explanation. You can make a list with three columns. In one column place those who are already allies. In column two list people who, with some explanation, might come to understand better. Column three is for those who will never get it, no matter what. Scratch them off of your list. What kind of relationship can you have with someone who will not give you even the basic respect of believing you? On the other hand, those in column two might be worth communicating with. If you can't meet with them in person, you could try writing a letter to them:

> "At first, I felt terribly misunderstood by my in-laws. I've spent some time working on this—looking at my own perceptions, etc. I wrote letters to better inform them of my situation and I feel much better now about the whole thing.
>
> —Twenty-four-year-old woman with
MCS married one year

If people don't come around even with much effort on your part, you will at least have the satisfaction of knowing that you tried. Move them to the third column, scratch them off your list and move on with your life.

> "I'm learning to put my health first. If I don't regain that, I have nothing. I'm less concerned about what others think. If they think I'm crazy, I don't waste time with them. Convincing some people about chemical allergies is like challenging them about politics. I've lost a few 'friends' but now know who the real friends are."
>
> —Sixty-one-year-old woman with MCS
for six years

Even if you are unable to reach an understanding with someone in the present, this does not mean that they will not understand at a later point. Even years later is better than never. You may be helpful in initiating a process that eventually raises someone's awareness to where they truly understand what MCS means for those who experience it.

Plug into MCS Support Groups

Others with MCS are often the best sources of information for people newly adjusting to living with sensitivities, and you may want to join a local support group. There are a growing number of local support and advocacy groups for MCS, and joining one will allow you to meet others struggling with similar problems. If you are unaware of groups in your area, you can phone the national Human Ecology Action League (HEAL) in Atlanta to see if there is a HEAL group in your area (see Appendix D for information on organizations). Keep in mind, however, that it is HEAL's policy to focus on education/support rather than advocacy or political action.

Take note, there is some etiquette you should observe when approaching others with MCS. Remember these people, like yourself, are struggling. They have limited time, energy, and resources. Therefore you want to be careful to give and take, appreciate what is given, and take care not to depend on any one person for too much help. Also, it is important to understand that peoples' triggers differ and, in sharing support, what is helpful to you may actually make others ill. For example, an air purifier that is helpful to one person may trigger a reaction in someone else.

For Significant Others

This section is for loved ones, partners, and significant others who want to support a partner with MCS, but who recognize that it is no easy task. The following suggestions may offer you some help.

Find Out What Your Partner Really Needs

If you can talk frankly with your MCS partner about what they really need and what degree of independence can be retained, you may save yourself some effort and support your partner's functioning at the same time. For example, one woman's husband yells, "Handkerchief, handkerchief, really stinky!" at her every time they encounter smells (such as auto exhaust) out in public. This is her cue to breathe through several layers of her cotton handkerchief until the smell passes. His wife feels that it is no longer necessary for him to yell "handkerchief" because (a) she is able to tell for herself when there are noxious fumes, and (b) she holds her breath sometimes instead of whipping out a handkerchief because it is subtler, and (c) she is doing better, and is better able to tolerate mild exposures without becoming ill. It is irritating to have someone yelling "handkerchief" when you are doing fine, are in the middle of an activity (such as a conversation with someone else), and are already handling the problem anyway (by holding your breath). Of course, if she becomes ill from the exhaust, he has to suffer the consequences of her irritability, and this may be part of the motive (besides caring for her) for his unwelcome eruptions.

Because you do have to suffer the effects of any chemical-induced mood changes, or do have to do extra work when your loved one is ill, you probably don't relish the idea of leaving anything to chance. This is understandable. But there may be some areas in which your MCS-afflicted loved one can assume more responsibility, or where certain interventions are no longer necessary because circumstances have changed.

Be Assertive About Not Bringing Toxins into the House

In addition to removing any toxins from your home over which you have control, you will have to be assertive with any family or friends whom you invite to your home. It should go without saying that anyone who is going to "stop by" should be told that they cannot wear fragrances, etc., in your home. Forgetting to convey this information, or feeling discomfort about being clear about this, will cause illness in your partner and jeopardize their health. Therefore, if you have customers, clients, friends, family, or other folks coming to your home, it is imperative that they be informed about the necessity to be fragrance-free.

Offer Whatever Assistance You Can

You may have some skills that will help your loved one and yourself cope with a difficult situation. Gathering information is a primary task for the person coping with MCS. Can you find articles and resources that will help your loved one find medical care, safe products, and so forth? Legwork is another area in which you can help. Can you do the grocery shopping, gas up the car, run errands that are too toxic for your loved one? If there are children in your family, someone has to communicate with the schools, often in an environment that is intolerable for the person with MCS. Can you attend school activities and teacher conferences? If your loved one is limited regarding reading, can you gather important resources and read them, find a reading box, get books on tape, etc.?

Of course, the risk here is that the instrumental tasks can become overwhelming and take up all of your time. Organizational skills may become very important to cope with so many demands when you have limited time and energy. But there may be other people who can help as well. Do you have a friend who could help with shopping? Is someone good with resources? Try to enlist others' help, as it is good for them to learn about MCS, and you may be able to return the favors with resources you do have. For example, at some point you will probably know a lot about the pesticides your friends are using around their children, and you may be able to educate them as to the dangers.

Have a Way of Coping When Your Loved One Has a "Brain Reaction"

Neurotoxic reactions can be frustrating to both people in a relationship, and you will need a way to respond when you know that your partner or loved one is reacting. Unfortunately, saying something like, "You are just reacting now, so I won't take you seriously" probably won't cut it. It's a lot like being told, "You have PMS so anything you say this week will be disregarded." But you may be able to ask gently, "You seem extra upset, are you reacting?" People with MCS have to take responsibility for sorting out when they are reacting so as to minimize impacting others with their negativity. However, it is not always easy or even possible to know during the reaction that it has been chemically triggered (or incited by food). And once a negative irritable cycle begins, it is hard to break. So you may need an internal coping strategy of your own in order to get through.

Get Some External Support

It will be a long time before any good research is done on MCS caregivers, seeing that the scientific establishment can't even agree that MCS exists. The majority of research on caregiving has been done on Alzheimer's caregivers and this has highlighted the tremendous burnout that those who care for an ill loved one for an extended period of time can experience. Although MCS is different from Alzheimer's, (there are some similarities) the stress induced in the caregiver may be the same. You may need some external support from a clergy person, spiritual advisor, friend, counselor, or someone who understands something about MCS. Of course, this eliminates 90 percent or more of the population, but some people are teachable.

Recognize Your Own Losses

It is also important to recognize what you have lost as a result of your loved one having MCS. Possible losses for partners include financial security, mobility, social interactions, spare time, hobbies, lifestyles, and many others. Which losses are you mourning? Do you need some outside support for this, such as a counselor or friend? Which losses are no big deal? Are there any that you can do something about? For example, if you have a hobby that uses paints or solvents, do you have a little shed in which to work where the chemicals will not impact your loved one? (Of course, you may have to change your clothes before entering the house to avoid bringing chemical odors inside.)

Don't Let Go of Your Own Growth

You can't live completely for another person or give up everything because your partner is limited. If your partner were in a wheelchair, you would not stop walking. In the same vein, you might want to preserve for yourself some activities that your partner cannot do. You may have to shower, change clothes, or invoke other precautions so as not to contaminate your environment when you get home, but you need some outlet for yourself. This will not only support you, but also make you more interesting to others both in and out of the home. I would suggest trying to preserve some community involvement, friendships, and activities for yourself. This will help your loved one as well, for you may be a lifeline to the outside world, and your loved one may enjoy hearing about what you were able to do.

Stay Connected to Others

Staying connected is one of the toughest challenges for those with MCS and their families. There may be times when you really are too ill to have contact with people except on the phone (even if they are being supportive). It is important, however, to be vigilant and take advantage of opportunities for interacting with people for whom you care.

Chapter Twelve

Miscellaneous Pathways

You Are Never Really Stuck

There is always a way out of a maze, even if that maze is based on learning how to better cope with a chronic illness, such as MCS. This chapter offers a collection of techniques that may help you to improve your quality of life, take better care of yourself, enhance your self-esteem, and generally cope better.

Nurture Yourself

Any type of chronic health problem demands increased self-nurturing. With MCS, however, self-nurturing is even more important because the stresses are so pervasive and cumulative. Therefore, nurturing yourself is one of the best things you can learn to do to improve your health and well-being.

Following are some self-nurturing suggestions that may help you to live better with being chemically sensitive. Some of the suggestions come from my experience, some come from the experience of others with MCS, some from the work of Jennifer Louden (1992), and some suggestions come from other sources. My hope is that at least one suggestion will work for every reader—even if only in a small way.

Write New Scripts

Both men and women with MCS must write new scripts for themselves in terms of the roles that they are *expected* to play versus the roles that they actually are *able* to play. In our culture, gender roles especially can affect the healing process. Women, for instance, often are expected to give of themselves without concern for their own needs, i.e., parents, children, and partners come first. With MCS, this becomes impossible; you must give yourself permission to be a woman who uses her time and energy to meet her own needs. Likewise, cultural stereotypes demand that men be "breadwinners," physically strong, tolerant of chemical irritants, and never emotionally vulnerable. These stereotypes can negatively affect even healthy men; they also have been criticized for supporting violence, disallowing men's feelings, and emphasizing economic success over personal characteristics. Our Western models of masculinity have supported imperialism that to this day continues to steal land from Native Americans and others, a military industrial complex that has all but broken the global ecosystem, and a lack of tolerance for any other mode of being (e.g., non-industrialized societies are seen as "backward"). Multiple chemical sensitivity demands that you write new scripts for what is considered healthy male and female behaviors.

Make a Comfort Journal

Remember the appeal of coloring books, stickers, paste, scissors, and other little means to creativity? Louden (1992) suggests that you have "a safe place where you can doodle, compose, paste, and jot [i.e., write] anything that relates to your ideas of self-nurturing." This is not a journal about good art per se, but rather a place for you to express yourself and enjoy it. You can use whatever media are safe for you, including magazines, paints, string, yarn, pencil, leaves, anything.

Keep your journal near your bed or in another location where you can look at it easily at any time. Your journal should make you feel good. It is a good idea for it to be private, although you may wish at certain times to share it with others. I have a journal in which I draw images of what I want to come true. For example, I have drawn journals in which I want to publish future MCS articles, books that I want to write, and gardens that I want to grow. I have also drawn pictures of me eating dinner with people I want to get together with, animals I would like to have, and my dream farmhouse. In your comfort journal, you can draw pictures of yourself when you are healthier, make lists of items for events that you hope will come true, save mementos of activities in which you did participate, and more.

Comfort Box

Louden (1992) suggests keeping a special box filled with items that make you feel good. They can be visual (e.g., pictures), beautiful (e.g., crystals), humorous (e.g., gag gifts), cuddly (e.g., stuffed animals), or anything else you choose. When you need to rest and/or feel better, you can take out your comfort box and play with the items in it.

Reading Children's Books

Another suggestion of Louden's (1992) is to read children's books. She says that reading books written for children can provide comfort and a fresh perspective, and can recharge your imagination. You might want to get some old books from friends or from the library that have already been off-gassed. You can read them to yourself and look at the pictures for diversion and rest.

Positive Self-Attribute List

When you are feeling well, make a list of everything you love about yourself. Include everything of which you are proud, especially your positive character traits, such as caring, intelligent, sensitive, loving, enthusiastic, artistic, etc. Then, when you are feeling badly, read the list to remind yourself what a good person you are. Don't forget to remember that you were *thinking clearly* when you wrote the list.

Pleasure Program

Make a list of activities in which you can participate and would enjoy (Louden 1992). (You can use the upper-left corner of the anti-isolation activity grid from chapter eleven.) Take out your calendar (or make one) and actually schedule time for these activities so that there is at least one activity each day that you look forward to doing. Scheduled events can be as simple as taking a bath or as special as going on a favorite, safe outing. Other activities can include visiting friends, taking a walk, talking on the phone with a friend who makes you feel good, seeing a video, playing with your comfort box, expressing yourself in your journal, praying, and so forth.

Create a "Done" List

Louden (1992) suggests creating a "done" list just before you go to bed. That is, instead of flogging yourself about yet another day in which you didn't accomplish what you wanted, make a list of everything you did accomplish. You might be surprised by seeing and recognizing what you did do and be better able to appreciate yourself because of this. You should include every activity on your "done" list, such as "took all my supplements (all 102 of them!)", made dinner, read about reflexology, refrained from getting crabby after an exposure, planted one nice flower, made one phone call, etc.

Write a Letter to Yourself

When you are feeling well, write a letter to yourself that you will read while you are having a chemical reaction. It can include anything that will help you deal best and cope with an exposure, including soothing statements, encouragement, cautions regarding situations about which you want to be careful, and more. Keep the letter handy so that you can read it when you need to. Write a letter that is appropriate for you. Here is a sample letter:

Dear _____ (your name),

You've had a bad exposure. It's too bad and it's not fair, but it will wear off in _____ hours/days. Right now you need to know that you have to be good to yourself. The exposure will wear off. Get away from any further exposure even if you feel confused. Go straight home, take powdered vitamin C, and sit with your comfort box. Be extra careful driving, and warn family members that you may be a little irritable. Tomorrow you will feel better.

Use Affirmations to Change the Way You Think

Although affirmations are not an end-all cure, they can be used to restructure the way you talk to yourself which, in turn, influences how you think of yourself. Affirmations can be used in many ways. One is simply to write down positive sayings for and about yourself and display them in places where you will see them. Affirmations can relate to specific issues on which you are working, e.g., being nurturing, taking time for yourself, etc. You can open your cabinet and see a sign that says, "I am taking great care of myself and feel better because of it." Use affirmations to bring your thinking toward what you would like for yourself as well as to reinforce *how* you would like to think.

You can also use affirmations in a corrective manner. Be aware of what you say to yourself. For instance, do you ever say or think any of the following statements?

- I'm stupid.

- I'll never be better.

- MCS has taken everything.

- I'm ugly now.

- I have nothing to offer.

- I am useless now that I don't work.

- What good am I to my family?

If you find yourself making a negative statement such as those listed above, write it down in a notebook in the left hand of two columns. Directly across from the negative statement, write a more realistic and positive statement in the right column. For example, if you have written that you said, "I'm stupid," you might write in the right column, "I'm coping intelligently with a difficult situation." If you want to be more encouraging to yourself, you can say something like, "My own personal genius is becoming more apparent every day." (Stop laughing.) Another example would be to replace the negative statement, "MCS has taken everything," with a positive affirmation such as, "I still have the gifts of intellect, faith, love, and hope" (or some other appropriate statement that lists your particular gifts). You get the idea.

Keep your notebook with you and write down negative statements and their corrective positive affirmations. If you want to, you can wear a rubber band (if you're not allergic to the rubber) on your wrist and snap it every time you catch yourself saying (or thinking) a negative statement about yourself. The truth is, you know that these negative statements are not true. What *is* true is that although MCS can cause neurological damage, it sets your priorities straight, provides deeper understanding of environmental issues, creates empathy for others with chronic illnesses, and teaches you how to live more cleanly. Does this sound like stupid?

Reread the statements of people regarding their spirituality and identity in chapter ten. Does this sound like MCS has taken everything? Cindy Duehring won the Alternative Nobel Prize. Does this sound like she was useless because she didn't engage in traditional employment?

Be Your Own Perfect Loving Parent

There is nothing wrong with talking to yourself as you would like to be talked to. Your inner voice can sound like a loving parent that is encouraging, kind, and supportive. Try saying things to yourself such as, "Oh, honey, you got a lot done today. Pretty good for the obstacles you were faced with." Or, "You sure are working hard to make a contribution. How many people have a heart so big that they spend the little bit they have to contribute to the bigger picture?" Or, "Now take your vitamins. I know they're a pain, but you need them and deserve to have them." Clear enough, right?

At first, you might feel stupid talking to yourself in this way. If this becomes second nature to you, however, wouldn't you rather hear these types of comments than abusive statements that originate out of frustration? Sit down and write what you would like a loving person to say to you in your situation. Then, say it to yourself. Doesn't it feel better than saying, "I'm stupid"?

Other Cognitive Techniques for Coping

Here are other coping techniques that were suggested by participants from all phases of my research:

"I remind myself that tomorrow will not be the same as today. If I need to cry, I cry. If I need to sleep all day, I sleep. I do not worry if I cannot sleep at night. I get up and do something interesting and useful."

—Fifty-eight-year-old woman with MCS for thirteen years

"I have an informal routine that involves [doing activities in] five to ten minute increments. Energy allotment is the name of the game! It is precious and scarce, but it is a satisfying challenge to accomplish so much with that teaspoon of energy! If you saw my little garden you would not know it was a 'five minute a day' garden. Then, I do five minutes of housework, etc. I do a little bit of drawing, a bit of reading (depends on my brain function on any given day.) Cooking food always gets top priority. Next: Keeping clean. A phone call a day keeps the blues away, so that is next. . . . So, at the end of the day I've had a varied and satisfying day. These five minute increments are interspersed with rest periods. The first five minutes of the day is the most important, however. I always start the day with a positive, hopeful bit of reading (I make affirmation signs and put them all over the walls so it's easy to find inspiration at a glance) and a prayer for guidance ([I] . . . dump my complaints and worries on God first thing in the [morning] so I don't have to carry them around. That takes energy!)"

—Fifty-one-year-old woman with MCS since childhood

"I practice a viewpoint . . . that if I was completely without sensitivities it would be like having an inability to feel pain. I would be
around harmful substances all the time without being able to sense
it. (I know when to leave an area that's toxic because my hands—if
[I'm] touching it—feel "hot." My feet go numb and bluish). I hate
being sensitive, but I don't like pain either. For a lot of people,
[having this viewpoint] would be like being in hell and saying, 'At
least it's not cold here.' But, it works for me (sometimes)."

> —Forty-five-year-old woman with MCS
> for five years

"I make time to be sick. When I make plans to leave home, socialize, [go to] doctor's visits, drive, etc., I plan nothing for [the] following day or two. I allow myself 'down time.'"

> —Forty-six-year-old woman with MCS
> for twelve years

"Ingenious practice? A good sense of the absurdity of the human
condition and a friend who makes me laugh.

> —Forty-year-old woman with MCS for
> two years

Setting Limits, Saying "No"

Having MCS means that you can no longer do the number of things
you were once able to do. This means that you must prioritize. Be aware,
people will not stop asking you to do things that require your time and
energy just because you have MCS. (After all, most people don't even know
what MCS is.) Therefore, to survive, you will have to get good at saying
"No." If there's anything MCS will do for you, it will teach you to set priorities. Boring and obligatory activities seem all the more so when you are feeling badly; and you will reconsider exposing yourself to a bunch of junk just
so someone else can be satisfied.

At some point, you will have to learn to say "No" without worrying
about others' approval. Louden (1992) makes a good point about assertiveness. She says, don't bother looking to the other person to make it okay for
you to say "No." After all, they want you to say "Yes." Watch other assertive people and see how they say "No." They usually don't apologize, worry
about what others will think, or take time to wonder if they are being "fair."
If it doesn't feel right to them, they say "No." You can practice saying "No"
to one request a day. You can learn to say, "I'll think about it." Listen to
your body. If you are becoming tense as the person makes their request, it's
a pretty good indicator that you don't want to say "Yes."

Creating a Comfort Network

Louden (1992) offers the following activity as a way of clarifying—for yourself—who the supportive people in your life are and expanding your support system. There are eight steps to creating a comfort network.

1. *Determine who supports you.* First ask yourself the following questions to identify the strengths and weaknesses in your support system. (Feel free to adapt the questions to your situation.)

   • Name three people you get in touch with when you are feeling depressed.

   • Do these people usually make you feel better?

   • Who energizes you?

   • Whom do you like to play with?

   • Name two people you would contact in a crisis. Do you feel you could count on these people to be there for you no matter what, and that they would not make you feel guilty or needy? Would they bring you food if you were ill? Would you feel comfortable giving them your house key?

   • At work, who do you seek out when you need honest feedback? Do they help you? Can you trust them?

   • With whom would you like to discover new things? With whom would you enjoy traveling?

   • Is there someone with whom you can discuss spiritual ideas and concerns?

2. *Discern who is comforting and who is not.* Recognize people's strengths and ability when you call on them for support. One friend may be good at humor, but be unable to give comfort. It is important to call on the right people at the right times.

3. *Pick people you trust.* Discover what trust means to you. Write in your journal for fifteen minutes about the issue of trust. Then, assess whether the people you are close to embody the qualities of trust.

4. *Listen to your body.* How do you feel when you are around a friend? Ask yourself if you clench your jaw during phone conversations or breathe shallowly around certain people. If you feel nervous or fearful, or trapped or crazy around someone, this is good input for you in making decisions as to whom you should spend time with.

5. *Be sure your expectations are realistic.* Louden says, "If you feel abandoned and rejected by the people in your life, ask yourself if you are

expecting others to take on your feelings to cure you. Don't blame yourself, just check to see what your expectations are." With MCS, there is a chance that the desperate part of you wants more from others than you are aware of—or than people usually give one another. Knowing this can help.

6. *Strengthen your comfort network.* Once you are familiar with the information in the steps above, you can assess the weaknesses in your network and perhaps come up with some solutions for strengthening it. Do you need someone to listen, someone to laugh with, someone smart to talk to? Louden says to use every situation as a chance to make contact, including the neighborhood, the gym, work, etc. (You might have to settle for the health food store, the doctor's office, and the park.) She says to pick three people with whom you would like to strengthen your relationship and write down one step you could take to do so. With MCS, of course, this is all the harder, but it may not be impossible. Take one step today.

7. *Ask for friendship.* Louden suggests directly asking for friendship even though it is a risk. Avoid thinking that no one would want to spend time with you and risk saying something like, "I like you. I'd like to spend more time with you."

8. *Do not always unload on the same friend.* This is crucial in MCS. Although there is always something to complain about, you will have to think about how the other person feels when they hang up the phone or when they go home from seeing you. If you expect someone to always support you, then their needs are not being met. Caregivers get burned out. Louden suggests having a list of five people you can call when you need extra support. Start at the top and go as far down the list as you have to until you reach someone.

Animal Companions

Animals can put you in touch with the natural world. Although you may not be able to tolerate certain types of animal hair or fur, some people are connected to and feel better around animals. There may be a way you can spend time with animals or even have an animal companion. If not a dog or a cat, then perhaps a turtle or a fish. Or, maybe you can have a small and beautiful aquarium or terrarium with your own lizard friends.

If you can't have a pet, perhaps you can spend time with your neighbor's dog or cat. Or, if you live in the country, even a cow. (Cows are fascinating animals who get even less respect than people with MCS do.) Those of you who love animals might want to read some books by people who have special relationships or who have had healing experiences with animals. (See Appendix C for further reading.)

Gardening

Perhaps you can nurture some medicinal plants, grow your own organic produce, or tend to certain types of flowers that make you feel good. It is sad that chemicals are driving many people with MCS indoors and away from the natural landscape. Assess whether it is possible for you to have some tomato plants in pots on your sunny porch, or a small plot of organic flowers that will provide you with beauty, exercise, fresh air, and a connection with the land. If you can't have a plot, perhaps you can have one potted plant either indoors or outside. If you can tolerate it, something green and alive adds a vibrant, healthy energy to your life.

Learn to Sew with Organic Fabrics

There are many sources for organic cotton and hemp fabrics. If you are able to tolerate fabric, you might want to learn how to sew. You can make yourself some beautiful things to wear or to use in your home. (See Appendix C for product sources for organic sewing materials.)

Invent Something Needed by the MCS Community

You might have some idea for something that you can make and sell to others in the MCS community. Can you make useful masks, aprons, a new type of air purifier, or a safe skin lotion? Many people with MCS have started small home businesses and are providing others with needed services. Perhaps you can add your own invention to the list and sell it through MCS newsletters. Remember that many creative and enterprising people began simply. For example, the MCS-safe builder John Bower began by trying to make a safe home for his wife Lynn. Can you invent an MCS-safe product and sell it?

Improve Your Intellectual Knowledge

Is there some subject that you would like to study? Perhaps you are interested in history, the English classics, architecture, or botany. If you have time and are able to read, this may be a great opportunity to pursue leaning. (Think of all the people who have gotten college degrees while serving time in prison.) You may be able to read aired-out books, peruse the Web, or borrow resources at your local library.

Nurture Your Spirituality

Do you believe in the benefits of spirituality but have trouble making a real connection? There are countless inspirational books that can help you to nurture the spiritual aspect of yourself. Depending on your beliefs, you might refer to the Christian section, the New Age bookshelf, or the Eastern mystic readings at your local bookstore or library. Illness can be an impetus for further spiritual development. Many people who receive comfort and guidance from a spiritual source are adamant about it saving their lives and making their illnesses bearable. (See chapter ten for more on spirituality.)

Inspiring Reading

Although part of coping with MCS is acceptance, there also is always hope. There are quite a number of books written about people who found unexpected help—even miracles—in their darkest hours. These books provide inspiration, hope, and appreciation for the small miracles in your life. Perhaps some authors will help you to see your situation from a new vantage point. See Appendix C for a listing of books that offer positive, inspiring, and healing information, but do not resort to simplistic "think your way out of your problem" kinds of approaches.

Turn Avoidance Trips into Retreats

Many people with MCS must vacate their premises periodically to avoid chemical exposures from paving, pesticiding, construction, and other developments. In her book, *The Women's Retreat Book: A Guide to Restoring, Rediscovering, and Reawakening Your True Self—in a Moment, an Hour, a Day, or a Weekend,* Louden (1997) provides suggestions that will allow you to turn desperate escapes into nurturing retreats. Some of her strategies include bringing special items with you that feel comforting, seeing the getaway as a spiritual retreat, devising rituals to do when you are alone, and viewing the exposure as a message (rather than as a threat) that it is time for you to have a retreat.

PART IV

DISABILITY, POLITICS, AND ACTIVISM

Chapter Thirteen

Disability Issues

Workplace Accommodations and Applying for Disability Benefits

Facing the reality of not being able to continue working is painfully difficult. Consequently, some people who are very ill with MCS push themselves to continue working much longer than they should, and their bodies often pay the price in increased disability. On the other hand, many chemically sensitive people are forced out of jobs prematurely because of their employers' refusal to provide appropriate accommodations.

My own bias is that if there is any way of making your work environment safe, remaining in the workforce allows you to keep your income, benefits, work-related self-esteem, contacts with other people, and sense of being productive. Deciding whether you have the option of continuing to work may be easier if you understand something about the Americans with Disabilities Act (ADA).

The Americans with Disabilities Act

The employment provisions of the ADA apply to all employers with fifteen or more employees, including private employers; labor unions; government and nonprofit institutions, departments, and agencies; public transportation systems that receive federal financial assistance; and all public entities that provide public transportation.

Although you are not automatically covered by the ADA just by virtue of having MCS, you may be covered on an individual basis (as with other disabling conditions). To qualify individually, you must meet one of the three prongs of the definition of "handicap" as defined in both Section 504 of the 1973 Rehabilitation Act and the ADA. These prongs are:

1. Having a physical or mental impairment that substantially limits one or more of the major life activities

2. A record of such an impairment, or

3. Being regarded as having such an impairment (ADA 1990, Sec. 3).

Workplace Accommodations for MCS

Although employers sometimes argue that the accommodations required for MCS are so inclusive they are impossible to adhere to, this is usually not true. If you are fortunate enough to have your own individual workspace (office, classroom, etc.), you have many immediate opportunities to improve the quality of your work environment. You can use an air cleaner, specify less toxic cleaners, and reduce the amount of dust, fresh paper, smoke, and fragrance in your personal workspace. You can also request that no toxic paints, pesticides, or other chemicals be used in your individual office. You can unplug or turn off equipment and lighting that emit electric or magnetic fields if they trigger any symptoms. Changing airflow and heating is more difficult. If your workspace is taking in toxicants from other parts of the building, you may have to ask to relocate your office.

Accommodations may not be as easy to control if you share workspace or common areas with others. In this case, you will have to ask for help with some of the problematic exposures. Air fresheners, for instance, may add unwanted toxic fragrances to bathrooms, but it may not be too difficult to talk employers into using the new citrus-based fresheners once they see how effective they are. Simple baking soda and fragrance-free kitty litter, changed on a regular basis, will also absorb odors. If you want to use alternative air fresheners, you may have to buy the first container and ask your employer to order it from then on. The citrus-based products are sold at most health food stores. Some of the same companies make citrus-based cleaners. If you are sensitive to ammonia, chlorine, or solvent-based cleaners, you may be able to get your office cleaning staff to do a trial with these products or other safe cleaners (see Appendix B for product sources). With paints, you may have to ask for advance warning so you can prepare to be out of the office for a period of time after painting. Or, you can try and arrange that your office use totally safe paints. Milk paints are the least toxic, but hardest to work with, and they do not cover enamels well. It may be easier to convince employers to use some of the lower or no volatile organic compound (VOC) paints (see Appendix B for product sources). Regarding pesticides, you may be able to speak with the person who manages pest control and provide them with information on integrated pest management (IPM). This management system uses the least toxic solutions for bug problems, with toxic applications always used as the last line of defense. Specific suggestions for workplace accommodations are listed on page 234.

The Fragrance Problem

Fragrance on co-workers is a difficult issue. Some co-workers may not be sympathetic to your need for a fragrance-free space in which to work. The least threatening strategy for gaining some cooperation may be to have individual conversations with co-workers. Some people may understand right away when you explain that you become ill from fragrances. However, you must be very clear about what it does to you. Many people interpret a complaint about fragrance to mean that you simply find it irritating. Also, bear in mind that some people wear fragrances because they are attempting to cover up a medical condition, or what they perceive as their own body odor, and they will be uncomfortable disclosing this information. For example, co-workers with bowel or bladder control problems may feel that they are unable to stop wearing fragrance and may be ashamed to tell you why or to discuss alternatives. Explaining that it causes you debilitating symptoms may help. There are many studies that demonstrate the harmful effects of fragrance, and that show how many people in the population complain of illness caused by perfume. These studies, combined with clippings about some of the fragrance-free sites and activities now in place, may help to convince co-workers that your complaint is justified. The following may be helpful.

Studies that Find Fragrance Harmful

- Anderson and Anderson (1998) allowed groups of mice to breathe one of five commercial perfumes for one hour or "zero-grade medical air." Three of the perfumes caused airflow limitations suggestive of asthmatic-like constriction. All five perfumes caused signs of being toxic to the nerves or nervous tissue (i.e., neurotoxicity) that worsened with repeated exposures.

Effects of the perfume varied by dose and included changes in breathing patterns, and indications of neurotoxicity, including altered posture and gait, twitching and tremors, and exaggerated responses to stimuli. Some of the perfume-exposed mice developed limb paralysis and/or convulsions; some lapsed into coma; five mice died. None of the mice in the control group died. Furthermore, air tests found a large number of toxic chemicals in the perfumed air, including benzene-dicarboxylic acid.

- Lorig and Schwartz (1988) found that fragrance alters the human electroencephalogram (EEG) pattern, and that similar fragrances can have very different patterns. The effects from nose breathing were greater than those from mouth breathing. And, fragrance levels in room air were able to stimulate the nervous system, thus affecting EEG patterns, even when fragrance was not detectable through odor.

Fragrance-Free Organizations

- The University of Minnesota School of Social Work became fragrance-free in 1997. Both faculty and students who enter the building are asked to wear no fragrance.

- The National Women's Studies Association's annual meeting has been completely fragrance-free since 1997.

- The Association for Women in Psychology's annual meetings have been fragrance-free since 1997.

- The executive committee of Division 35 (Psychology of Women) of the American Psychological Association has had fragrance-free meetings since 1996.

How to Request Accommodations

To begin, you may decide to informally ask your immediate supervisor for the accommodations that you feel would help you to function safely and productively in the workplace. You can provide physicians' letters and explain your problem to the best of your ability. If your documentation can state that you are sensitive to—or become ill from—chemicals, and that it threatens your health to be exposed to them, this will be helpful. These letters should be tactful, tasteful, and not reveal too much personal information. You need to maintain your dignity at work. (For example, giving your employer a letter stating that you have toxic encephalopathy, which means brain damage, may not be exactly what you want your documentation to say.) The letter also should be tailored to you as an individual. Some physicians, for instance, use form letters that may request MCS office accommodations to include products that may be a problem for you (e.g., vinegar).

It is best to put your request in writing. Your employer is not required to provide any accommodations if you do not request them. If you encounter resistance to getting the accommodations that you need, you will need to speak with those who have more authority until you receive help. Depending on the structure of your workplace, you may save a lot of time and energy by speaking to someone with a lot of authority right at the start. At the least, you need to talk to someone who has enough authority to implement changes once convinced to do so.

You can also write a "Request for Reasonable Accommodation." This legal document states that you have a disability covered by ADA, and that: "In accordance with Title II of the Americans with Disabilities Act and section 504 of the Education Act, I am in need of the following accommodations for my disability in order to be safe working in . . ."

You can then list your needed accommodations. Be judicious, however, and ask only for what you really need so as not to be interpreted as asking for the impossible. Toni Temple (see activist profile in chapter fourteen) reminds people with MCS that it is important to be reasonable in requesting accommodations. Remember that employers are not required legally to make expensive renovations. An employer does not have to make an accommodation that imposes an "undue hardship" on the operation of the business. Undue hardship means "significant difficulty or expense" when taking into account (on a case-by-case basis) the structure and resources of the institution or workplace.

Although you may be unable to perform some minor functions of your job, you must be able to perform its "essential functions" to qualify for ADA accommodations. If you are a typist, for example, and sustain an injury that renders you unable to type at all, then you are unable to perform the essential function of your job and your employer does not need to modify your job for you. However, if you are unable to stand over the photocopy machine, and this is a minor part of your job, then your employer must accommodate your need.

Many MCS accommodations can be made easily and with little expense. Limiting smoke and perfume in the workplace is not costly or difficult. Using less toxic air fresheners or paints, likewise, is not cost-prohibitive. Providing an air cleaner for employees is also a reasonable strategy that is fairly easy to implement. The booklet *Multiple Chemical Sensitivities at Work: A Training Workbook for Working People* by the Labor Institute (1993) is a helpful workbook that details possible interventions for MCS. You can purchase it to give to your employer. Although some suggestions for accommodations are listed below, the booklet may lend credibility to your request.

Once you receive cooperation, looking ahead to prevent future mishaps is critical. If you know that some process, such as painting or spraying, is being considered, finding out when it will be done and what chemicals will be used may save you from another toxic insult.

Specific Workplace Accommodations That May Be Helpful in MCS

1. Work near a window that opens rather than in a sealed area of a building.

2. Reduce the fragrance that co-workers use if possible.

3. Eliminate the use of toxic pesticides and implement the substitution of less toxic alternatives, such as boric acid for ants and roaches.

4. Initiate flexible work hours that allow you to leave during highly toxic exposures, e.g., painting, and/or to work during off-hours to avoid photocopy and other office fumes, and rush hour traffic.

5. Receive notification of impending pesticiding, painting, and construction/repair that may generate fumes or cause other harmful effects.

6. Eliminate "air freshener" in bathrooms, install fans, open windows, or use nontoxic alternatives.

7. Relocate your work area to a safer part of the building.

8. Place an air cleaner in your work area.

9. Vent the photocopy machine appropriately.

10. Use less toxic cleaners and eliminate strong smelling ammonia, solvent, phenol, or chlorine-based solutions.

11. Delegate errands to toxic areas, photocopying, and other small nonessential tasks to an employee who does not have chemical sensitivities.

12. Minimize the amount of time spent under fluorescent lights or in the vicinity of any transformers, electric cable, computers, or other electromagnetic field sources that trigger symptoms.

Applying for Disability: Receiving Assistance When You Can No Longer Work

It is possible that regardless of how hard you attempt to "hang on," you may reach a point when you are no longer able to work. This may be temporary or permanent, but unless you are independently wealthy, you may find yourself in the position of having to apply for disability compensation. There are several types of disability compensation available, including private disability insurance (if you have a policy), the Social Security Administration's Disability Income and Supplementary Security Income, and workers' compensation.

Private Insurance

In addition to health insurance, many employers offer disability insurance for a modest fee. If you have the opportunity to purchase this insurance, it can be an excellent investment. Read the policy carefully to be sure that no conditions that resemble MCS are excluded. If the policy does not exclude MCS, purchase the highest level of coverage possible. Some policies allow you to choose a premium based on what portion of your current salary would be paid to you monthly should you become disabled.

Having disability insurance does not mean that the insurance company will not try to avoid payment. Private insurers have access to the same detractors who testify for employers against people applying for any other types of compensation for MCS. However, purchase of the insurance (along with excellent medical records and documentation of symptoms experienced at work) will lay the groundwork for future benefits should you ever become disabled. If your employer does not offer disability insurance, you may be able to purchase it privately.

Social Security Administration Benefits

The Social Security Administration (SSA) provides Social Security Disability Income (SSDI) for people who are disabled to the point of being unable to work. The two and a half million people who apply to the SSA each year for disability benefits must deal with the state agencies called Disability Determination Services (DDS). The DDS conducts disability determinations for the SSA. Disability Insurance (DI) and Supplemental Security Income (SSI) are the two major benefit programs for people with disabilities. These two programs define disability as "the inability to engage in any substantial gainful activity by reason of a severe physical or mental impairment that is medically determinable and is expected to last at least twelve months or result in death." Established in 1956 by Title II of the Social Security Act, SSDI provides monthly cash payments to severely disabled workers. Similarly, SSI, which was established by Title XVI in 1972, provides monthly cash payments to aged, blind, or disabled people whose financial resources are below a required threshold.

Qualifying for Benefits

You do not have to be completely and totally disabled to qualify for SSDI, only unable to engage in paid work. But apply as soon as possible after you become disabled. It takes at least sixty to ninety days to process your initial claim. The qualifying process involves filing an application and supporting documentation through a local field office that then forwards the materials to a state Disability Determination Services (DDS) office.

A DDS examiner then works with a medical or psychological consultant to study your documentation to make a determination. Additional data may be requested. (**Note:** At this level the applicant does not have any personal contact with any of these professionals.) If the application is denied, the applicant can ask DDS to reconsider. A new examiner/consultant team then reviews the application. If your application is denied a second time, the next step is an appeal to an Administrative Law Judge (ALJ) in the SSA Office of Hearings who will hold a hearing where the applicant can testify and present new evidence. If denied at this level, the applicant can appeal to SSA's Appeals Council and then bring suit in federal court.

The SSA is supposed to use the following five-step sequential evaluation process to determine whether an applicant qualifies for benefits:

1. Is the applicant engaging in substantial gainful activity? (The answer must be "no.")

2. Does the applicant have an impairment that has more than a minimal effect on the applicant's ability to perform basic work tasks? (The impairment must be expected to last twelve months or result in death.)

3. Does the applicant's impairment meet or equal the medical criteria for an impairment in SSA's listing of impairments? (This list includes over 150 categories presumed to meet the severity test. You can bet that MCS is not on it.) If the impairment is not listed or the condition does not match listed criteria, then it must be the "medical equivalent" of one of the listings. Criteria for mental impairments are more subjective and focus more on subjective evaluation of the person's functional limitations than those for physical impairments, which are supposed to be documented more by medical fact. (Some conditions, however, must be assessed by functional limitation, e.g., musculoskeletal conditions. But awards for musculoskeletal conditions are infrequent. MCS falls into the category of impairment that is difficult to document by medical fact, and therefore proving functional limitation is crucial.)

4. Comparing the applicant's Residual Functional Capacity (RFC) with the physical and mental demands of the applicant's past work, can

the applicant perform his or her past work? If medical evidence does not substantiate a condition of adequate severity in SSA listings, the adjudicator must determine what the applicant can still do in a work setting. The examiners must use "all relevant medical and nonmedical evidence," such as statements from others about the applicant's symptoms. If it is determined that the applicant can still perform past work, the claim is denied.

5. Can the applicant perform other work in the national economy? This is determined using the RFC, age, and educational and skill level of the applicant.

The application process is standard, but leaves room for complex decision making by the adjudicators. For example, if the person cannot be deemed disabled on the basis of medical evidence only, the adjudicator must then decide if the applicant can perform prior or other available work despite their condition. The SSA's medical vocational rules suggest that older, less educated, and less skilled people are more likely to be given benefits. (See discussion of this process later in this chapter under "Is the Application Process Fair?"

Workers' Compensation

Workers' compensation is a system of insurance to which employers contribute money to cover wages and financial damages for those injured on the job. In exchange, workers' compensation laws protect some employers from lawsuits by employees. Employees who are eligible for workers' compensation are not able to sue their employers for a greater benefit. However, they are able to sue other parties, such as architects, manufacturers, and building owners. In addition, there are some exceptions to employers' protection. If employers are also the building owners, they are not protected from lawsuits. If they intentionally expose workers to unsafe conditions (they do not have to have intended harm), or if the illness would not normally be expected as a result of that employment (e.g., toxic exposure is not expected in offices), then the employer is not protected from lawsuits. Your workplace has the forms you need to file for workers' compensation if you believe you were chemically injured on the job.

MCS and Disability Compensation

Dubin cites two legal cases where disability benefits were awarded for MCS and three cases where they were denied. Dubin cites *Slocum* v. *Califano* as one of the first cases in which disability under the Social Security Act was awarded for MCS. The plaintiff had to live an isolated chemical-free lifestyle and was debilitated for days following simple chemical exposures. In this case, benefits were awarded and were retroactive to the onset of the sensitivities some ten years earlier (Dubin 1994). In *Kouril* v. *Bowen*, a woman was granted disability benefits on appeal because of the "disabling effect" of ordinary chemicals and the combined effect of her many health problems. The court cited the standard requiring that a person be "unable to engage in substantial gainful activity," and reiterated that total incapacity is not required to acquire disability compensation (cited in Dubin, p. 13). The three denied cases that Dubin cites all involve court skepticism regarding medical evidence of disability acquired through "environmental" medicine.

We sent an additional questionnaire to those who indicated in Phase I that they had applied for disability compensation for MCS, that asked about the conditions under which people became disabled, diagnoses used in filing the application, and the responses of the courts to their petitions. For more information, see Appendix A, "Research Methodology."

Stresses of the Application Process

The application process is extremely stressful, as applicants must often face skeptical examiners with unsafe offices and struggle to maintain their self-esteem despite acquiring incorrect and stigmatizing psychiatric labels. They must also endure severe financial problems during the waiting process, and come to terms with a new self-definition that does not include work. How could it not be stressful under such conditions? According to respondents, the most difficult parts of the application process are the appointments with Social Security Administration (SSA)–appointed medical examiners. These appointments are challenging because SSA office environments are rarely safe and skeptical examiners seldom know anything about MCS.

People often are humiliated and frustrated by psychiatric labels that render their physically caused complaints invisible and invalid. Interestingly, psychiatric labels can be assigned at any point in the application process, even if the applicant's personal physicians provided only physically based diagnoses. For example, only seventeen people in my study filed for disability with a psychiatric diagnosis included in their petition (either in combination with MCS or as a stand-alone classification). Twenty-seven, however, were granted disability benefits for psychiatric reasons. When an SSA-chosen expert assigns a psychiatric diagnosis, this diagnosis can be used for disability eligibility even if none of the applicant's personal health providers believe the applicant has a psychiatric diagnosis. For example, one woman filed for disability for chronic fatigue syndrome (CFS) and was granted disability for paranoid schizophrenia.

Some people choose to allow the use of psychiatric diagnoses in filing because of their financial desperation. One woman decided to "accept a psych[iatric] diagnosis rather than starve" and gained benefits on her first attempt. Likewise, another woman who had endured a long wait for benefits chose to cope with adjusting to a psychiatric diagnosis rather than fight to prove physiological impairment. She says, "It took one and a half years to accomplish my being granted disability benefits, during which time I became homeless due to no employment, no income, and depleting my savings."

One woman who successfully acquired Social Security Disability Income and work insurance (but not workers' compensation) after filing three times for Social Security benefits, four times for workers' compensation, and three times for work disability, describes the process as:

> "Worst fight of my life. Pure hell. I gave into PTSS [posttraumatic stress syndrome] as it was the only way to get disability.... We have spent over $200,000 getting medical care and diagnosis for disability. Became homeless ... My husband was under such pressure fighting for my rights that he had a heart attack and double bypass."

—Twenty-four-year-old woman with
MCS for one year

Not every applicant knows what diagnosis is used to determine disability. Some know only that the Social Security Administration has "determined them to be disabled." MCS was not the only reason for discrimination in the application process. One woman said she was finally granted Supplemental Security Disability Income after five applications in a ten-year period because she was "too old to fill scarce job slots." Physicians did no laboratory tests, documentation was scarce, and on each new application, she was sent to a psychiatrist. Legal Aid had refused to help.

Because of lack of income, many disability applicants live with their parents or extended family during the application process and risk further health decline because of the chemicals in the home environment. Some applicants have no permanent place to live, and survive on porches or in recreational vehicles or cars.

Documenting Invisible Disabilities

The challenges of proving an invisible disability are considerable, especially because "not looking sick" may prevent the MCS applicant from receiving consideration or from being seen as needing help. It is a frustrating fact that people can be more sympathetic when your handicap is more obvious. Nonetheless, in a court situation, you have the difficult task of convincing a judge about the reality of your invisible health condition.

Respondents used some of the following strategies to help them legally prove the reality of MCS. Some people recorded their symptoms through detailed written descriptions of their reactions. One woman sent a videotape to the judge who was deciding her case that was recorded while she was experiencing a chemical reaction. Another individual who had been denied benefits after three appeals had friends and neighbors testify as to her decline in health since becoming chemically sensitive. This same woman also provided the judge with photographs of her safe bedroom and car with air filters. One respondent even reported having had a life-threatening reaction while she was in court, which convinced the administrative law judge (ALJ) that she really was ill.

However you choose to document your symptoms, it needs to be concrete and detailed enough to help a judge understand that chemical exposures lead to disabling symptoms. One woman with MSC explains:

> "[It is] best to explain, in detail, how you are disabled, i.e., 'when I am around perfume I get dizzy and lose my memory and sometimes lose coordination,' etc. They usually deny first claim[s] and insist you can find a place to work [that] is 'safe.' You must reply *why* it is not safe for you, how you have no control over what others wear and use, etc. List each item and what it does to you in detail. . . ."

You might want to make a list of the chemicals you are exposed to in a normal working day, including the identification, severity, and duration of each symptom caused by the chemical reaction. You can make the case that you cannot control exposures in the workplace—they are inevitable. And cumulatively, the symptoms you are exposed to at work keep you debilitated to the point that it is impossible for you to function.

The level of persistence needed is sometimes astounding:

> "Getting disability and work[ers'] compensation benefits while suffering from MCS-related pain has only been obtainable through tenacious persistence. They (workers' comp and the private carrier) *will* stop benefits and will only be persuaded by well-organized appeals."
>
> —Forty-one-year-old woman with MCS
> for six years

In a sense, it is a full-time job just to apply for benefits, and the effort must be seen in context of your long-term health and survival. The process will require collecting extensive medical documentation, educating Social Security Disability Income (SSDI) officials and examiners, and making numerous phone calls. Some people even contacted their state senators for assistance. It is very difficult to do this type of work while you are feeling poorly, but even if there is no one to help in the process, you must find a way to get it done.

Physician Assistance

Obtaining documentation from physicians regarding your MCS may be the most important component of the disability application process. It is essential that the documentation be from doctors who are knowledgeable about and supportive of chemical sensitivity. Being certain that your physicians will testify or provide written statements for a hearing is also important. Of course, this in itself is a hardship for people with MCS, as their medical needs are often reported to be unmet (Engel, Gibson, Adler, et al. 1996). In addition to the difficulties of finding physicians who are educated about MCS, you have the added obstacle of coping with their office environment. Nonetheless, reports from physicians are extremely important. Be sure to review any physician reports before they are submitted. Even with excellent documentation, it will be challenging to win MCS-related disability cases.

Be aware: Documentation varies widely. Well-documented physician reports must include some general MCS education as well as a statement that the applicant is disabled to the point of being unable to engage in substantial gainful activity. On the other hand, there are some reports that even a sympathetic judge would not take seriously. For example, in one instance, a physician scratched two sentences on a prescription pad something along the order of: "Please grant disability to _____ . She can hardly walk from place to place let alone work." Needless to say, this woman was not granted benefits.

A physician's letter needs to be serious. It should be written or typed on professional letterhead and detail the reasons why you should be considered for disability benefits. I suggest that you explore this issue when you first begin seeing a physician, even if you are not currently disabled. Ask the physician what they would do to help you if you ever become disabled, and what type of documentation/report would be submitted. Knowing ahead of time that your physician would desert you when you needed their assistance can save a lot of heartache. There are physicians (even MCS experts) who want no part of the disability application process. One physician told her patient that she would no longer be able to treat him if he went on disability.

At the very least, your physician needs to be aware of the process used by the Social Security Administration (SSA) in determining disability, particularly regarding the emphasis on functional capacity. If your medical documentation can explain in detail what you can and cannot do, and how your ability to work is compromised by chemical exposures in the workplace (and that these chemical exposures are in *every* workplace), this will help the Disability Determination Services worker to see that your Residual Functional Capacity is low.

The Single Photon Emission Computed Tomography (SPECT) is one medical screening procedure admissible in court and it shows objective evidence of physical brain damage. Although this procedure is expensive and difficult to obtain because so few practitioners use it for MCS, some applicants (particularly those who have had one massive exposure likely to cause neurological damage) have sought it out to cut through some of the medical denial.

Is the Application Process Fair?

A recent report by the General Accounting Office (GAO) (1997) suggests that the process of determining disability qualification has not been fair. For example, the report found that 65 percent of those who apply for Social Security Disability each year are denied. One-third of these appeal to an administrative law judge (ALJ), and two-thirds of these eventually get benefits. Overall, approximately 49 percent of those who apply receive benefits; 71 percent of awards are made at the initial determinations or reconsiderations and 29 percent are made on appeal. The differences between the likelihood of being awarded benefits at the initial determinations (by DDS) and at the ALJ level has brought the Social Security Administration (SSA) under scrutiny both from within and outside of the organization. The Government Accounting Office report explored the fact that ALJs are more likely to grant benefits. Although ALJs work for the SSA, safeguards protect their independence. For example, SSA management does not control their pay or subject them to performance appraisals. This independence allows ALJs to reverse decisions made by DDS without retribution. According to the Government Accounting Office (1997) report, the following four reasons account for the discrepancy in benefit awards granted by the DDS and ALJs:

1. Residual Functional Capacity (RFC) is often assessed differently, with ALJs finding many more people to have severe limitations in the workplace. The classification that the person's RFC is "less than the range of sedentary work" often leads to receiving benefits. ALJs rated 66 percent of cases as such while DDS saw less than 6 percent of applicants as fitting this category.

2. Although the DDS has medical or psychological consultants determine RFC, an ALJ may or may not respect these findings, and has the authority to determine RFC independently. ALJs may request that an Independent Medical Examiner (IME) see an applicant, but they rarely do. IMEs were involved in only 8 percent of cases in which benefits were awarded at the ALJ level. (This has probably worked in favor of those with MCS.)

3. The reasons for denial at the DDS level are often not clearly explained in the paperwork given to the ALJ. This encourages the ALJ to start from scratch in making a determination. This probably

works in favor of those with MCS also, but is targeted for change as part of SSA's attempt to make the process more congruent at the two levels. SSA plans to require that reasons for denial be clearly indicated so that they can be better used as "a solid foundation for subsequent appeals." (This will likely make it more difficult for people with MCS to obtain benefits at the ALJ level.)

4. New evidence can be presented at the ALJ level and in approximately 75 percent of the appealed cases it is. The ALJ level is the first opportunity applicants have to testify in person as to their impairment, and this personal testimony allows the ALJ to judge the person's credibility. (This probably works in favor of most MCS applicants.) Applicants also may engage the services of an attorney at this stage, and attorneys are financially motivated to obtain awards. In addition, 10 percent of people applying for benefits switch to a mental/psychological diagnosis for the hearing.

According to the General Accounting Office report the disability determination process has been under scrutiny since 1994 with SSA aiming to "make the right decision the first time," thus saving time and money.

Some of the planned changes include more clearly indicating any reasons for denials, sending a number of applications back to DDS rather than ALJs for appeal, and encouraging ALJs to engage the services of independent medical examiners. In fact, a 1996 ruling reinstates a policy that an ALJ must use "expert medical opinion" in demonstrating that cases that do not match disorders on their lists are actually equivalent in severity. None of these changes will help those with MCS. However, the SSA plan to conduct a "predecision interview" with a disability examiner before rejecting an application will give the MCS applicant the opportunity to speak to someone in person.

Medical Evidence and Opinion

Adjudicators must determine disability from medical opinion and evidence. Medical opinion may be gathered from physicians or psychologists who have ongoing relationships with the applicant, clinics or others who have treated the applicant shorter term, and consultants. Medical evidence can include medical history, clinical examination findings, laboratory test findings, diagnostic statements of disease based on signs and symptoms, and treatment suggestions and prognoses (expectations as to probability of improvement). Statements from physicians as to what the person can do in the workplace are also needed as medical evidence. These statements should detail the person's limitations for performing workplace tasks, interacting with co-workers, understanding and carrying out instructions, and stamina for workplace stress.

One important issue to consider is the weight that is accorded to medical opinions, especially given that MCS and those who treat it get very little institutional respect. The SSA is supposed to consider the following factors when deciding what weight to give a medical opinion:

1. More weight is to be given to a physician who examined the patient than to one who didn't. (Therefore, avoiding hostile examiners is very important, because the fact that they saw you will give their testimony more weight.)

2. A physician who has a treating relationship should be given "controlling" weight, if the opinion is well supported by the documentation (i.e., consistent with the medical evidence).

3. Weight given should be commensurate with the length of relationship, number of medical visits, and extent of examinations and testing performed or ordered by the physician. (See your physician regularly and leave an appropriate paper trail, if possible.)

4. An opinion is given more weight if it is supported by evidence (e.g., lab tests) and is clearly explained.

5. Consistency with the case record should give an opinion more weight.

6. Specialists must be given more weight in their area of specialization.

Adjudicators must evaluate whether your condition *could* produce the symptoms you describe. For this task, you can submit statements from family, employers, and others in addition to medical evidence. Adjudicators are not supposed to reject a claim simply because the medical evidence does not clearly support your statements. To evaluate your pain and other symptoms, they should consider what factors aggravate pain and symptoms, what medications are used and their side effects, treatments used, and other factors. For MCS, you can see that, theoretically, it should be possible to gather statements from others, explain that symptoms are aggravated by unavoidable exposures in the workplace, document that medications are difficult to use due to sensitivities, and educate the examiner that treatment involves *no exposures*. This seems logical, but requires reasonable documentation from physicians, which generally has not been available to those with MCS.

It is important to understand that the reality of remaining on disability benefits long-term is an ongoing process and is not ever a "done deal." In fact, remaining on disability compensation may require periodic reviews when you will be required to demonstrate that you still are unable to work. Reviews often mean entering toxic offices, facing skeptical examiners, having expensive testing, and a renewed bout of stress, much as in the original application process.

Beyond Disability: Damage Suits

You may decide that your workplace was instrumental in robbing you of your ability to support yourself, and therefore you may decide to file a lawsuit for further compensation. You will need to find out the statute of limitations regarding toxic exposures in your state. If the claim is a workers' compensation claim, it must be filed within twelve months of the incident, or within twelve months of the time that you found out the incident was responsible for your negative health consequences. You must notify your employer's insurer within thirty days of the incident. Without this notice, there is no case. Therefore, Baiz (1997) suggests that you use a written notice with return receipt requested.

If the incident is not a onetime exposure, but rather an extended repeated series of exposures, then occupational disease laws may be more appropriate than workers' compensation, which is for work-related accidents. Baiz says that under the Occupational Disease Act, you must file a claim to your employer, its insurer, or the Department of Labor within two years from the date you knew or should have known that your disability resulted from an occupational disease. In the event that death results, your beneficiaries have one year to file a claim.

With legal advice and help, toxic tort lawsuits can be filed on a variety of bases. Although success depends on a wide number of factors (locale, attorney, judge, jury, your documentation), Plunkett (1993) shows that there are a number of ways that legal theory supports gaining compensation for workplace-engendered MCS. She reports that most states have had plaintiffs win cases for sick building syndrome or MCS on the basis of negligence, strict liability, breach of contract, express or implied warranties, and fraud and misrepresentation. Each is mentioned here, not as legal advice, but to allow you to assess whether you would like to consider the matter with an informed attorney.

Negligence

Negligence is failing to exercise the level of care that a reasonable person would exercise to protect others against unreasonable risk of harm. Personal injury cases from indoor air pollution are often based on negligence. Proving negligence requires that the defendant owed a "duty of care" to the plaintiff, that the duty had been breached, and that the breach resulted in harm.

Strict Liability

Strict liability refers to liability for damage from a dangerous activity, and does not require negligence as a factor. In strict liability, reasonable care could not have eliminated the risks. For example, products that are dangerous by manufacture or design are often the targets of indoor air pollution lawsuits. Plunkett (1993) says that to succeed, a plaintiff "must demonstrate that he or she was injured by a defective product which was unreasonably dangerous because of its manufacture, design, or lack of warning" (p. 9). Strict liability applies to manufacturers, engineers, architects, contractors, and others, and can be targeted at heating systems, glues, photocopy chemicals, and any other toxic materials to which people are exposed in the workplace.

Breach of Contract

Breach of contract and express or implied warranties can be between builders or sellers of homes/buildings and buyers. Express warranty is a representation to a buyer whether in written, verbal, or other form. Injuries from indoor air pollution may be the result of a breach of warranty because sold items are implied by law to have the warranties of merchantability and of habitability. That is, they are fit to be sold, and fit to be used for the purpose for which they are sold (e.g., homes are meant to be lived in). If carpets emit noxious fumes or mobile homes have unsafe levels of formaldehyde, then the warranties of merchantability and habitability have been breached. Plunkett (1993) cites a case where a family was granted $16,203,000 from urea formaldehyde particleboard manufacturers because of the breach of the implied warranty of merchantability. The family was able to prove that:

1. The formaldehyde levels in the home were beyond recommended limits.

2. The particle board was the source of the formaldehyde.

3. Serious health effects had resulted.

The warranty of habitability requires that severe damages occur—a home may not merely be an irritant. Although it is more difficult to successfully sue over habitability for commercial buildings, many argue that commercial buildings also fall under the warranty of habitability.

Fraud and Misrepresentation

Misrepresentation involves false statements—either fraudulent or innocent—by builders, sellers, or brokers. It is more difficult to prove fraudulent misrepresentation, as you must prove that the defendant knowingly made a false statement with the intent of getting you to rely on it, and that damage ensued to you as a result.

Other Legal Theories

Plunkett (1993) mentions other legal theories that may be used to recover damages for MCS, but which are pretty much untested in indoor air pollution cases. One is *nuisance*, which involves interference with or invasion of property. Nuisance cannot be used simply for personal injury, but it may be combined with negligence or strict liability. Under *risk of future illness*, a plaintiff may be able to recover damages for the increased risk of future illness as a result of a toxic exposure, but there must be some demonstrable damage present. For example, a person hospitalized for smoke inhalation following a chemical fire may then argue that they are at greater risk for lung disease. Even *fear of future illness* as a result of toxic exposure may be used in toxic tort litigation, and Plunkett cites several successful cases. Plunkett also says that battery might also be used in cases of toxic tort, although there are no known cases. Battery requires that the defendant intentionally caused harmful or offensive contact and that the contact occurred. Contact with a toxin can in and of itself constitute the injury. Contact with asbestos dust, radiation, and other toxins has been the subject of a large number of lawsuits. Plunkett says that battery may be easier to prove than negligence because battery places less emphasis on causation.

Documentation

To solidly document personal injury claims, Baiz (1997) advises the plaintiff to keep good records, including finding out as much as possible about the exposure, and keep a journal of symptoms, medical appointments, consultations, and therapy. He advises noting mental/emotional symptoms as well as symptoms more often thought of as physical. If there are witnesses to the exposure and the effects it had on you, provide names and addresses.

Although damage suits can consume tremendous resources on your part and be terribly stressful to initiate, they have the potential to put polluters on notice, and to prove that checks and balances sometimes actually work. Damage suits set precedents, making it easier for others who are injured by toxins to receive compensation, gain publicity for the issue of a safe workplace, and, if successful, provide you with compensation for some of what you have lost.

Applying for Disability Benefits

The decision of whether to apply for disability compensation is an extremely difficult one. On the one hand you have the difficulty of the process, and if adequate accommodations in your workplace can be made, it may be more beneficial to continue working. However, if your workplace is forcing you deeper and deeper into illness, then it may be necessary to receive benefits so that you can give your body the rest it needs. This area is so new, and interpretation of policy is in such flux, that little is certain about what will really work in the application process. Talk to other people who have applied for disability and determine what helped and what challenges they faced in the process. You can also gather any resources they may have that might help you. See Appendix A for some more information about the application experience of my research respondents. It may be less stressful if someone helps you through the process, and that person need not be an attorney. Many applicants have acquired benefits without legal representation. This legal arena may heat up in the next few years given that corporate interests already are attempting to exclude MCS from being covered by the Americans with Disabilities Act (ADA). The issue of compensation for damage by chemicals in a chemical-dependent economy cuts right to the heart of economic justice, power, productivity, and cultural issues.

For some, acquiring disability compensation is a step toward increased rather than decreased productivity. (See chapter fourteen.) Some people unable to work in traditional contexts have gone on to found organizations, edit newsletters, write books, support others, and foster important political and social change.

Chapter Fourteen

If You Can't Join
Them, Beat Them

Activism, Education, and Advocacy

People with MCS have had to become advocates for themselves to survive. Many have made tremendous contributions to education and policymaking regarding toxicants and health. To find out more about these contributions and to see how common political involvement might be for those with MCS, I asked people in Phase III of my study to respond to an eighteen-item scale designed to assess activism at various levels (See Appendix A for further research.). Included were items ranging from reading about MCS and attending support groups to more intensive types of work, such as doing research, establishing support groups, and editing newsletters and books.

People with MCS make significant contributions to others with the condition and to environmental education and policy. For instance, some have produced educational materials, initiated legislative actions, and secured various types of accommodations for others with MCS. Individuals with MCS have also founded many support groups and networks. Activists who have experienced firsthand the harm caused by toxic chemical exposures are in positions to advocate for the prevention of further spread of this condition and, in some cases, make the toxicology literature accessible to the greater public. To communicate their accomplishments and increase public awareness of environmental hazards, chemically sensitive activists have used a variety of resources and channels, including World Wide Web sites, radio spots, and television interviews. There is a lower level of activism among MCS survivors who are employed outside the home. This may be because most of their available energy is channeled into maintaining jobs that involve ongoing exposures and other MCS-related challenges.

There is a relationship between an individual's level of activism and the severity of their condition. Manzo and Weinstein (1987) found that those who have been harmed by the environment are more likely to be active. Some people find new motivation and make significant contributions by becoming politically active in the emerging grassroots movement of people with chemical injuries. As Glendinning (1990) has stated, these technology survivors first become empowered through self-education, and then extend this educational process to others.

Even though the process is challenging, activist work brings attention to the voice of a marginalized group of people who have been either ignored or delegitimized by inadequate health care systems. People who have experienced chemical injuries are the most qualified to help others understand the condition. Unfortunately, powerful interests purposely counter messages from this disabled community with false assurances of safety and erroneous characterizations of the chemically injured as somaticizers.

Economic interests dictate that to continue a chemically dependent lifestyle, we must not acknowledge the culpability for negative health effects from chemicals. Conventional medicine is unable to help because it is so embedded in the dominant economic/industrial structure that adopts and supports new technologies in the name of production, regardless of their consequences. Some of these technologies (e.g., nuclear power) are associated with consequences that will be salient for thousands of years (Mander 1991; Mies 1993). Those disabled by chemicals are thus in conflict with the dominant culture that values only measurable commodities: reducing human effort into "labor," defining the natural world by its "resources" or "raw materials," and labeling the act of caring for others as "women's work."

Health is measured against profit in "risk assessment," and human health and natural ecosystems are seen as fair trade-offs for convenience and increased production. The Interagency Workgroup on Multiple Chemical Sensitivity (1998) echoed these statements in their policy recommendations of the Predecisional Draft *Report on Multiple Chemical Sensitivity*. The report states that, "Increased scientific knowledge about MCS and the role of environmental chemicals will inevitably be put into the context of benefits and risk" (lines 1882-1883). Can you imagine a group of federal agencies making such a statement about AIDS, cancer, or multiple sclerosis?

Industrial culture continually attempts to convince us that chemicals bring convenience, save lives, and improve our ability to provide and transform "resources" (e.g., "ADM—Supermarket to the world.") Thus, characterizing chemicals as problematic in *any* way—let alone as causes of illness—is going strongly against the grain of society.

Consequently, the far-reaching influences of the chemical industry have rendered those who live with the consequences of chemical injuries as some of the *only* voices able and willing to provide information and to motivate others to fight for a healthy, nontoxic environment. The increasing number of people who have been killed from being directly exposed to thousands of volatile chemicals calls for immediate action to ensure our safety in the future. This process of activism was articulated by Wilkinson and Kitzinger (1994) who cited Winnow (1992) in relation to breast cancer prevention: "Real prevention would mean changing fundamental social structures. It would mean going after the tobacco industry, stopping the pollution of our environment, providing quality food."

People who are injured by chemicals experience firsthand the unforeseen consequences of Western industrial exploitative culture. Chemical sensitivity/injury is thus a warning to and a critique of the Western obsession with production and profit. Ironically, such injury is a condition that prohibits any continuance of a chemical-laden lifestyle for those who experience it. Following are some examples of the personal triumphs and contributions made by MCS activists. I hope they will inspire you. These activists are not all physically healthy. In fact, some highly effective MCS activists work from their beds, are virtually unable to speak, are totally housebound, and have had periods of homelessness. Yet, they persist and inspire and educate others. The late Cindy Duehring, for example, was unable to speak while she was suffering from MCS because the human voice caused her auditory-induced seizures. During her lifetime, however, she greatly contributed to the MCS community.

MSC Heroines

I asked some of the people who have made very strong contributions to the MCS community to answer questions about their activism. The questions were written with the help of Susan Molloy. My goal was to help others understand what has been done and hopefully to inspire more people to contribute in spite of their disabilities. Some answered the questions exactly as they were asked. Others submitted statements in different formats. Therefore, some of the following descriptions are very structured questions and answers, and some are less structured. I have expanded some of the information where individuals sold themselves short or were very brief.

Cynthia Wilson

Cynthia Wilson is founder of the Chemical Injury Information Network (CIIN), a tax-exempt, nonprofit support/advocacy organization that is run by chemically injured individuals primarily for the benefit of others who are chemically injured. She founded CIIN in May 1990, and serves as the executive director and chairperson of the board. The primary focus of CIIN is education, credible research on multiple chemical sensitivity, and the empowerment of chemically injured individuals. The organization publishes the monthly newsletter *Our Toxic Times* and has more than 5,000 members in thirty-four countries.

In 1994, CIIN merged with the Environmental Access Research Network (EARN) (directed by Cindy Duehring). As the research division of CIIN, EARN was responsible for the administration of one of the largest existing private libraries on chemical health issues. Its primary focus was to make scientific, medical, legal, and government literature available to health care professionals, expert witnesses, attorneys, and lay people. The *Medical & Legal Briefs* and *Environmental Access Profiles* newsletters were both published by EARN. (The newsletter archives are maintained by CIIN.)

Considered a leading organization worldwide for chemical health problems, CIIN fields more than 500 requests per month for information on toxic health problems. The newsletters are invaluable resources for the MCS community. In my opinion, it would be hard to overestimate Wilson's contribution to the knowledge of the relationship between chemicals and health. Many MCS activists see her as the leading voice on some of these issues. Her constant, informed, and organized presence is a source of security for many.

Wilson wrote the book *Chemical Exposure and Human Health*, which reviews the effects of more than 300 chemicals and cross-references symptoms with possible chemical causes. In addition, she and Cindy Duehring were commissioned in 1994 by the Chemical Impact Project to write a white paper. The sixty-five-page report, *The Human Consequences of the Chemical Problem*, was presented to Vice President Al Gore, First Lady Hillary Rodham Clinton, Secretary of the National Institutes of Health Donna Shalala, and the Centers for Disease Control and Prevention (CDC). The CDC peer reviewed the paper and found it to have "merit," and a conference was convened to discuss the health issues raised by the paper. The Agency for Toxic Substances and Disease Registry called it "powerful and well researched." The Special Assistant to the President requested extra copies to distribute and Senator Conrad Burns (R-MT) requested an extra copy to present to the Senate Committee on Labor and Human Resources.

Wilson currently has the goal of completing research on the role of aminolevulinic acid as a possible mediator of reactions to inhaled chemicals. She has contributed to many projects, including the Chemical Impact Project; National Coalition for the Chemically Injured; the 1994 Conference on MCS (as a planning committee member and presenter), which was hosted by the ATSDR; and the 1999 conference on Gulf War Syndrome (as an MCS panel member), which was hosted by the CDC.

Lynn Lawson

For forty years, Lynn Lawson suffered from increasingly severe and frequent headaches, including so-called common migraines. Until Theron G. Randolph, M.D., correctly diagnosed Lawson in 1986 as chemically sensitive, she thought her condition was incurable. (Randolph discovered in 1951 what he later called "the chemical problem.") Once Lawson learned which chemicals, products, and foods were causing her problem, it took one year for her to improve her health 80 to 90 percent, by avoiding chemicals and building up her immune system through supplements and better eating. At present, she does public relations work and edits a bimonthly newsletter, *Canary News*, for her Chicago-based support group, MCS: Health & Environment. Here are her answers to my questions:

When did it occur to you that you should help in regard to MCS?

As soon as I was diagnosed, I knew I needed help in dealing with this complex condition, so I joined the local support group and became active. For three years, I was public relationships chair for the Human Ecology Action League (H.E.A.L.) during which time I received a letter about perfumes published by "Dear Abby." The letter brought more than five thousand responses to H.E.A.L. My biggest disappointment was in trying to get several dozen celebrities to speak out against chemicals for Earth Day 1990; none responded to my mailing.

Actually, I have been an environmentalist ever since I read Rachel Carson's *Silent Spring* in 1962 and realized why robins were dying in our neighborhood. After the first Earth Day, in 1970, I taught a popular environmental rhetoric course for two years at the University of Illinois. Little did I know then that my headaches were pollution-related. In April 1990, my essay, "We Are All at Risk," won second place in the Unitarian Universalist magazine, *World's*, environmental essay contest. Since then, I have had several articles on MCS published in the Northwestern University's Center on Aging newsletter and in a Chicago area free magazine called *Conscious Choice: The Journal of Ecology & Natural Living*.

In 1994, the Noble Press published my 488-page book, *Staying Well in a Toxic World: Understanding Environmental Illness, Multiple Chemical*

Sensitivities, Chemical Injuries, and Sick Building Syndrome. Now published by Lynnword Press, it is in its fourth printing. I wrote my book for two reasons: to warn people of the dangers from modern chemicals and to validate EI/MCS as much as I could. Also, I tried to answer two irksome questions for myself: Where have the public health people been? And why haven't the environmentalists been doing anything about human health?

The publication of my book gave me more opportunities to educate the public through several dozen book signings, a dozen or so radio talk shows (from the comfort of my living room), a few TV sound bites, and other presentations and appearances.

What goals do you have?

- To keep on writing my newsletter as long as I am able.

- To continue networking with other groups and trying to reach the general public.

- To get the governor of Illinois to sign a proclamation recognizing May 10 through 16, 1999 as MCS Awareness Week. (He did.)

What projects have you made contributions to?

In 1990, when I took over the support group newsletter and renamed it *Canary News*, the group had 160 members, with only one living outside of Illinois. It now has close to 400 members, more than a third of whom are national and international members; an additional 200 people receive complimentary, exchange, or introductory copies of the newsletter. In the five years that I coordinated the group, I wrote an MCS Access Checklist and a brochure explaining MCS. I also do a yearly update of our thirty-nine-page Resource Guide and started what is now an extensive lending library and a service for mailing informational pieces on request.

For Earth Day 1995, our group presented an all-day public program on environment and human health that featured, as the speaker, William Rea, M.D., of the Dallas Environmental Health Center, and showed videos, such as public television's *Bad Chemistry*. The program was attended by more than 150 people. At Earth Day 1997, we showed videos of the all-day Washington Toxics Coalition conference, "Chemical Exposure and Disease: Is Our Environment Making Us Sick?" Earth Day 1997, however, was attended by only a handful of people.

Also in 1997, for the thirty-fifth anniversary of the publication of *Silent Spring*, we organized an all-day event called Healthier Environment Education Day (HEED), at which we networked with other groups, such as those for fibromyalgia, chronic fatigue, and endometriosis, in offering information to the general public. It was attended by more than fifty people. Also in 1997, several of us testified about toxic chemicals dangerous to our health at the Chicago hearing of the EPA's Endocrine Disrupters Screening and Testing Advisory Committee.

1998 was an active year. In May, two members went to our state capitol to give a presentation at the 14th Annual Disability Rights Conference, sponsored by the Coalition of Citizens with Disabilities in Illinois. Two others attended a state candidates forum, sponsored by several disability groups, and presented a packet of information about MCS to the two women candidates for lieutenant governor. In October, three of us were physically active: we rallied and marched in downtown Chicago against Monsanto with a small but vociferous group called the Chicago Coalition to Ban Genetically Engineered Food. All three of us carried large posters saying, "Ask not just what you can do for the environment; ask what the environment is doing to you." This kind of activity is a first for our group; actually, it proved to be quite exhilarating.

Our main ongoing project is our hospital education project—an attempt to make hospitals safer for us, other patients, and staff. To date, members have given presentations at four large local hospitals. We had fairly notable success at one, which now provides substantial accommodation for chemically sensitive support-group members.

Is there anything you wish you would have done differently in terms of expenditure of energy or resources?

For events such as HEED, it is very important to have plenty of publicity, but I suspect that no amount of publicity would have brought more people to our second Earth Day presentation. Most people still do not make the connection between the environment and human health—until they get sick and are properly diagnosed, of course. The public health people are showing signs of coming around, but the large environmental groups still focus their substantial resources on the natural world, not people. I recently sent some of the flyers from our two Earth Day events to a group working on Earth Day 2000 for their "archives," but I added that I had pretty much given up on them. Maybe I'll change my mind.

Do you have any advice for people who have newly found out they have MCS, or who are currently at a very low point?

Be aware that you can get better, as I did, by avoidance, supplements, and improving your diet, as described in my book. Several surveys have shown that avoidance and diet are by far the most successful "treatments" for most people. Listen to what your body tells you; realize that we are all different in our symptoms and exposures; and find a doctor who will listen and work with you in finding the causes of your particular set of symptoms. Then you must avoid as much as possible.

Do you have solidarity or support with/ from other activists?

Very much so. I exchange newsletters with about fifty other support groups and related organizations and I am in frequent contact with other activists by phone, fax, regular mail, and e-mail. One of the compensations of having this illness is the many wonderful new friends I have made worldwide.

Have you received any recognition for your work?

My chief reward has been hearing that my writing or my work has helped someone. I have been fortunate in the expressions of appreciation I have received for my newsletter, my work with the group, and my book. When my book was first published, a friend organized a marvelous picnic in my honor. A support-group member tried to get the *Chicago Tribune* to review the book, but was told, "We do not review self-help books, only books with literary merit." Interestingly, a few months later the Chicago-based Society of Midland Authors invited me to join their group—on the basis of literary merit.

Mary Lamielle

Mary Lamielle is founder and director of the National Center for Environmental Health Strategies (NCEHS), a nonprofit organization that for more than twelve years has focused on solutions to environmental health problems, with an emphasis on indoor air quality and outdoor toxins, chemical sensitivities, and environmental disabilities. Lamielle's pioneering work has helped to bring visibility to public health problems of those who are ill and disabled because of low-level chemical and environmental exposures. She is currently a member of the President's Committee on Employment of People with Disabilities, and has served on invitation-only committees for a number of federal agencies, including the disability policy summit meeting sponsored by the National Council on Disability. She has published numerous articles and has lectured and presented workshops for a broad range of audiences around the country. Lamielle is the recipient of several awards, including the Carleton Lee Award from the American Academy of Environmental Medicine and the Indoor Advocate of the Year by IAQ Publications. Through the NCEHS, Lamielle provides clearinghouse services, technical assistance, educational materials, workshops, policy development, research, support, community outreach, and advocacy for the public and those injured by chemical and environmental exposures in the home, at school, at work, and in the community. Requests to the center for information may include as many as 1,000 per month. Lamielle's advocacy includes numerous testimonies before Congress, has been covered extensively by media, and has been significant in achieving recognition of chemical sensitivities as a public health problem.

Elaine (Malafarina) Tomko

Elaine (Malafarina) Tomko submitted her own statement, and was very emphatic that it is not her, but the members of the Ecological Health Organization (ECHO) who deserve the credit for the successes and progress being made in Connecticut. Here is her statement:

Elaine (Malafarina) Tomko is a woman disabled by Multiple Chemical Sensitivity who has been active in the Ecological Health Organization (ECHO) since its inception in January 1992. ECHO is a non-profit support, education, resource, referral, and advocacy organization for people with multiple chemical sensitivity, others who are sensitive to chemicals in the environment, and those who care about the prevention of chemical injuries. It is one of the first organizations in Connecticut linking environmental issues and public health. Its goals are to provide information and support to people with MCS and others sensitive to chemicals, to educate the public about MCS, to collaborate with other organizations on issues of the chemically sensitive, to advocate for public policies that promote the health and welfare of the chemically injured and prevent chemical injuries, and to encourage medical research on MCS. Tomko has served as executive director of ECHO for many years and in spring 1998 was elected president. Tomko has also edited the ECHO newsletter since fall 1992.

Tomko believes that it is very important for everyone with MCS to become actively involved in support groups for several reasons, including to gain and share useful information to cope effectively and successfully with this illness, and to positively direct their feelings and act constructively to educate others about the illness.

She is motivated by the many phone calls she receives from people with MCS or with symptoms of MCS who are looking for treatment or searching for ways to cope with the condition. Her hope is that through the activism of groups like ECHO, people disabled by chemical exposures will find the help they need, whether health care, legal referrals, safe housing, or workplace accommodations.

The success of ECHO is due to its officers and board of directors willingly devoting their time and talent to the organization. Through cooperation, consensus, and negotiation, ECHO, as an organization team, works toward evaluating, identifying, and accomplishing its goals.

Accomplishments of ECHO Since Inception

Since 1992, ECHO has had the support of its members for the many projects it has undertaken and accomplished, including:

1. Producing a report, "How to Accommodate the Worker with Multiple Chemical Sensitivities," at the request of the Connecticut State Office of Protection and Advocacy for People with Disabilities in

spring 1992. More than 800 copies have been distributed to date by that office, by ECHO, and by the president of the Connecticut State AFL-CIO. It has also been distributed to state agencies, labor groups and other disability rights groups. Tomko and President Linda Thompson wrote the report.

2. Publishing a twelve-page newsletter distributed quarterly to more than 200 members and the public since 1992. Tomko is the editor.

3. Initiating (and cosponsoring with twenty other environmental, labor and community organizations) a "Conference on Human and Planetary Health," with 150 people attending in spring 1994. ECHO received a $2,000 grant from Citizens Clearinghouse for Hazardous Waste to hold the conference. People at the conference were introduced to the new disease syndrome, Multiple Chemical Sensitivity, and to ECHO's approach to stopping the spread of this preventable disease. The conference was the first smoke- and fragrance-free statewide environmental event in Connecticut, allowing injured workers and people who are disabled with MCS to attend.

4. In November 1994, Carolyn Wysocki, M.A., M.H.S.A., and ECHO support group facilitator, presented a workshop on "Multiple Chemical Sensitivity and Accommodations of the Worker Under the Americans with Disabilities Act" at a conference on Indoor Air Quality sponsored by the Connecticut Council on Occupational Safety and Health (Connecti-COSH). The conference drew sixty people from diverse backgrounds, including machinists, teachers, health professionals and trade unionists who were all keenly interested in the health problems associated with indoor air pollution. The Labor Institute's curriculum workbook, *Multiple Chemical Sensitivities at Work*, was distributed to conference participants. Wysocki used the video, *Multiple Chemical Sensitivity: An Emerging Occupational Hazard*, produced by the Labor Institute, which accompanies the workbook for her presentation. She also wrote a handout on accommodations for people with MCS under the Americans with Disabilities Act (ADA) definition and developed a paper, "ADA Title I Accommodations for People with Multiple Chemical Sensitivity," for distribution and use at conferences on accommodations needed for people with MCS. Wysocki is presently working on a new brochure, "ADA Access Guidelines for Conferences, Workshops, and Meetings for Planners and Attendees," so people with MCS can attend these functions safely.

5. The ECHO Speakers' bureau has reached college students and faculty members, state agency managers, centers for independent living directors, rehabilitation services managers and staff, and the

Northeast Rehabilitation Association's members. The bureau's purpose is MCS education, accommodations in the workplace, and coverage of this illness under the Americans with Disabilities Act. ECHO has published and updated an "ECHO Resource Guide" given to all members who have a membership subscription. It contains research articles on MCS by doctors, articles of practical information on how to live with this illness, and resources for products helpful to people with MCS. In 1997, ECHO President Wysocki authored the first ECHO Brochure, "What is MCS?—Multiple Chemical Sensitivity," which has been distributed to more than 2,000 people to date. In spring 1998, through the efforts of Wysocki, the Governor of Connecticut issued a Proclamation designating May 11 through 17, 1998 as Multiple Chemical Sensitivity Awareness Week in the State of Connecticut.

Ann McCampbell, M.D.

Ann McCampbell is a physician who has been disabled with MCS for ten years. She chairs the MCS Task Force of New Mexico and is president of the board of MCS Referral and Resources. In 1994, she cofounded the Healthy Housing Coalition, a nonprofit organization that helps people with MCS find housing and promotes healthier building. She served on its board through 1998. Here are McCampbell's answers to my questions:

When did it occur to you that you should help in regard to MCS?

As soon as I knew I had it. I kept remembering a phrase from a well-known self-help group that "no matter how far down the scale you have gone, you will see how your experience can benefit others." I don't think I would have survived without others helping me and I vowed to return the favor whenever my health allowed.

What goals do you have?

My goals are to help people with MCS and prevent others from getting it through education, advocacy, legislation, and whatever else it takes. I have a particular interest in educating the medical profession about MCS.

What projects have you made contributions to?

In 1996, I organized and moderated a Town Hall Meeting on MCS for the New Mexico Governor's Committee on Concerns of the Handicapped. As chair of the MCS Task Force of New Mexico, I have drafted legislation, testified before legislative committees, prepared background materials for MCS lobbyists and speakers, drafted pesticide notification regulations, participated in an MCS prevalence study working group, and submitted testimony to the National Institutes for Health. I also wrote an MCS brochure with the New Mexico State Department of Education, co-wrote a resolution adopted by the City of Santa Fe to reduce pesticide use and adopt an Integrated Pest Management (IPM) program, and revised my 1992 booklet "Multiple Chemical Sensitivity."

Is there anything you wish you would have done differently in terms of expenditure of energy or resources?

Not really, although my friends and loved ones tell me I should work less!

Do you have any advice for people who have newly found out they have MCS, or who are currently at a very low point?

For those new to MCS: Get away from chemicals!

For those at a low point: I understand.

For both: You're not alone and we care about you!

Do you have solidarity or support with/from other activists?

Yes, lots. We at the task force have a core group of ten to fifteen people and a mailing list near 500. We are working with other environmental and disability groups in New Mexico. I also am well connected nationally with a lot of other advocates.

Have you received any recognition for your work?

Yes, I get thanked all the time. My task force co-workers also nominated me for Certificate of Recognition by the New Mexico Commission on the Status of Women in New Mexico (1997) for making outstanding contributions to the status of women in New Mexico, and the FRIEND'S Award honoring individuals coping admirably with major health problems (1998). (I didn't win.)

Susan Molloy

Susan Molloy is a well-known MCS/disability advocate who edited the *Reactor* newsletter for years. She is well versed in disability issues, and has made a national contribution to education and advocacy for MCS. Here are her answers to my questions:

Please write a little description/introduction of who you are and your current position.

Currently, I work fifteen hours per week for the Independent Living Center (ILC) in Prescott, Arizona. I work from home—from bed if I'm having a rough time—on the ILC newsletter and fielding questions from people with MCS. I serve on the Board of Arizona Technology Access Program as well, and try to help other MCS people with their efforts. I'm especially impressed and encouraged by Rhonda Zwillinger's "Dispossessed Project" and by the Electrical Sensitivities Network that Lucinda Grant has put together. It's a challenge to establish disability rights and accessibility within the greater community. We are fighting for our right to live, to have a future together in relative safety.

When did it occur to you that you should help in regard to MCS?

I didn't ever actually think of it in terms of "helping." In 1981, when it became clear I was in immediate danger of dying, it seemed as though I'd been captured into some kind of underground gulag in some sort of covert, undeclared war. We had no legal rights or political vehicle through which to defend ourselves. The only way I knew to survive was to quietly, diligently seek out trustworthy people with whom to work who could encourage each other—similar to seeing if there's anyone able to respond from the next cell block or the next foxhole without drawing so much fire that we're all put out of business right away. We had a hand we didn't know how to play in a high stakes game, and there was no choice but to proceed. It was hard. It's still hard, but now this war is no secret. People with this disease don't all have to live such a totally underground existence anymore, thank God. Sometimes people can get help before they've lost all their resources and all their relationships. I didn't set out to "help" people—my motivation is more akin to self-defense with a significant mutual aid component.

What goals do you have?

I want to work hard, have a good time. I want us to have enforceable legal protection, to stop the assaults and abuses against us, and for us to have healthy choices in housing. I want to earn a black belt, play with my dog, help out friends, and grow in spirit.

What projects have you made contribution to?

I organized and edited the *Reactor* newsletter in California for eleven years, and turned our best articles into the *Best of the Reactor*, a book that Environmental Health Network (EHN) sells. It includes the language of our bills, and all our legislative, policy, and housing efforts both nationally and in the state of California. We've actually done some pretty fair work. Hundreds of MCS people's best efforts to build our own culture are in that book. I helped EHN get started, and with political advocacy for the Ecology House project in San Rafael. Moving to the high desert, and establishing my own peculiar little household in our community in East Snowflake has been a lifesaver— there's so much to invent, retrofit, customize, and try regarding structures, protection, and social change.

Is there anything you wish you would have done differently in terms of expenditure of energy or resources?

Yes. I overemphasized the value of educating personnel within government agencies, and spent too much time in development of information to share with them. For the most part, they don't learn and won't help until they are sick, threatened, or paid to do so. It used to encourage me when we were even asked for help, or for our opinion, and I was very sincere about forwarding our issues through education. But "education" alone changes nothing unless there is some serious muscle behind it. We should have been more disruptive, demonstrating, been much more forceful. Then again, we aren't done yet, are we?

Do you have any advice for people who have newly found out they have MCS, or who are currently at a very low point?

Get out of the line of fire now before you get sicker. Avoidance is our only choice until the medical research gets up to speed—do not give away your resources trying to buy a cure. Don't get stuck in an urban area unless you are very well-to-do. Keep things simple. Trust God.

Do you have solidarity or support with/from other activists?

Yes, I love them very, very much.

Have you received any recognition for your work?

In 1994, I was awarded the Resourceful Women Award, which assisted rural activists within economically disadvantaged communities, and leadership on behalf of economic and social justice. They allocated $5,000 which went into making my house, and $7,000 seed money with which to establish a grant writing scholarship fund for low income people with disabilities here in northeast Arizona.

Irene Ruth Wilkenfeld

I, Irene Ruth Wilkenfeld, see myself as a "wounded healer," defined as an individual whose healing knowledge comes from personal experience with her own wounds. My life was irrevocably changed when, in 1969, I was chemically injured and left chronically ill because of a workplace exposure. My occupation may surprise you. I was not employed in what is generally accepted as a "high-risk" industry. I was a teacher. I had just been hired to work in a brand new, state of the art, energy-efficient, climate-controlled, suburban middle school in New Jersey. There, I was exposed to chlordane (a pesticide used as a termiticide that has since been banned in the United States) and to formaldehyde and other volatile organic compounds that are ubiquitous in building construction and furnishing materials. Within just three months, I was bedridden. I thought my life was over.

For fifteen years I searched aimlessly and in all the wrong places for the cause of my long laundry list of debilitating physical complaints. I put my faith and trust in mainstream medicine. That trust was shattered and betrayed. Isolated, ostracized, and unable to work, I at first thought I was a victim of some unknown medical conundrum. Now I know that every victim is really a survivor who does not yet know the extent of her power. Now I know that my suffering was really a doorway to my transformation; and that doing my research into what I now call the Sick School Syndrome, recording the case histories of others injured in contaminated classrooms, and sharing these stories, is my *dharma*, my higher purpose in life. Now I use my wounds and my case histories as doorways to educate the educators, empower and help find accommodations for those who previously felt disenfranchised after developing MCS, and to prevent additional school-based injuries. Safe Schools, my home-based consulting service, founded in 1987, is now my vehicle to promote environmental health literacy in schools nationally and internationally.

When did it occur to you that you should help in regard to MCS?

After fifteen years of that aimless and unproductive search for the trigger responsible for my devastating illness, I met Diane Hamilton, the founder and longtime president of the state-wide H.E.A.L. of Louisiana chapter. The moment I understood the nature of my injury and its relationship with my employment in that "toxic terrarium" of a school, I promised [Hamilton] and myself that as soon as I was physically able, I would devote my professional life to detoxifying our nation's schools. But first I would have to become a student and educate myself about this complex illness that had almost succeeded in erasing my life as I had come to know it. I spent years devouring everything I could find about MCS and now have an office with twenty-seven filing cabinet drawers, some 3,000 books, and an ever-growing collection of case histories totaling more than 2,800. Each of the clients associated with these case histories has endured a personal struggle for recognition, validation, accommodation, and competent care. And, like my own school-based chemical "assault," each of these injuries could have been and should have been avoided.

Soon it became very clear to me, from my meta-analysis, that the Sick School Syndrome (one piece of the MCS puzzle) was a pervasive, insidious problem, a public health crisis, a sentinel health event, an ecotastrophe and a national disgrace. I had no choice. I became compulsive about sounding the alarm about our toxic schools.

What goals do you have?

I am reminded of a quote that I collected years ago: "We are all of us angels with just one wing . . . we can only fly, embracing each other." I work every day to live up to this goal.

As my health allows, I now travel throughout the United States and Canada, presenting my "in-serve" training workshop entitled *The Sick School Syndrome: When Learning Becomes Lethal.* I alert my audiences to the fact that our schools are in deplorable condition and that these conditions put vulnerable youngsters in harm's way. (Some teachers deserve hazard pay.) My take home message is reflected in an old Lakota Indian saying, "Mi taku oyasin," which means, "We are all interconnected." We are one with our environment and with each other. What we do to the planet, we ultimately do to ourselves. Each presentation seeks to educate attendees that our bodies are permeable and behave like barometers of our environment.

As a former teacher, I am angry, frustrated, and embarrassed by the pervasive level of denial about the validity of MCS and the Sick School Syndrome. But each day, I remind myself that I must be tenacious and plant the seeds that will eradicate this psychic numbing and autistic reaction to this environmental health threat and replace it with a commitment to make every school a citadel of safety.

What projects have you made contributions to?

- I have presented workshops and lectures in a variety of contexts, including school districts, conferences, and professional meetings. For example, in 1992 I was a guest faculty lecturer at the 27th Annual Meeting of the American Academy of Environmental Medicine (Lincolnshire, IL). I presented at workshops for the Kitchener-Waterloo and the Wellington school systems in Ontario Canada, which are now recognized innovators in accommodating MCS students and teachers in their ECO classrooms. I was the keynote speaker at a conference sponsored by the New York State United Teachers Union and the American Lung Association, speaking on "The Vulnerable Brain."

- I have a chapter in *The Healthy School Handbook*, published in May 1995 by the National Education Association's (NEA) Professional Library. I have published numerous articles about the Sick School Syndrome in such publications as *The Environmental Physician (AAEM), Informed Consent, Our Toxic Times, Indoor Pollution Law Report, The Townsend Letter for Doctors,* and *The New Reactor.*

- I was the founder and president of a H.E.A.L. chapter, editor of the chapter newsletter, and president of a state chapter of CIIN.

- I have submitted testimony to a Board of Regents at the New York State Department of Education at a Public Hearing on Environmental Quality in the Schools; to the Maryland State Legislature's Environmental Matters Committee on the issue of pesticide notification in schools; to the Maryland Department of Agriculture on pesticide notification; to the United States Occupational Safety and Health

Department (OSHA) for their proposed revised Indoor Air Quality Guidelines; to the United States Department of Transportation, on their proposed aircraft disinfection policy; to the United States Environmental Protection Agency (US EPA), on their draft document entitled, "Improve Your School's IAQ" (now called Tools for Schools); and to the State of Minnesota's IAQ Initiatives for Schools (on environmental audits). I was recently tapped as a resource by the office of Sen. Barbara Boxer (D-CA) to help identify environmental health hazards faced by children for a piece of draft legislation entitled "The Children's' Environmental Protection Act" (CEPA). I was also invited by Barry L. Johnson, Ph.D., then assistant surgeon general, to offer a critique of a draft report prepared by the ATSDR's Child Health Initiative entitled, "Healthy Children—Toxic Environments: Acting on the Unique Vulnerability of Children who Dwell Near Hazardous Waste Sites."

- I have worked with teachers nationwide to help them integrate environmental health issues into their classroom activities.

- I routinely give media interviews and have appeared on radio and TV broadcasts nationwide.

- I gave a presentation about the hazards of pesticides at an Adjudicatory Hearing of the Louisiana Department of Agriculture and Forestry after I was exposed to a misapplication of Dursban TC (while in a doctor's office). I won my claim against both the applicator and the pest control company.

Is there anything you wish you would have done differently in terms of expenditure of energy or resources?

I regret that I wasted fifteen years trying to find answers to my health problems in the mainstream, medical community. I was misunderstood, misdirected, and occasionally abused by practitioners who are uninformed about environmental illness. My path would have been much easier had I used my energies and resources, earlier on, to network with MCS survivors. I have also since recognized that my chances of being perceived as a professional are enhanced when the school district/officials contact me, rather than my behaving like Don Quixote and flailing at every windmill (sick school) I become aware of.

Do you have any advice for people who have newly found out they have MCS, or who are currently at a very low point?

I wholeheartedly believe that vigilant avoidance is the cornerstone of healing and prevention. I would urge all newly diagnosed MCSers not to jeopardize their health by participating in any treatment protocol that does not endorse avoidance. I would encourage these new patients to educate themselves about their illness until they begin to feel like an "expert" in their own case. And, I would strongly suggest that they connect their sense of isolation and ostracism. I try to alert patients to the wisdom of listening to their bodies. "Your symptoms are gifts," I tell them. Ignoring your symptoms, or trying to mask them with palliatives, is like removing the batteries from your smoke detector. I remind them, too, of the concept of "biochemical individuality." Just as we all look different and have different fingerprints, so too are we different biochemically. Just because a treatment worked for your MCS friend, doesn't mean it will necessarily work for you. And finally, I caution against allowing others (especially those in a position of authority) to label or define them.

Do you have solidarity or support with/from other activists?

And how! One of the greatest gifts this illness has given me is a huge pool of friends and contacts worldwide. I could quite literally fly into any state and a dozen foreign countries, knowing that I have a supportive friend in each "port."

Have you received any recognition for your work?

When clients for whom I have advocated, choose to travel three and four hours to hear me speak, when I am in their general geographic area and they arrange luncheons for me ... their "applause" and their hugs are all the reward I need. Their words of thanks and their letters of endorsement reenergize me and propel me to strive even harder to continue my consultation, activism and advocacy. (See Irene's website at: http://www.head-gear.com/SafeSchools)

Peggy Wolff

I am a woman with MCS who has been the chairperson of the Environmental Health Coalition of Western Massachusetts (EHCWM) since 1995. This grassroots organization has a more than 200 person membership consisting of people with MCS, CS, and others concerned about sensitivity. The EHCWM was funded by the EPA, Region 1, and the Community Foundation of Western Massachusetts to increase the public's awareness of MCS and other health problems caused by environmental hazards and to improve communication within the MCS community. Presently, we have a seven-member board of advisors and four study/action groups. The study/action groups focus on issues related to:

1. Emergency care and hospitalization—preparing guidelines, creating an emergency medical kit, and hospitalization accommodations for people with MCS

2. Health care—preparing a list of health care practitioners (primarily practitioners in Western Massachusetts) who are experienced in managing MCS and/or willing to accommodate people with MCS

3. Housing issues—a pamphlet for the public on home health hazards and "safer" alternatives

4. Schools—supporting teachers with MCS, joining with other environmental groups on the Healthy Schools Network throughout Massachusetts, and seeking accommodations for teachers, students, and parents with MCS

When did it occur to you that you should help in regard to MCS?

Almost immediately after my own illness was finally labeled. Having been a nurse for more than thirty years, I had no idea why I was so sick; neither did all the health care practitioners (conventional and alternative) who I saw prior to being diagnosed by a friend with MCS. I soon realized that few people in the health care professions knew much about MCS.

What goals do you have?

My goals are to fund myself and a handful of other people disabled with MCS through grants so that the work of the EHCWM can continue. Each of the four study/action groups mentioned above has goals specific to the area of concern. I am committed to supporting other environmental groups, especially environmental health groups, so that we can all work together to improve the quality of air, water, and soil of our planet. I am also committed to continuing my work as a psychotherapist/stress management therapist.

What projects have you made contributions to?

Cosponsored an Indoor Air Quality (IAQ) in schools conference, which was attended by more than 200 people, including teachers, administrators, school nurses, and people with MCS. Created resource lists about health, schools, homes and MCS.

Is there anything you wish you would have done differently in terms of expenditure of energy or resources?

I would have liked to spend more time on grant proposals from large foundations so that the EHCWM would be well funded for a few years. I'm working on having more and more people actively involved in the EHCWM so that the work is distributed among more people.

Do you have any advice for people who have newly found out that they have MCS, or who are currently at a very low point?

Trust that this health condition is a great teacher, although not an easy one! Know that there are ups and downs and remind yourself when you are down that "This too shall pass." Don't take on all the burden of the downs, but take responsibility when possible to encourage your whole self to heal. Healing is more important than curing a disease. Seek out people with MCS who are making progress. Seek out health care practitioners referred to you by people with MCS who have been helped. Minimize blame of self and of others. Read relevant books, papers.

Do you have solidarity or support with/from other activists?

Yes, I have actively sought out a group of people (board of advisors, other environmentalists, friends) who are most supportive. I don't want to, nor can I, do this work alone. My interdependency with others has been an important lesson.

Have you received any recognition for your work?

Getting grants was a most important means of recognition, especially from the EPA. Each time I am asked to join with other groups/individuals I know my work is being recognized/honored. Writing articles on MCS/CS for professional nurses, publishing newspaper articles on MCS and writing letters to the editor have given my work some visibility.

Toni Temple

Toni Temple has accomplished a tremendous amount of work in education about accommodations for MCS. Before becoming chemically sensitive, Temple was attending college and receiving good grades, working full-time as management director for three state trade organizations, raising her children, and participating actively in her community. After an exposure to zinc chloride through furnace ductwork in her home, Temple's life changed drastically. Although she is totally disabled, suffers from afflictions other than MCS, and can leave her home only with a respirator, she still manages to be an active and effective agent for change in regard to accommodations for those with MCS. She is currently heading a national campaign called "Healthier Hospitals on the Horizon," which came about from her book, *Healthier Hospitals* (Temple 1996). Temple founded the Ohio Network for the Chemically Injured, and served on the steering committee to found the National Coalition for the Chemically Injured. She has written numerous articles for newsletters and other publications, such as "New Meaning for Access," and has also appeared on television and radio shows to speak about MCS. Although the bill was not passed, Temple lobbied on behalf of Ohio House Bill 389, which would have mandated that physicians receive education in toxicology and nutrition. Here are her answers to my questions:

When did it occur to you that you should help in regard to MCS?

After many months of trying to find appropriate medical help and being incorrectly diagnosed so many times, I was very frustrated because no one was listening to what I was saying about what was causing my health problems (i.e., the chemicals). It wasn't until some time later when I was a patient at the Dallas Environmental Health Center that I learned everyone with MCS was being treated the same way (i.e., told they were "depressed"; no one listening; abused by families, friends, employers, and physicians, etc.). I listened to the same story over and over again from other MCS people and realized that most of them did not know what to do to fight the stigma and physicians' diagnoses of mental illness. I knew, by talking to these people, that they were no more mentally ill than I was. They were just ill and needed someone who could understand what they were going through. I met people who were teachers, nurses, airline stewardesses, men from the Valdez Oil spill cleanup crew, a lawyer, and many other intelligent people. I wanted so badly to help them, but at that time, I could not even help myself. Somehow, I knew then that I had to do something although, at that time, I did not know what I would do.

What goals do you have?

I am planning my next book, *The Ostrich Syndrome*, which will be directed to the general public. I am hoping it will create a better understanding that all products on the market are not safe and that we must educate ourselves. Health is our responsibility and preventing illness is possible. My notes are ready to go, although I am having difficulties with finding the time to write and I am still searching for the proper way so I do not turn people off from reading it. No one really pays much attention until they get sick, so I am looking for the magic way to get attention.

I have started drafting my "Talk to Toxic Toni" column. It will be similar to "Dear Abby," only it will be about environmental issues related to preventing illness and the measures one can take when the environmental contaminants are known to be causing health problems. I am very fortunate to have physicians, a pharmacist, and many other experts to back me up when I write the column. The column has been put to pasture temporarily due to my current health problems, but I am hoping I can return to it soon.

I invented the Protecto-Zone (disability accommodation booth for those with MCS, asthma, etc.). [The Protecto-Zone is a booth that purifies air, yet lets in sound for use by those with MCS in concert halls and other public arenas.] Case Western Reserve University School of Engineering has completed this prototype for the booth. I also have goals for public education classes.

What projects have you made contributions to?

I wrote *Healthier Hospitals*, a book that has been instrumental in helping hospitals offer safer accommodations for those with chemical sensitivities. Paired with staff education, the book has been accepted by and used as a guideline for many hospitals in making environmental changes in their milieu.

Is there anything you wish you would have done differently in terms of expenditure of energy or resources?

I would never again waste my time trying to convince someone who has a mind-set against MCS (including family and physicians, employers, etc.). I have learned to go over heads and find people who are willing to listen and who can do something about the problems we are experiencing.

So many people with MCS will consume numerous hours of their time complaining to each other about no one believing them or accommodating their health needs. They share abuse stories with each other (which are all probably true). Yet these very same people complain that they are too sick to call or write to a federal representative or an agency that could address some of the difficulties they are experiencing. Disability agencies, such as the Independent Living Centers and the state's Governor's Council on People with Disabilities, are good places to start (they can hook you up with other community agencies who may be able to help). Different agencies can help with different issues.

I used to think that because I was sick and had obvious health problems (blood clotting, anemia, etc.) that everyone would believe me and help me. Not so. The squeaky wheel does get oil and we need to be heard. Make sure you spend your time wisely and don't ever permit anyone to place you on the defensive or talk you into thinking you are depressed or need dangerous medications.

As to resources, I spent too much money trying to "cure" myself of MCS. There is no cure. When, or if there is a cure, the word will travel like wildfire. Many of us have been guinea pigs and have spent money we can ill afford to spend. If I had to do it all over again, I would immediately start the organic food, home environment cleanup, and self-education on MCS, and not waste time going from physician to physician, treatment center to treatment center, test after test, etc. Meeting others at these centers, however, is what helped to validate me, educate me, and get me started on the right path. However, a word of caution: Many well-intentioned people with MCS offer medical advice to each other which may be dangerous. Some with MCS have other health problems as well and may be on medications that can interact with seemingly "innocent" cures, such as vitamin C.

Due to prior health problems, I learned to check everything out before I tried it (and I still ran into problems at times). Even though those with MCS are angry at physicians, they must find one they can trust who can supervise any vitamin taking, make sure nutritional requirements are being met, etc., and be there for you in case of other unexpected health problems, such as an erupted appendicitis or injuries caused by an auto accident.

Do you have any advice for people who have newly found out they have MCS, or who are currently at a very low point?

- Believe in yourself, your instincts and, most of all, listen to what your body is telling you. (Many times we pretend we don't hear what our body is telling us, e.g., in a store we know we are uncomfortable, but stay until we get "used to it," then react later.)

- Don't be intimidated by others in any way and don't argue with them. Give them a list of books on MCS to read and ask them to continue their discussion after they have educated themselves.

- If your MCS reactions cause you to be unable to perform life functions, such as breathing, walking, learning, working, etc., you are covered under the Americans with Disabilities Act and have a legal right to be accommodated in the workplace, in public places, etc. You must ask for this accommodation in writing (or someone may deny that you ever asked). [See chapter thirteen for more information.]

- Stop wasting time and energy looking for a magic cure. Tend to your nutritional and environmental needs instead. Get plenty of rest and avoid stress as much as possible because it exacerbates symptoms.

- Recognize that any disease has low points and bad days. Don't try to fight it. Rest or do whatever will make you feel better and remember that not every day is this bad.

- Help others. It really helps give you a sense of purpose when you feel you don't have one.

- Keep busy whenever you can. Don't sit and think about your problems.

- Limit your "complaining" time. Don't pull each other down by constantly having negative conversations. Try to talk about other things.

- Keep a diary. Be a detective and find patterns. You can discover what foods, places, etc. could be triggers for worsening your MCS symptoms.

- Educate yourself as much as you can about MCS and its effects on your body. Everyone is different and what works for one doesn't for the other. Most doctors are currently not trained at all in the area of toxicology and nutrition and you will have to bring certain facts to their attention.

- Support each other and the MCS support groups in any way you can. Do your fair share of writing and working on projects and don't leave it to just the few who have had to work so hard. There is strength in numbers. If enough people complain to the right parties about MCS, we will get help.

- Let your support group know when something they have done works. If there is no support group, start you own. Let local newspapers know of your successes and support groups. Create the "Joneses" that everyone else can follow, rather than criticizing those who don't help us.

- Educate others about MCS. Asking for accommodation and help without education won't work because people do not know what we need unless we tell them. Pretend you are listening to someone with MCS. What could they say that would convince you? Don't be unreasonable in your requests. One woman in our support group was offered a private office to prevent perfume exposure. She demanded that everyone quit wearing perfume instead. The law requires *reasonable* accommodation. We must be reasonable.

- Don't ever give up. Total failure is impossible. Keep trying. Success will come. Combined efforts will hasten the success.

- Find a support system. You need someone who will point out the positive things you can do and who will not let you dwell on the negatives. Someone who will help you find solutions.

Do you have solidarity or support with/from other activists?

I have a tremendous network of friends and activists both within the MCS community and with many who work in other disability areas. They have helped to spread the work I do (I do not have a computer with Internet access) and make it available to others. They come through for me when I need someone to lean on and get me through the difficult times. It would be great if we could all meet someday (in a safe place)! I have friends I have never met who are now my adopted family because of the strong bond between us.

Have you received any recognition for your work?

While I have never done any of my work for recognition, I am pleased to say that I received many beautiful letters and comments about my *Healthier Hospitals* book, including from the Vice President, First Lady, and the [county] Board of Health, as well as my hospital. This type of recognition and feedback is important because it lets me know that what I am doing is being accepted by the community. If this is so, then I am helping others with MCS.

Recognition comes when something I am doing "works" and someone lets me do it (i.e., being allowed to educate children in a grocery store with a contest that teaches them about safer food or having the library in our area routinely print booklists on MCS).

When I first started out, it was to convince everyone that MCS existed and was a "legitimate" disease. I thought if the controversy and discrimination would end, then everyone could go about the business of finding a cure or a pill, etc. I now realize it is not quite as simple as that (as evidenced by the long fight of the tobacco industry), and that I will not be able to "retire" from this work quite as quickly or easily as I once thought I would be able to do. It seems that my activism has also given me a reason for living and has kept me using the skills I have.

The recognition that is so important to me is the phone calls I get from people letting me know that because of the information and help I gave them, they were able to have their employers successfully create a "safe office room" so they could continue to work without further health damage. Courts have provided reasonable accommodation or excused people from jury duty. There have been too many success stories to list them all here. We successfully get these positive "stories' in the newspapers, on TV, and on the radio. We now have credibility in this entire area and, to me, that is real recognition of my work. When I came here, no one knew what MCS was and because they now know, many, many people are being helped, understood, not discriminated against, and believed. That was my goal.

Alice R. Osherman

Alice R. Osherman, 66, has been ill for more than thirty-five years. It took twenty-five years and seeing many unbelieving physicians before she was diagnosed with MCS. The first illness she had was celiac disease, a problem of gluten intolerance, which then expanded into fibromyalgia, chronic fatigue syndrome, and multiple chemical sensitivities.

While earning her Bachelor's of Arts degree in her early thirties, Osherman was exposed to chemicals while she was working on a cadaver for an anatomy course. In 1975, during a medical test, she went into anaphylactic shock, and had a near-death experience. During that experience, she bargained with her Higher Power, promising that if she lived, she would work on something important, though she did not know what it would be. She lived, and after learning about MCS, she knew that it would become her life's work.

As a gerontologist (working with the elderly), Osherman owned her own business in which she provided seminars for major corporations on all aspects of preretirement planning. However, in 1991, she had to go on disability benefits once she was unable to work in new buildings, or to tolerate clients' scented products. In 1994, she became active on a steering committee that formed the National Coalition for the Chemically Injured (NCCI); she currently is the treasurer of that coalition. Additionally, she is on the board of directors and hospital education chair of MCS: Health & Environment, and is the group leader for an MCS support group she founded in Florida.

Here are Osherman's answers to questions about her life and MCS:

What goals do you have?

To gain recognition for MCS, to help those who do not know what their illness really is, to teach them to understand it, to have doctors and hospitals learn about and accommodate for MCS, and to work on having NCCI become a voice for the MCS community.

What projects have you made contributions to?

Created the Project Information Bank for NCCI for the purpose of sharing successful projects and how to do them; and developed a seminar/program, "Making Hospitals Safer for Patients and Staff: Understanding How Low-Level Chemicals Can Affect Your Health." Organized volunteers with MCS, chronic fatigue syndrome, fibromyalgia, asthma, lupus, and multiple sclerosis to hand out information at May CFIDS Awareness Day events.

Is there anything you wish you would have done differently in terms of expenditure of energy or resources?

I wish I had started earlier and that I was able to do more. Having something worthwhile to work on diminishes my concerns about how I am feeling. Since being involved in helping others does have a positive effect, it often is my only reason for getting out of bed in the morning.

Do you have any advice for people who have newly found out they have MCS, or who are currently at a very low point?

First, know you are not alone! While it is unfortunate that our numbers keep growing, many who have been ill for some time are willing to share what has been helpful to them. It is very important to clean up your living space, and get rid of anything that might be suspect. Make lists of creative ways to use your past life experiences in a way that helps others. Transferring those skills can be very satisfying, especially when you find that what you once thought you had to give up is not really gone forever.

Do you have solidarity or support with/from other activists?

Some of my best friends are those who are very involved in working on education, recognition, and offering support and encouragement. However, many of us feel there is a need for more involvement, no matter how little, by others who are ill, as burnout among activists can be a problem.

Have you received any recognition for your work?

The recognition for my work comes when someone says thank you for the help or for just taking the time to listen. Hearing positive comments on my letters to the editor on related topics is a kind of recognition. Asking me to be part of this book is an acknowledgment that these efforts have some worth, and makes me very proud indeed.

Personal Advocacy and Activism

You can see that many people with MCS, even if they are seriously disabled, have made tremendous and important contributions to advocacy, education, legislation, and social action around the issue of environment. This chapter provides only a small sample of the people who have dedicated their energy and resources to making things better for others. There are many people not represented here because of space considerations, because I do not have contact with them, because they are not as visible, or because they chose not to write about themselves. Janet Dauble of Share, Care and Prayer, Rev. Linda Reinhardt of the Jeremiah Project, and Rhonda Zwillinger of the Dispossessed Project are just three other examples of visionaries who have made outstanding contributions. Their contributions have been invaluable, as will be the contributions that you may be able to make each day, even if they are not organized on a community or public level. Because MCS is such a demanding teacher, you probably now have skills that were developed from coping with it that can benefit others. I hope that reading about the work of this small sample of activists will inspire you to figure out where you can make your contribution. It is impossible to turn on the TV or step out of your house without seeing an environmentally related need. Perhaps as you improve and learn to live with MCS, you will be able to fill one of those needs.

Chapter Fifteen

Final Comments

Understanding the Cultural
Response—What We Are Up Against

I used to think that people with MCS got treated badly partly because their ailments were invisible. That opinion changed in November 1995 when *Life* magazine ran a cover photo of a Gulf War veteran holding his malformed child. The President's Commission on Gulf War Syndrome concluded that the veterans' problems were caused by stress in spite of the highly visible birth defects and illnesses afflicting their children, the fact that their sperm is caustic, and that their ailments appear to be even casually transmitted. Partners report the sperm to be caustic, but no one will test it.

Even an inquiry by an initially sympathetic Congressional committee did not conclude that veterans had been made ill by chemical exposures. Gulf War veterans, like Vietnam War veterans, have waited years for benefits, medical care, and a respectful audience; and their wait continues.

This is exactly the same kind of disrespect and dismissal endured by those with MCS. I believe that people with MCS are an inconvenient cog or threat to the economic/industrial system that makes decisions based on profit and "risk" assessment, and has little or no respect for life and the environment. To study this system is to experience anger, frustration, and temporary feelings of helplessness. But understanding the system also provides a realistic idea of what anyone who opposes industrial capitalism is up against. To truly understand the system, you must stop naively hoping that chemical companies will do the right thing willingly, learn to rely on yourself for your own protection, and eventually align with others to make changes through education and activist work. (See chapter fourteen for a discussion of activism among those with MCS.)

The Environment Is the Bottom Line

To my mind, neither the emergence not the overlooking of MCS is all that surprising given the way that corporate industry has treated the environment and those without power. Minorities and poor people have lived for decades with environmentally induced cancers, birth defects, and high levels of chemicals in their children's bodies. Native Americans endure political manipulation by industry and government to coerce them to accept nuclear dumps and storage facilities. Hispanic migrant workers live and work (in many cases without access to health care) in constant proximity to mutagenic, carcinogenic, and embryotoxic pesticides that threaten their health and that of their children.

Lax (1998) says that when viewed holistically and in context, "MCS is a product and problem of contemporary capitalism" (p. 737). Historically it has been possible, even easy, for middle-class Americans to hide from the consequences of our treatment of the environment. Factories are constructed in inner-city neighborhoods, toxic waste is dumped into the oceans, and outlawed pesticides are shipped to "developing" countries. Middle-class Americans leave their polluted cities to vacation in as yet uncontaminated areas. Eventually there will be no place to hide as pollutants migrate to all parts of the globe. Arctic people are storing high levels of PCBs and other hormone-disrupting chemicals in their fat tissues not because these chemicals are used in their region, but because the contaminants migrate north in water currents, air streams, and in the bodies of birds and fish who consume them by eating fish from contaminated rivers.

Often, when people suffer corporate or government-induced environmental injury it is not an "accident" per se. Much of the dumping and polluting is done illegally with full knowledge of the consequences. Jerry Mander (1991) discusses the fact that corporations have all of the rights but none of the responsibilities of individuals. In fact, corporations are "legally obliged to ignore community welfare" (p. 123) as they could be sued by shareholders if they ever failed to put profit motives first.

Although they can be sued by those who have been injured, the individuals who make the key harmful decisions are immune from any personal liability. Having the company pay a settlement is often deemed preferable and cheaper to changing damaging practices. For example, we know that cigarette companies have known for years that tobacco is addictive and that they even manipulate nicotine levels to make some brands more addictive.

Everyone needs to better understand the motivations and behaviors of economically driven institutions and become fully aware of the manipulation used to market toxic products. Often, when problems are identified, instead of truly cleaning up their practices, companies hire public relations firms to refashion their public images into environmentally concerned entities. Industry officials anticipate and head off information likely to concern citizens in regard to chemicals. Responding to just the proofs for *Our Stolen Future* (Colborn, Dunanoski, and Myers 1997), a book on the global effects of hormone disrupting chemicals, a public relations firm of a chemical corporation said:

> Quite honestly, my first reaction is that this might be a cause of genuine concern to women and the general public. Even though this issue affects virtually every segment of the population, women are affected in a direct way: the issue plays into the concern of many women's organizations that breast cancer research is underfunded. . . . Up to this point, the general media have not shown much interest in this issue. With the release of Colborn's book, however, this may change.

The memo goes on to encourage the pesticide and chlorine industries to feature women spokespersons, produce women-oriented fact sheets, and conduct media outreach to women's magazines. Is this why we now see so many women scientists on commercials? (See Appendix C for further reading.)

MCS victims are a direct challenge to chemical technology and hence to profit as usual. Having the nerve to complain that perfumes and other pollutants make you directly ill often puts you in an extremely precarious social position. After all, you are asking for building redesign (You want air?!); changes in ingredients in perfumes, paints, waxes, and cleaners (You object to inhaling degreasers into your brain tissue?!); modern farming techniques to be reconsidered (You want safe food?!); and serious research on human health effects be conducted before the production and release of any new products.

Under the General Agreement on Tariffs and Trade (GATT) any national, regional, or local legislation that can be seen as interfering with trade can be challenged. The MCS person is a challenge to the dominant company line that prescribes more chemicals, less health care, and growing corporate power. People debate whether environmental damage can be rectified or whether we have come so far that things will never get better. Chemically sensitive people are a very important part of this debate. The challenge of having to respond to MCS propels people into soul-searching, political activism, aiding others, and many other activities. It makes sense that MCS is a warning of what is to come if we continue arguing rather than acting in regard to environmental cleanup. Having MCS, you know something that is both illuminating and painful through personal experience. The world will never look the same again. The innocence of consumerism disappears once you become aware of its consequences. Having MCS means having to redesign an entire life, complete with purpose, actions, script, and props. It is probably the hardest thing you can do, but you have to do it. I hope that this book has been able to help a little with those tasks. I wish you great MCS friends, a spiritual connection, your own good purpose, a sense of humor, inner strength, and a connection to the planet Earth.

—Pam Gibson, 1999

Appendix A

Research Methodology

Between 1992 to 1997, my students have helped me to collect more than forty pages of information from each of more than 300 people with MCS in four separate data collections. Information was collected via mail surveys, and each respondent was assigned a number to maintain confidentiality; their names were kept in a locked closet accessible only to me. *For the protection of the study participants, names are no longer able to be associated with numbers or with the data.* Some people responded to all four phases, some to only one or two, and some joined the study in 1997.

Phase I

In Phase I (1993) people provided demographic data, including age, gender, length of illness, level of perceived disability, the safety level of their workplace and home, their partner status, and their partner's opinion of their MCS. Respondents also completed three standardized instruments to measure quality of life—the Herth Hope Scale (HHS) (Herth 1991), the Personal

Resource Questionnaire 85 (PRQ85) (Weinert 1987) to measure social support, and the Psychosocial Adjustment to Illness Scale Self-Report (PAIS-SR) [Derogatis 1986], a self-report scale measuring seven life domains including health care orientation, vocational environment, domestic environment, sexual relations, extended family relations, social environment, and psychological distress.

Open-ended questions requested that respondents explain how limited they were as a result of MCS, what activities they wanted to engage in but couldn't, if they had a doctor who was knowledgable about MCS, whether they believed they had ever been harmed by inappropriate medical treatment, whether they had ever received a psychiatric label for MCS, whether they had experienced any significant personal growth as a result of having MCS, and what they thought should be done to make life less difficult for those with MCS.

Demographics

A total of 305 people responded to Phase I—32 percent from the Chemical Injury Information Network (CIIN), 19 percent from an ad in the National Ecological and Environmental Delivery System (N.E.E.D.S.) newsletter, 16 percent from the ad in the *Human Ecologist*, 7 percent from the National Center for Environmental Health Strategies, 6 percent from support groups, and 2 percent from physicians' offices. Eighteen percent learned of the study from other sources (probably from others with MCS/CI), and 0.7 percent did not respond to the question asking where they learned of the study. The final convenience sample of 305 self-identified people had a mean age of 46.8 years (ranging from age 23 to age 79).

Women comprised 80.3 percent of the sample (n=245). People reported having MCS for a mean of 15 years, but did not attribute their suffering to MCS for a mean of 7.5 years. Participants included 282 Caucasians, fifteen Native Americans, three Latina/Latinos, two Asian Americans, and two who identified themselves as "other."

Respondents reported experiencing varying levels of chemical sensitivities including mild (12.8%), moderate (31.1%), severe (39.3%), and totally disabled (15.7%). The average reported decline in annual income for participants after developing MCS was $17,761 (from approximately $27,000 to approximately $9,000). Here is a profile of the total sample characteristics for 305 initial respondents and 209 continuing participants in the 1993 and 1995 studies, repectively:

Table 1: Participants with Self-Reported Sensitivity to Chemicals

	Initial 1993 Sample n=305	1995 Sample n=209
Gender (% women)	80.3	82.3
Mean age in 1993	46.8	45.0
% Caucasian	92.5*	91.9**
% Employed in 1993	31.5	34.4
% Employed in 1995		34.0
% In intimate relationship	61.3	51.7
Personal income in thousands	13.3	16.3
Household income in thousands	35.7	37.2
% Citing one sensitizing exposure	42.3	49.0
% Citing pesticide as sensitizer	27.1***	24.5***
Years with MCS (1993)	14.4	14.7
Age became ill	32.0	32.3
One-year medical costs in dollars	5,784	5,899
Total medical costs in dollars	34,783	35,258
Cost to make home safer in dollars	27,816	27,974
% Who had doctor educated re: MCS	72.1	73.7

---

* Other groups represented include Native Americans (4.9%), Latina/Latino (1.0%), Asian (.7%), and "other" (.7%).

** Other groups represented include Native American (4.8%), Latina/Latino (1.0%), Asian (1.0%), and other (1.0%).

*** Of those who had one identifiable exposure.

Hope

The Herth Hope Scale (HHS) (Herth 1991), a respected instrument used to measure hope as an index of well-being (Foote, Piazza, Holcombe, et al. 1990; Herth 1991; Raleigh 1992), consists of thirty items each scored from 0 (never applies to me) to 3 (often applies to me). The highest possible score is 90. Average level of hope in Phase I MCS respondents was 65.8. Below are the scores found with other populations by the author of the scale, Kay Herth. You can see that MCS respondents had low levels of hope compared with the adult well group and older adult populations.

Adult Well Group	80
Older Adult	72
Elderly Widowed	54

Social Support

The PRQ85 has two parts. In part 1, participants were asked to mark who they would turn to for help in ten life situations, and to mark their level of satisfaction with help received on a six-point scale ranging from "very dissatisfied" to "very satisfied." This is what people said:

Table 2: Percent of Respondents Reporting Support Needs in the Last Six Months and Satisfaction Level with Help They Received

Situation	% Answering "Yes"	Level of Satisfaction with Help Received *
Had a crisis?	62.0	4.23
Needed help caring for an extended family member?	17.4	4.26
Had a concern about a relationship with spouse, partner, or intimate other?	40.3	4.01
Needed advice for a problem with a family member or friend?	52.1	4.49
Had financial problems?	53.8	3.76
Felt lonely?	77.0	4.43

Been sick and unable to carry out usual activities for a week at a time?	55.4	4.31
Been upset and frustrated with the conditions of your life?	80.3	3.96
Had problems with work in or out of the home?	54.4	3.77
Needed someone to talk to about day-to-day personal concerns?	87.5	4.59

---

* 6 = greater satisfaction, and 1 = lesser satisfaction.

For help with these situations, respondents reported turning to various support sources in this descending order: friends in 4.7 of the possible ten situations, spouses in 4.5, professionals in 2.9, children in 2.3, other kin in 2.9, spiritual advisors in 1.6, support groups in 1.2, neighbors in 1.0, and no one in 0.6.

Perceived support was measured by part 2 of the PRQ85. The instrument has twenty-five items rated on a seven-point scale with highest possible score being 175 and lowest 25. Respondents scored between 58 and 174 on perceived social support with an average of 125.9. This score is lower than scores of other groups measured with this scale, which ranged from 139 to 149 in middle-aged and older adults. Foote, Piazza, Holcombe, et al. (1990) found PRQ means of 141.13 in forty people (32 women; 8 men) with multiple sclerosis (mean age = 48.2). White and Richter (1990) found a mean of 131 in a sample of 134 women with diabetes mellitus who were similar in age to the present sample.

Women reported higher levels of perceived social support than did men. Women's average score was 127.7 and men's was 118.6. People who were more fatigued reported lower levels of social support. Those whose health had improved in the last two years had higher levels of support than those who had worsened; those who said they had improved in their health had a mean of 131.18, and those who reported deterioration had a mean of 119.69. Neither severity nor length of illness was related to perceived social support.

Part of the problem with maintaining relationships had to do with barriers that were created due to the restricted number of safe locations for social interaction. Here are the limitations spontaneously mentioned when respondents were asked how limited they were:

Table 3: Limitations of People with MCS

Item/Area	Limitation	% of Respondents (n=305)
Church	Can't attend church at all	11
Driving	Drive only in low traffic areas	14
	Drive only with air filter in car	17
	Drive only with mask or respirator	11
	Some days cannot drive at all	7
	Cannot drive at all	7
Malls	Malls only for a very limited time	21
	Malls only wearing a mask	2
	Cannot go to malls at all	25
Movies	No movies at all	8
Restaurants	Restaurants rarely	23
	No restaurants at all	19
Socializing	No one enters home with fragrance	5
	No one enters home at all	2
	Can socialize only outdoors	2
	Cannot socialize at all	4
General	Must carry oxygen at all times	10
	Cannot ever be around perfume	41
	Cannot walk outside freely	7
	Was housebound in past	4
	Totally housebound now	8

Note: These percentages were compiled from an open-ended question and represent bare minimums regarding how many people have this limitation. That is, people had to specifically mention the limitation to have it count.

Table 4: Thwarted Goals of People with MCS

Thwarted Goal	% of Respondents (n=305)
Want to work	56
Want to pursue education	25
Want to pursue hobby	33
Want to travel	22
Want to visit family	9
Want to attend church	8
Want to nurture others (e.g., attend children's activities)	4

Note: Again, these are activities specifically mentioned and represent minimums. Medical treatment is covered in chapter six, and personal growth in chapter ten.

Phase II

Of the 305 people in Phase I, 288 were willing to be involved in further research. Late in 1993, 268 of these 288 people returned surveys that explored how people had become sensitive, their occupation at the time, the consequences for their work, whether they had moved, how much money they spent on health care and cleaning up their residence, whether they had applied for workers' compensation or disability benefits and whether it was granted, how they were treated by family members, and whether or not they had children. Women without children were asked if MCS had anything to do with their decision not to have children. Respondents were also asked about the number of medical and psychological providers they had seen and how they had been treated. Final questions dealt with whether they had ever been housebound, if their health had improved, and the results of any treatments they had tried.

Of the 268 Phase II respondents, 135 believed they had been made sensitive by one identifiable exposure, 64 said that they had not, and 67 did not know. The most commonly cited exposure thought to initiate MCS was pesticide (n=35) followed by remodeling (n=13) and workplace renovations (n=8). Listed below are the chemical exposures thought by respondents to have caused their chemical sensitivity in the 135 people who blamed one exposure. Exposures are listed as respondents described them. If MCS was attributed to renovations without specifying chemicals, it is listed as such. If carpeting was specified, then the exposure is listed as carpet. An exposure was listed as remodeling even if it occurred in the workplace if it involved purchasing new items, such as furniture, carpet, and paint. If actual construction was involved, then it was listed as renovations. Many people felt that they had become ill from a long series of exposures rather than as a result of one identifiable occurrence, and they are not listed in this table.

Table 5: Chemical Exposures Reported to Cause Chemical Sensitivity in 209 People

Exposures in combination with poor ventilation (sick building)	n
Remodeling	5
Trichlorethylene	5
Duplicating chemicals	2
Dust control product	1
Herbicide trifluralin for cotton	1
Photochemicals	1
Photochemicals and exhaust fumes	1
Photocopy, remodeling, and pesticides	1
Exposures alone	
Pesticides	35
Remodeling, and/or new carpet	13
Workplace renovations	8
Formaldehyde	7
Anesthesia	4
Diesel fuel oil	3
Carbon monoxide	2
Natural gas	2
Paints, varnishes, turpentine	2
Poor ventilation (no specific chemicals mentioned)	2
Aerosol spray	1
Acrulein	1
Air freshener	1
Amalgam dental work	1
Antibiotic use	1
Boiler room spill (ethanol and glycol)	1
Bus fumes	1
Carpet cleaner with benzene butyl compound added	1

Carbonless paper	1
Carbon monoxide in auto (defective fresh air intake)	1
Chemicals used to clean chickens in poultry processing plant	1
Copy machine fumes	1
Electromagnetic fields	1
Fiberglass dust	1
Glutaraldehyde (used to disinfect surgical instruments)	1
Injection molding chemicals	1
Lacquer (industrial)	1
Manufacturing chemicals for prostheses/orthotics	1
Mercury from having all oral fillings removed	1
Methyl isoamyl ketone	1
MTBE gasoline additive	1
Perfumes	1
Petroleum distillate used to undercoat air conditioner in workplace	1
Petrochemicals coming through air-conditioning system	1
Rayon plant (near home)	1
Red dyes in work uniform and remodeling	1
Secondhand smoke in workplace	1
Silicone breast implants	1
Tile adhesive	1
Zinc chloride (water softener chemicals in heating ductwork)	1

Combinations, miscellaneous:

Pesticide and formaldehyde	3
Books and formaldehyde	1
Formaldehyde and linoleum adhesive	1
House fire, ammonia/bleach combination, hair perms	1
Long-term Lysol use and fuel oil spill in basement	1
Newspaper ink and bleach	1
Passive smoke and workplace renovations	1
Pesticide leak and work construction	1
Toluene, xylene, acetone	1

Table 6: Occupation at the Time of Developing MCS for 209 People with Self-Reported Sensitivity to Chemicals

Occupation	n
Homemaker	29
Secretary/clerical	24
Student	22
Teacher	17
Nurse	15
Social worker, psychologist, counselor	9
Sales, misc.	8
Owner of small retail business, misc.	7
Computer programmer/analyst/software designer	6
Health care worker (X-ray, cardiology, physical therapy, recreational therapy, independent living director)	6
Management (office, personnel)	6
Bookkeeper	5
Financial associate/planner	5
Retired	5
Restaurant worker	5
Chemist	4
Engineer (electrical, mechanical, process)	4
Factory worker	4
University professor	4
Banker or teller	3
Mechanic	3
Painter	3
Artist	2
Benefits worker	2
Budget analyst	2
Civil servant	2
Domestic	2
Farmer or rancher	2
Hairdresser	2
Journalist	2
Librarian	2
Museum worker (curator, editor)	2
Photo lab technician	2
Public relations	2
Tailor/Sewing machine operator	2

Typesetter	2
Accountant	1
Administrative assistant	1
Applications examiner for licensing land mobile radios	1
Auction clerk	1
Contractor, home renovations	1
Copy editor	1
Department store makeup artist, perfume promoter	1
Dental hygienist	1
Director of reading clinic	1
Educational curriculum developer	1
Eligibility worker, Dept. of Social Services	1
Health planner	1
Hotel clerk	1
Human resource worker	1
Injection mold worker	1
Insurance claims processor	1
Interior designer	1
Job service interviewer	1
Media instructional assistant	1
Memorial home employee	1
Minister	1
Navy program analyst	1
Office manager	1
Operation manager	1
Photographer	1
Piano teacher	1
Physician	1
Planning analyst	1
Police dispatcher	1
Private school director	1
Realtor	1
Research assistant	1
Service rep	1
Store clerk	1
Technical assistant	1
Trade organization administrator	1
Truck driver	1
YMCA desk employee	1

Of the 268 Phase II participants, 205 (76.5%) reported having lost or having had to quit a job because they were unable to tolerate the chemicals in the work environment. People spent an average of $27,816 to redo their homes. Many had moved repeatedly in search of safe homes. When asked how safe their current home was, 5 percent of participants replied that their home was "very safe," 36 percent said it was "mostly safe," 44 percent said it "should be better," 11 percent said it was "mostly unsafe," and 5 percent said it was "not at all safe."

Thirty-five of 64 women without children said that MCS had been a factor in this decision. Women had foregone childbearing because they felt that their health was too damaged to carry a child (n=10), for fear it would worsen their own health to carry a child (n=19), because medical offices were inaccessible (n=18), because of MCS-induced financial problems (n=18), and to avoid passing on chemical sensitivity to a child (n=24). Some women reported more than one reason.

(See chapter eleven for a discussion on relationships with family members; chapter six and seven, respectively, for more information on medical providers and treatments that have been tried; and chapter nine for psychological providers.)

The Disability Addendum

Of the 305 people in my initial study, 151 had applied for disability benefits or worker's compensation. In 1995, these respondents were mailed a short questionnaire asking them to detail their attempt to gain compensation.

Participants were asked several questions about the disability benefits application process, including what health labels were used on their applications, whether disability benefits were granted, under what label(s) disability benefits were granted, what medical evidence was used, whether they used legal representation, how long the process took, what evidence they thought was most helpful in court (if granted), and what obstacles they encountered in the process.

Questionnaires were returned by 104 respondents (75 women and 29 men) with a mean age of 45.5. Over half (n=66) reported developing MCS as a result of one identifiable chemical exposure, and 47 people reported that this occurred in the workplace. Most (n=97) reported having already lost or left their jobs because of their sensitivities.

The Filing and Granting Process

Of the 104 people who filed for disability benefits, 51 had filed once, 22 twice, 20 three times, 3 four times, 5 five or more times, 1 was not sure, and

2 did not answer this question. (Appeals and hearings were counted as additional filings for the purposes of this study.) Fifty-nine participants were awarded disability benefits, 13 were denied at the time of the study, cases for 31 individuals were still pending, and one response was unclear. Of the 59 people who received disability income, 29 were awarded on first petition. The average cost of obtaining disability benefits was $2,060, it took an average of twenty-three months to obtain, and the average award was $12,702.

People used a wide variety of labels in the application process: some used MCS-related conditions (48 people filed under labels such as multiple chemical sensitivity, environmental illness, toxic encephalopathy, and sick building syndrome); some filed under other diagnoses, even though MCS was their primary health problem (n=23); and 29 people used a combination of MCS and other labels. These additional labels included psychiatric problems (n=11), respiratory illness (n=10), musculoskeletal dysfunction (n=7), chronic fatigue immunodeficiency syndrome (CFIDS) (n=5), immune disorders (n=4), circulatory problems (n=3), gastrointestinal disorders (n=3), and others (n=17). Types of medical evidence provided by filers for disability benefits are presented below. Most commonly submitted test results were blood work (primarily immune panels and blood screen for chemicals) and brain scans.

Table 7: Medical Evidence Included in Application for Disability Compensation

Procedure	n
Any Type of Blood Work	55
Immune Panel	40
Blood Screen for Chemicals	27
Viral Tests	6
Chemical Antibodies	5
Autoimmune Antibodies	3
Activated Lymph Profile	2
Cholinesterase Level	1
Other Blood Work	7
Any Type of Brain Scan	22
MRI	10
SPECT Scan	8
PET Scan	2
CT Scan	1

Allergy Tests	11
Neuropsychological Examination	9
EEG	8
EEG with Evoked Potentials	7
Challenge/Provocation Neutralization Testing	6
Chemicals in Fat Tissue	3
Liver Profile	3
Pulmonary Function Tests	2
Thyroid Tests	2
Hepatitis	1
Double Blind Booth Test	1
Other	8

Attorneys represented 60 people in the filing process, and 44 people represented themselves. Of the 29 people who were granted disability benefits on their first petition, 10 used the aid of attorneys, and 19 did not. Those who did use attorneys had to search extensively for someone educated or experienced regarding MCS. One respondent said, "I approached over twenty lawyers—none which would accept my case, though most said I had a case and should keep trying!"

The labels under which disability compensation was granted are presented below. The primary category under which compensation was granted was MCS; psychiatric categories were second.

Table 8: Labels Under Which Disability Compensation Was Granted

Labels	n
MCS Related*	44
Psychiatric**	27
Chronic Fatigue Immunodeficiency Syndrome	7
Musculoskeletal	3
Circulatory	2
Immune Related	2
Respiratory	1
GI	0

| Did Not Know | 9 |
| Other | 10 |

---

* Includes labels such as multiple chemical sensitivity, environmental illness, toxic encephalo-pathy, sick building syndrome, sensitivity to fumes, multiple allergies, chemical allergy, multiple hypersensitivities, etc.

** Psychiatric labels include: depression (n=7), posttraumatic stress disorder (n=4), conversion disorder (n=2), schizophrenia (n=2), somatoform disorder (n=2), anxiety disorder (n=2), affective disorder (n=2), schizoid personality disorder (n=1), dementia (n=1), "emotional" (n = 1), global assessment of functioning scale = 50 (n=1), and unspecified psychiatric (n=2).

Phase III

In 1995, the two-year follow-up study (Phase III) collected information from the 209 people who could be contacted. Respondents were again asked about employment, partner status, and income, and asked to complete three instruments of measures of life satisfaction—the Satisfaction With Life Scale (SWLS) (Diener, Emmons, Larsen, et al. 1985), the Life Satisfaction Index Z (LSIZ) (adapted from Neugarten, Havighurst, and Tobin's 1961 Life Satisfaction Index A, as cited by Wood, Wylie, and Sheafor 1969), and the Congruity Life Satisfaction Measure (CLS) (Meadow, Mentzer, Rahtz, et al. 1992).

In addition, I designed a measure that looked at activism, and asked further questions about the accessibility of medical help. One open-ended Phase III question related to how the person's identity had been affected by having MCS. Demographics of this sample are included in Table 1 along with the Phase I sample. Satisfaction with life was generally low. Activism results were as follows:

Scores on the activism scale ranged from 0 to the highest possible score of 18. When given 1 point for each item, the average activism score for this sample was 6.9 on the MCS Activism Scale, which means that people had been involved in an average of seven of the listed activities. Most people had done personal reading (n=207), and more than half had attended support groups (n=117). Table 9 lists the percentage of respondents who engaged in each activity. Level of activism was not significantly related to age, gender, income, length of illness, or course of illness. Activism was positively related to education (with more educated people being more involved in activism), severity of condition (with people more severely injured engaging in higher levels of activism), and with having lived in unusual circumstances, such as a tent, trailer, porch, or RV. Activism was negatively related to working outside of the home (with people able to work being less active than those unable to work). This is probably because they had less available time for activism.

People's efforts were concentrated toward educating the public about chemicals in ambient air, helping to pass legislation to protect the public from the negative effects of common chemicals, mandating education of medical personnel in regard to toxicology, improving health care service delivery for people with chemical sensitivities, and acquiring both recognition of the condition chemical sensitivity/ injury in the mainstream medical community and training physicians regarding treatment.

Table 9: MCS Activism Scale Results in a Sample of 209 People with Self-Reported MCS/CI

Sometimes having an illness or a disability leads to involvement with others around educational or advocacy issues. In response to your condition, have you:

	% Answering Yes
1. Done personal reading of books, articles, newsletters, or other materials to educate yourself regarding MCS/CI?	99
2. Joined an organization that published a newsletter that dealt with MCS/CI (e.g., CIIN, HEAL, NCEHS, NYCAP, etc.)?	84.2
3. Supported other people with MCS/CI in a nonprofessional capacity?	89.5
4. Attended any meetings of a support group?	56
5. Taken an active role in a support group?	43.5
6. Written an article for a newsletter/publication?	36.8
7. Engaged in letter-writing campaigns in relation to MCS-related issues?	56
8. Organized other citizens to take a stand on an environmental issue that was related to MCS?	32.1
9. Been an officer of a support/advocacy group for those with MCS/CI?	23
10. Spoken publicly about MCS-related issues?	34.9
11. Done a media interview in relation to MCS?	28.7
12. Advocated for legislation beyond letter writing that would affect those with MCS?	22.5

13. Engaged in original research (data gathering and collating and reporting) in relation to environment or MCS?   32.5

14. Started/headed a local advocacy or support group for MCS?   18.2

15. Worked with others with MCS in a professional capacity (as a physician, consultant, counselor, etc.)?   15.3

16. Edited a newsletter or publication devoted to MCS/environmental issues?   12.9

17. Written a book/technical report on the topic of MCS/environment?   9.1

18. Started/headed a national advocacy/educational/ support group for MCS?   4.8

Phase IV

Some new people were added to the study in Phase IV and data were collected at this point from 254 people. Again, demographics were collected, but this survey dealt primarily with the types of chemicals people reacted to and the kinds of reactions they experienced. In addition, the Sickness Impact Profile (SIP) (Bergner, Bobbitt, Kressel, et al. 1976; Bergner, Bobbitt, Pollard, et al., 1976) was used to measure illness-engendered dysfunction in everyday life. The SIP looks at respondents' assessment of their limitations in functioning that are caused by illness. Patrick and Deyo (1989) summarized the literature on the use of the SIP with a number of chronic illnesses.

Comparing my data with that of Patrick and Deyo, we find that MCS respondents demonstrated more dysfunction than patients with angina, Crohn's disease, rheumatoid arthritis, chronic lower back pain, and oxygen dependent chronic obstructive pulmonary disease. The only conditions in Patrick and Deyo's data bank showing more dysfunction than MCS on the SIP are non-responding chronic pain and amyotrophic lateral sclerosis.

The most serious problems for MCS respondents from my study were shown in the categories of work, alertness behavior, and recreation and pastimes. Considerable impairment was also shown on sleep and rest, social interaction, home management, emotional behavior, and mobility. (See Gibson, Rice, Dowling, et al. 1997 for more information.) The details of the Phase IV data collection are in the process of being revised for a nursing journal.

James Madison University MCS/CI Research Team Publications

Journal Articles

Gibson, P. R. 1999. "Social Support and Attitude Toward Health Care Delivery as Predictors of Hope in People with Multiple Chemical Sensitivity." *Journal of Clinical Nursing* 8(3):275–283.

Gibson, P. R., J. Cheavens, and M. L. Warren. 1998. "Social Support in People with Self-Reported Sensitivity to Chemicals." *Research in Nursing & Health* 21(2):103–115.

Gibson, P. R. 1997. "Multiple Chemical Sensitivity, Culture and Delegitimization: A Feminist Analysis." *Feminism & Psychology* 7(4):475–493.

Gibson, P. R., J. Cheavens, and M. L. Warren. 1996. "Multiple Chemical Sensitivity/Environmental Illness and Life Disruption." *Women & Therapy* 19:63–79

Gibson, P. 1993. "Multiple Chemical Sensitivities/Environmental Illness: Invisible Disabilities." *Women and Therapy* 14:171–185. Also printed as a chapter in M. E. Willmuth and L. Holcomb, eds. *Women with Disabilities: Found Voices*. 1993. New York: Hayworth Press.

Conference Presentations

Gibson, P. R. 1999. Failing to Accommodate Sensitive Populations: Individual and Cultural Consequences. In M. Lamielle, chair, *Worker Power, Health, and Accommodation in a Global Economy*. Symposium delivered at the joint APA/NIOSH Conference on Work, Stress, and Health '99: Organization of Work in a Global Economy March 11-13, Baltimore, MD.

Gibson, P. R., M. A. White, and A. Earehart. 1998. Integrating Chemical Stressors into Paradigms for Women's Health. In R. Ackerman, chair, *Chemical Exposure and Women's Health*. Symposium delivered at the 106th Annual Convention of the American Psychological Association, August 15-18, San Francisco, CA.

Gibson, P. R., J. M. Lane, S. Ostroff, and L. Placek. 1998. Disability-Induced Identity Changes in People with Multiple Chemical Sensitivity. Poster delivered at the 22nd National Conference, Association for Women in Psychology, March 5-8, Baltimore, MD.

Gibson, P. R. 1997. Multiple Chemical Sensitivity, Illness and Culture: On the Margins of Health Care. In P. Gibson, chair, *Marginalized Health Problems and Women: Fibromyalgia, CFIDS, and Chemical Sensitivity*. Symposium delivered at the 105th Annual Convention of the American Psychological Association, August 15-19, Chicago, IL.

Gibson, P. R., V. M. Rice, E. Dowling, D. B. Stables, and M. Keens. 1997. The Phenomenology of Multiple Chemical Sensitivity at Four Levels of Severity. In P. Gibson, chair, *Multiple Chemical Sensitivity: An Emerging Social, Environmental and Medical Issue.* Symposium delivered at the 105th Annual Convention of the American Psychological Association, August 15-19, Chicago, IL.

Gibson, P. R., M. A. White, and V. M. Rice. 1997. Life Satisfaction in People with Invisible Disabilities: Chemical Sensitivity/Chemical Injury. Poster delivered at the 21th National Conference, Association for Women in Psychology, March 6-9, Pittsburgh, PA.

Gibson, P. R., V. M. Rice, and D. M. Stables. 1997. Invisible Disabilities and Social Action: The Case of Multiple Chemical Sensitivity. Poster delivered at the 21th National Conference, Association for Women in Psychology, March 6-9, Pittsburgh, PA.

Gibson, P. R. 1996. Measuring Adjustment to Illness in People with Multiple Chemical Sensitivity. Poster delivered at the Annual Meeting of the Southeastern Psychological Association, Norfolk, Virginia, March 20-23.

Engel, L. R., P. R. Gibson, M. E. Adler, and V. M. Rice. 1996. Unmet Medical Needs in People with Self-Reported Multiple Chemical Sensitivity. Poster delivered at the Annual Meeting of the Southeastern Psychological Association, Norfolk, Virginia, March 20-23.

Crowley, C., and P. R. Gibson. 1995, March. Chemical Sensitivity: People, Controversies, Legalities. Poster delivered at the Annual Meeting of the Southeastern Psychological Association, Savannah, Georgia, March 22-25.

Cheavens, J., P. R. Gibson, and M. L. Warren. 1994. Social Support and Isolation in People with Multiple Chemical Sensitivities. Paper delivered at the First Annual Conference of the Southern Regional Chapter of the Association for Women in Psychology, Hilton Head, South Carolina, October 28-30.

Gibson, P. R., J. Cheavens, and M. L. Warren. 1994. Chemical Sensitivity/Chemical Injury: Life Impacts. Paper delivered at the American Psychological Association's Conference: "Psychosocial and Behavioral Factors in Women's Health: Creating an Agenda for the 21st Century" May 12-14, Washington, DC.

Cheavens, J., P. R. Gibson, M. L. Warren, and D. Pasquantino. 1993. Chemical Sensitivities: Patients' Views for Improved Access in a Technological Society. Poster delivered at the Annual Virginia Women's Studies

Association Conference: Women and Information Technology, James Madison University, Harrisonburg, VA.

Gibson, P. R., M. L. Warren, D. Pasquantino, and J. Cheavens. 1993. Limitations and Thwarted Goals for People with Chemical Sensitivities. Poster delivered at the Annual Virginia Women's Studies Association Conference: Women and Information Technology, James Madison University, Harrisonburg, VA.

Appendix B

Product Sources

Multiple Product Companies

Bio-Designs, c/o Allergy Resources, 557 Burbank St., Suite K, Broomfield, CO 80020. Phone: 303-438-0600.
   Water and air purifiers, bedding, supplements, personal care, cleaning, books, foods.

The Cutting Edge Catalog, P.O. Box 5034, Southampton, NY 11969. Phone: 800-497-9516; 516-287-3813 (NY Metro); Fax: 516-287-3112; e-mail: cutcat@cutcat.com; Website:www.cutcat.com
   Water and air purifiers, EMF detectors, radon and water test kits, Bau-Biologie Correspondence Course, books, other.

The Dasun Company, P.O. Box 668, Escondito, CA 92033. Phone: 800-433-8929.
   Organic fabric, zeolite, Golden Karre grapefruit seed extract cleansing solution.

Environmentally Sound Products, P.O. Box 214, 167 Main St., Eldred, PA 16731. Phone: 800-886-5432; Fax: 814-225-9922

Has cleaners (Citra Solv, Cloverdale), recycled paper products, cellulose bags, radon tests, EMF detector, and other handy things.

Harmony (formerly Seventh Generation), 360 Interlocken Blvd., Suite 300 Broomfield, CO 80021. Phone: 800-869-3446; Fax: 800-456-1139.

Harmony has laundry, dish, and toilet cleaners as well as recycled paper products like paper towels, napkins, tissues, and toilet paper. Harmony also carries energy-saving household products, natural cottons, and garden items. Be sure to read the details about each product. Detergents are coconut-oil based and nonfragranced, but the description of dishwasher detergent says "Seventh Generation dishwashing detergent does still contain a petroleum-based cleaning agent yet we feel this is a small price to pay for a phosphate and chlorine-free product that really works." Catalog is glossy, printed on recycled paper that contains 10% post-consumer waste.

The Living Source, P.O. Box 20155, Waco, TX 76702. Phone: 800-662-8787; 254-776-4878.

AFM paints, Denny Foil moisture and vapor barrier, personal care products, air purifiers, filter media.

National Ecological and Environmental Delivery System (N.E.E.D.S.), 527 Charles Ave. Suite 12-A, Syracuse, NY 13209. Phone: 800-634-1380; Fax: 315-488-6336.

Has a variety of supplements, personal care products, air and water filters, and you may be able to rent at first to test your tolerance of a particular filter. Be sure to investigate product ingredients for yourself.

Real Goods, 555 Leslie Street Ukiah, CA 95482-5576. Phone: 1-800-762-7325; e-mail: realgood@realgoods.com; Website: http://www.realgoods.com

Real Goods sells household items, energy-saving devices, solar power equipment, and books on building and alternative energy. Glossy catalog, comes often, mailing list is sold to others.

Safer Alternatives, P.O. Box 491663, Redding, CA 96049-1663. Phone: 530-243-1352; e-mail: safer@c-zone.net

Air purifiers, zeolite, cleaning and personal care (Granny's), cotton pillows, AFM paints.

Terresentials, 2650 Old National Pike, Middletown, MD 21769-8817. Phone: 301-371-7333.

Truly nontoxic hair and skin care, soap, makeup, books, pet care, shower filters, EMF meters. Clean, recycled, soy-based ink catalog. Small company with true environmental interest.

Tomorrow's World, 194 West Ocean View Avenue, Norfolk, VA 23503. Phone: 1-800-229-7571; Fax: 757-480-3148, Outside USA: 757-480-8500; Website: http//:www.tomorrowsworld.com

Very "clean" clothing catalog environmentally speaking. Included are organic cotton and hemp clothing; leather-free footwear; organic, unbleached cotton bedding; and energy-saving household items. Catalog is nonglossy, recyclable, and they don't deluge you with catalog after wasted catalog if you don't buy.

Bedding

furnature (listed in furniture section) has available totally organic adult and crib mattresses.

Heart of Vermont, P.O. Box 612, Barre, VT 05641. Phone: 1-800-639-4123; Fax: 802-479-5395.
   Heart of Vermont sells organic bedding, towels, and mattresses, as well as futon frames. Prices for double mattresses are $1300 for organic cotton and $1600 for cotton and wool.

Janice Corporation, 198 Route 46, Budd Lake, NJ 07828. Phone: 800-JANICES; Fax: 973-691-5459.
   Has untreated and some organic cotton clothing, underwear, fabric; bedding including mattresses; soaps, etc. Offers 100 percent cotton mattresses with no fire-retardants or other processing chemicals. Prices begin at $995 for an organic twin mattress.

Organic Cotton Alternatives 3120 Central Ave. SE, Albuquerque, NM 87106. Phone: 888-645-4452; Fax: 505-268-1323; e-mail: organic@swcp.com; Website: http://www.organic-cotton-alts.com
   Produces futons, mattresses, and pillows including nursery bedding in cooperation with two New Mexico organizations that train women in job skills and buy from only democratically organized artisan co-ops.

Tomorrow's World (listed as multi-product company) has both wool and organic cotton mattresses. Prices for twin mattresses start at $460.

Building

Environmental Construction Outfitters of New York, 190 Willow Ave., Bronx, NY 10454. Phone: 718-292-0626 or 800-238-5008; Website: http://www.EnvironProducts.com
   "State of the art building products, services, & technologies." . . . "We can either discuss a particular category with you or help your designer write complete specifications for your project."

Carpeting

Design Materials, Inc., 241 S. 55th St., Kansas City, KS 66106. Phone: 800-654-6451; Fax: 913-342-9826.
Has carpets of natural, renewable sisal (a durable fiber from the henequen plant of the Yucatan), and coir (a soil-resistant fiber from coconut husks). I was told when I called the company that their wool rugs "went through the normal process," but that there were no herbicides, pesticides, or moth-resistant treatments in the sisal or coir rugs. (However, some of these materials must be treated at port of entry if they are not in sealed containers.)

Naturlich Natural Home Catalog, P.O. Box 1677, Sebastopol, CA 95473. Phone: 707-824-0914; Fax: 1-800-329-9398; e-mail: nathome@monitor.net
Carpeting with all natural fibers, no formaldehyde, no stain-repellent, no flame retardant, no synthetic blends, minimal glues and offgassing. No 4-PC. More expensive than conventional toxic carpet, but beautiful, and you can get samples for a fee. All wool carpets except Nature's Carpet *do* have mothproofing added in the manufacturing process to qualify for the label "New Zealand Wool." Also has cork, linoleum, sea grass floor coverings, natural paint, and bedding including wool comforters and organic sheets.

Nature's Carpet from Colin Campbell & Sons, 1428 West 7th Avenue, Vancouver, BC V6H 1C1 Canada. Phone: 800-667-5001 or 604-734-2758; Fax: 604-734-1512; e-mail: showroom@colcam.com; Website: www.colcam.com
Untreated carpets. The cleanest carpet I am aware of. Targeted to chemically sensitive persons with no mothproofing, dyes or added chemicals. Backing is natural latex from rubber trees. The company says that the carpet never comes in contact with chemical pollutants in the manufacturing process (from sheep to finished carpet).

Note: AFM makes a product that can be used to seal carpets of questionable safety called AFM Carpet Seal. (See AFM Enterprises under paints.)

Carpet Testing

Anderson Laboratories Inc., P.O. Box 323, West Hartford, VT 05084.
Carpet testing. Videotape of mice exposed to carpet, fragrance, school air.

Children's Products

Natural Baby Catalog, 7835 Freedom Ave., NW, Suite 2, North Canton, OH 44720-6907. Phone: 1-800-388-BABY.

Has cotton (some organic) baby clothing and wooden toys among other things.

Cleaning Products

<u>Allens Naturally</u>, P.O. Box 514, Farmington, MI 48332-0514. Phone: 734-453-5410, 800-352-8971; Fax: 734-453-8325.

Allens products are biodegradable, use no animal ingredients, are not tested on animals, are free of dyes and perfumes, have recyclable containers, and are made in the U.S. They also offer a money-back guarantee if you are not satisfied, they are economical, and list all the ingredients for the products in their catalog. They offer laundry detergent (liquid and powder), fabric softener, glass cleaner, multipurpose spray cleaner, dishwashing liquid, dishwasher detergent, all-purpose cleaner, and fruit and vegetable wash. It is preferable, of course, to buy organic produce. But if and when you do use commercial produce, the vegetable wash will remove the *surface (and only the surface)* pesticides. The company does use some controversial ingredients. Their all-purpose cleaner contains: water, Cocamide DEA, and borax.

<u>Bon Ami</u>, which is available in most local stores, makes three products—cleaner in a round container made of a synthetic detergent and feldspar (the "gold" can usually sold at the grocery store), cleaning powder made of soap flakes and feldspar (in a rectangular container), and cleaning cake (same as the cleaning powder). These are tolerable to most people with severe sensitivities and can be used for scouring bathrooms, counters, stoves, pots and pans. Lynn Bower suggests using the cleaning cake for windows, and buffing off the film with a cotton cloth before it dries. You might prefer the rectangular container without the synthetic detergent.

<u>Ecover, Inc.</u>, P.O. Box 2205, Placerville, CA 95667. Phone: 530-295-8400; Fax: 530-295-8404.

Ecover is not sold through a catalog, but in stores. These products are biodegradable, are produced in an ecologically sound factory in Belgium, and come in recyclable containers. They produce products for cleaning dishes, clothing, floors, toilets, and glass. Ingredients in the Natural Dishwashing Liquid are: water surfactants based on vegetable oil, whey, citric acid, chamomile, and calendula extracts, herbal extracts, preservative, and salt.

<u>Erlander's Natural Products</u>, P.O. Box 106, Altadena, CA 91003. Phone: 626-797-7004

Soaps and other products.

General Notes

Some products to explore might be Ecover, Seventh Generation, and Nature Clean. If you are really in a pinch, cannot go to a store, and need something quickly, you can call Terresentials at 301-371-7333 and ask them to help you find something. Bi-O-Kleen makes a line of products that are essentially nonpolluting, although some have some natural citrus odor. Their glass cleaner contains hard surface surfactants and emulsifiers from coconut oil, linear sulfonate, natural vinegar, and filtered spring water and it works. There is no vinegar odor, no animal testing or ingredients, no alcohol, ammonia, EDTA, nonyl phenol, coloring or fragrance. Their laundry liquid is all derived from coconut, citrus, corn, and water.

Clothing

Globalwear, 3530 Southeast Hawthorne Blvd, Portland, OR 97214-5148.
    Phone: 503-236-9699; Fax: 503-236-0753.
    Hemp and organic cotton clothing.

Hempy's Earthwise Enterprise, 917 West Grape Street, San Diego, CA 92101.
    Phone: 619-233-HEMP; Fax: 619-233-1355; e-mail: earthwise@hempys.com;
    Website: http://www.hempys.com
    Hemp activewear and travel bags.

Organic Cotton Alternatives (listed in bedding) has organic wear.

EMF Meters

Available through Cutting Edge and Terresentials (both listed above under multiple product companies.)

Flooring

Daltile Corporation, 7834 C.F. Hawn Freeway, Dallas, TX 75217. Phone: 214-398-1411.
    Large selection of floor and wall tile, including ceramic, slate, stone.

Dodge-Regupol Inc., P.O. Box 989, Lancaster, PA 17608-0989. Phone: 717-295-3400, 800-322-1923; Fax: 717-295-3414.
    Natural cork floor tile.

Furniture

furnature, 319 Washington St. Boston, MA 02135-3395. Phone: 617-787-2888; e-mail: furnature@tiac.net
Environmentally sound furniture scaled to the level of sensitivity of the customer. The company is an offshoot of a family upholstery business. Mr. Fred Shapiro described some of his goals to me which included opening a chain of stores and employing those with MCS, and starting a nonprofit to provide money to MCS research. He said, "We have to help these kids."

Shaker Workshops, P.O. Box 8001, Ashburnham, MA 01430-8001. Phone 800-840-9121; Fax: 978-827-6554; e-mail: shaker@shakerworkshops.com
Handmade wooden furniture. Beautiful wooden pieces, quite expensive.

Note: Lynn Lawson recommends sealing offgassing furniture with Pace Chem sealers.

Gardening Supplies/Pest Control

Gardens Alive!, 5100 Schenley Place, Lawrenceburg, IN 47025. Phone: 812-537-8650; Fax: 812-537-5108.
Products for organic gardening and pest control.

Hair Products

Earth Science makes Pure Essentials, a fragrance-free shampoo and conditioner; however, ingredients include sodium myreth sulfate, wheat-germamidopropyl, betaine, DEA, hydrolyzed protein, and potassium sorbate. Available at health food stores.

Granny's Old Fashioned Products makes a no-fragrance shampoo (Rich & Radiant) and conditioner (Soft 'N Silky) that most can tolerate. However, it contains laureth sulfate and hydrolized vegetable protein. Available through N.E.E.D.S. and The Living Source.

Paul Penders has a shampoo and conditioner (Dutch Salon Formula) that contain herbs and natural ingredients. It has a very mild natural fragrance that, in my experience, does not persist in the hair. But the list of herbal ingredients is very long and you will have to check it for ingredients that you are sensitive to. Available at health food stores.

Simmons Natural Bodycare, 42295 Highway 36, Bridgeville, CA 95526. Phone: 1-800-428-0412, 707-574-6634; Fax: 707-574-6684.
Solar-powered company that prints catalog on recycled paper with soy-based ink. Many personal care products, some unscented.

Simple Skin Care Products offers fragrance-free shampoo and conditioner as well as a variety of other bath and personal care items.

Terressentials' (multiple product company) products are not tested on animals and contain no animal products. The company also uses no coconut-derived highly processed emulsifiers or surfactants, such as sodium lauryl sulfate, no synthetic stabilzers, like cocamidopropyl betaine, no hydrolized proteins (extracting the protein molecule can create MSG), and no petrochemical fragrances or colors. While their products are very clean, many do have essential oils for fragrance. But there is a fragrance-free hair cleanser that contains: saponified olive oil, extracts of citrus seed, nettle, linden flower, shavegrass, and natural vitamin E.

Heaters

Biofire Inc., 3220 Melbourne, Salt Lake City, Utah 84106. Phone: 801-480-0266; Fax: 801-486-8100.
Expensive but beautiful masonry heaters.

Tulikivi U.S., Inc., P.O. Box 4024, NY, NY 10023. Phone: 212-721-6722; Fax: 212-579-7432; e-mail: tuliaha@adiglobal.com; Website: http://www.tulikivi.com
Soapstone woodburning stoves, which hold and release heat over an extended period of time.

Winrich International Corporation, 8601 200th Ave., P.O. Box 51, Bristol, WI 53104. Phone: 414-857-7800, 800-755-8403; Fax: 414-857-7542.

Pellet Stoves

Woodstock Soapstone Co., Inc., 66 Airpark Road, West Lebanon, NH 03784. Phone: 800-866-4344; Fax: 603-298-5958.
Soapstone Woodburners

Macrobiotic Foods

Gold Mine Natural Food Co., 7805 Arjons Drive, San Diego, CA 92126. Phone: 858-537-9830; Fax: 858-695-0811.
Macrobiotic foods, kitchen supplies, books.

Makeup

Eco Bella offers lipsticks, eye makeup, and face powders. You can buy Eco Bella, Paul Penders, and a line called "Living Nature Lipsticks" from

Terressentials. Many health food stores also stock these products. However, sadly, I see a trend for stores to replace these healthy lines with cheaper, fragranced, and more contaminated products. In addition, I was informed that Paul Penders has reformulated their makeup to include less pure ingredients. Because of this, Terressentials will now concentrate on Eco Bella and Living Nature. Eco Bella is also available in health food stores.

Paints

AFM Enterprises, 350 W. Ash Street, Suite 700, San Diego, CA 92101. Phone: 619-239-0321; Fax: 619-239-0565. Call for information and a distributor. Low volatile organic paints. In the West, the products are carried by The Living Source.

Auro, Sinan Co., P.O. Box 857, Davis, CA 95617-0857.
No petrochemical solvents. The solvents are citrus-based and do have some odor, so you should be sure to test the products first.

Eco Design, 1365 Rufina Circle, Santa Fe, NM 87501. Phone: 800-621-2591. Natural Choice mail-order catalog. Has paints, thinners, oils from plant sources, milk-based casein paint, other household items. Be careful of many of the plant-based oils and paints, as they may still elicit reactions from persons with MCS. However, you may be able to tolerate them. Some petroleum solvent is added to some products.

Miller Paint Co., Inc. 317 SE Grand Ave., Portland, OR 97214. Phone: 510-233-4491.
Low biocide/no fungicide paints. Samples available. Contact is Gary Wellman.

Old Fashioned Milk Paint Co., Box 222, Groton, MA 01450. Phone: 978-448-6336; Fax: 978-448-2754.
Milk-based, chemical-free paint.

Other: Benjamin Moore Paints makes "Pristine" and Glidden I.C.I. offers "Lifemaster" and "Spreadmaster" as solvent-free paints.

Personal Care

Dr. Bonner's organic cleaner is 100 percent biodegradable, and phosphate-free. Simple Skin Care Products make bar soaps without added fragrance or dyes which can be purchased from The Living Source or Janice's.

Simmons Natural Bodycare, 42295 Highway 36, Bridgeville, CA 95526. Phone: 1-800-428-0412, 707-574-6634; Fax: 707-574-6684.
Solar-powered company that prints catalog on recycled paper with soy-based ink. Many personal care products, some unscented. Check ingredients, as some products are purer than others.

Terresentials (multiple product company) has a variety of products including a moisturizer called Moisture Cream made from cold-pressed African Shea butter, and vitamin E.

Pest Control

Gardens Alive!, 5100 Schenley Place, Lawrenceburg, IN 47025. Phone: 812-537-8650; Fax: 812-537-5108.
Has a wide selection of strategies for both indoor and outdoor pest problems.

Terressentials has D.E. and pyrethrum powder.

Pets

Natural Animal Health Products, Inc. P.O. Box 1177, St. Augustine, FL 32085. Phone 800-274-7387.
Cleaner products for pets.

Pressure Treated Wood

Chemical Specialties, Inc. (CSI), One Woodlawn Green, Suite 250, Charlotte, NC 28217. Phone: 704-522-0825.
Outdoor use wood without arsenic, chromium, or other EPA-listed hazardous compounds.

Purifiers/Air and Water

Ametek, Plymouth Products Division, 502 Indiana Ave. P.O. Box 1047, Sheboygan, WI 53081. Phone: 800-645-5427.
Water purifiers.

Aquathin Corp., 950 S. Andrews Ave. Pompano Beach, FL 33069. Phone: 954-781-7777 or 800-GO-2-RO-DI; Fax: 954-781-7336; e-mail: info@ aquathin.com; Website: http://www.aquathin.com
Large selection of water purifiers.

Austin Air Systems, 377 Main St. Buffalo, NY 14203. Phone: 716-856-3704; Fax: 716-856-6023.
Air purifiers.

E.L. Foust Co., Inc., P. O. Box 105, Elmhurst, IL 60126. Phone: 800-225-9549, 630-834-4952; Fax: 630-834-5341.
Whole-house and room air filters and water purifiers. You can request a HEPA that is all cotton with a minimum of other pollutants. Also sells books, face masks, and Dennyfoil aluminum reflective insulation vapor barrier, which can be used to seal off particleboard, plywood, and other substances that cause emissions.

General Ecology, 151 Sheree Blvd., Exton, PA 19341 Phone: 610-363-7900; Fax: 610-363-0412; Website: http://www.general-ecology.com
Water purifiers.

Multi-Pure Corporation, Las Vegas Technology Center, P.O. Box 34630, Las Vegas, NV 89133-4630. Phone: 800-622-9206; Fax: 702-360-3110; Website: www.multipureco.com
Water purifiers.

Pure Air Systems, Inc., P.O. Box 418, Plainfield, IN 46168. Phone: 800-869-8125, 317-539-4097; Fax: 317-539-4959; e-mail: pas@pureairsystems.com; Website: http://www.pureairsystems.com
Has whole-house air purification systems.

Reading Boxes

The Safe Reading & Computer Box Company, 4407 Swinson-Neuman Rd., Rhodes, MI 48652. Phone: 517-689-6369.
Reading boxes.

Saunas

Heavenly Heat, 1106 2nd St., Encinitas, CA 92024. Phone: 800-697-2862; Fax: 760-634-1268.

Solar Energy

Solar Energy International., P.O. Box 715, Carbondale, CO 81623. Phone: 970-963-8855; Fax: 970-963-8866; e-mail: sei@solarenergy.org; Website: http://www.solarenergy.org/
Offers publications, videos, training seminars.

Wall Covering

Crown Corporation, NA, 3012 Huron St., Suite 101, Denver, CO 80202-1032. Phone 800-422-2099 or 303-292-1313.

Has embossed cotton, wood fiber, and vinyl (not recommended) wall-covering. "Anaglypta Original" is mostly recycled paper. "Lincrusta" is made from linseed oil, chalk, sawdust, natural resins, wax, and "non-toxic inorganic pigment."

Flexi-Wall Systems, 208 Caroline Dr., P.O. Box 89, Liberty, SC 29657. Phone: 864-843-3104.
Manufacturer of Flexi-Wall, a gypsum-coated fabric that comes in a roll. Samples.

homosote COMPANY, P.O. Box 7240, West Trenton, NJ 08628-0240. Phone: 800-257-9491, 609-993-3300; Fax: 609-530-1584; Website: http://www.homosote.com
Formaldehyde-free wallboard made from recycled newsprint.

Water Testing

National Testing Laboratories, Inc., 6555 Wilson Mills Rd., Suite 102, Cleveland, OH 44143. Phone: 800-458-3330, 440-449-2525. Detailed water testing. Offers several levels of testing including a simple bacteria test, a lead test, a Watertest of 33 items, Watercheck of 74 items, or the Watercheck with pesticide option. Costs range from $35 for bacteria testing to $149 for Watercheck with pesticide testing option. Results take 12 to 15 days.

Appendix C

Further Reading and
Chapter Resources

Chapter 2

What Causes MCS?

Systemic Breakdown to Pollution:

See the following for a discussion of the effects of hormone disrupting chemicals on both animal and plant life:

Colborn, T., D. Dumanoski, and J. P. Myers. 1997. *Our Stolen Future: Are We Threatening Our Fertility, Intelligence, and Survival? A Scientific Detective Story*. New York: Penguin.

Somatization Disorder:

Contact Albert Donnay at MCS Referral & Resources, 508 Westgate Rd., Baltimore, MD 21229-2343. Phone: 410-362-6400; Fax: 362-6401 for the following handouts:

"Overlapping Disorders: Chronic Fatigue Syndrome, Fibromyalgia Syndrome, Multiple Chemical Sensitivity and Gulf War Syndrome" and "Somatization Disorder, Organophosphate Poisoning or Overlapping Syndromes of Chronic Fatigue, Fibromyalgia and Multiple Chemical Sensitivity."

Chapter 3

How Lives Are Affected by MCS

See the following two books for more in-depth narratives of life with MCS:

Zwillinger, R. 1997. *The Dispossessed: Living with Multiple Chemical Sensitivities*. Paulden, AZ: The Dispossessed Project. P.O. Box 402, 885 Gina Marie Blvd, Paulden, AZ 86334-0402.

McCormick, G. 2000. *Living with Multiple Chemical Sensitivities: Narratives of Coping*. Forthcoming from MacFarland.

Zwillinger's book is a photoessay that may do more toward demonstrating the life conditions of those with MCS than any words can. McCormick's forthcoming book tells the very interesting life stories of people with MCS in depth. (I read the book when I wrote its forward.)

Chapter 4

Making Your Home Safe

Relocation

You can purchase Johnson's twelve-page relocation booklet for $3, or the entire 9/18/96 booklet for $10. The cost to order all five of Johnson's newsletters that summarize her research on MCS treatments (described in chapter six) is $13 for MCS patients with severe financial difficulty, $16 for other MCS patients, and $25 for health care providers. Although newsletters are available individually, I suggest you purchase them all because it doesn't cost much more and there is a lot of good information in each one on treatment options. You can obtain these newsletters by sending your name and address and payment to: MCS Information Exchange, 2 Oakland Street, Brunswick, ME 04011.

Books

Davis, A. N., and P. E. Schaffman. 1996. *The Home Environmental Sourcebook: 50 Environmental Hazards to Avoid When Buying, Selling, or Maintaining a Home*. New York: Henry Holt and Company.

Goldman, B. A. 1991. *The Truth about Where You Live: An Atlas for Action on Toxins and Mortality*. New York: Times Books.

Pinsky, M. 1995. *The EMF Book: What You Should Know About Electromagnetic Fields, Electromagnetic Radiation, and Your Health*. New York: Warner Books.

Scher, L., and C. Scher. 1996. *Finding and Buying Your House in the Country*. fourth Edition. Chicago, IL: Real Estate Education Company.

Weinhold, B. 1997. *Rating Guide to Environmentally Healthy Metro Areas*. Animas Press, P.O. Box 9094, Durango, CO 81302-9094. Available from Animas Press, P.O. Box 9094, Durango, CO 81302-9094.

Carpet

"EPA Poisons EPA: My Sister's Story," 1997. Video of the EPA carpet debacle by Terese Svoboda. Available from Svoboda/Bull Productions, 56 Ludlow St., New York, NY 10002. e-mail: sbull@el.net

Carpet testing and videotapes of mice reacting to carpet (and perfume and school air) are available from Anderson Laboratories, P. O. Box 323, West Hartford, VT 05084. Fax: 802-295-7648. Booklet on carpet issues $15.

Building/Creating a Safe Home

Kourik, R. 1986. *Designing and Maintaining Your Edible Landscape Naturally*. Santa Rosa, CA: Metamorphic Press.

Marinelli, J., and P. Bierman-Lytle. 1995. *Your Natural Home*. New York: Little Brown.

Pearson, D. 1996. *The Natural House Catalog*. New York: Fireside.
This book is a broad overview of environmentally friendly buildings, products, organizations, and resources. Extensive resource list, e.g., there are sixty-seven companies listed just for paint.

Rousseau, D. 1997. *Healthy by Design: Building and Remodeling Solutions for Creating Healthy Homes*. Point Roberts, WA: Hartley & Marks.
Described as an "architect in a book" how-to manual for siting, heating, ventilating, water, materials, finishes, etc.

Rea, W. J., and J. Enwright. 1988. *Your Home, Your Health, & Well-Being: You Can Design or Renovate Your House or Apartment to Be Free of Outdoor and*

Indoor Pollution. Berkeley, CA: Ten Speed Press.
Covers material, hazards, design, and other topics.

Rousseau, D., and Wasley, J. 1997. *Healthy by Design: Building and Remodeling Solutions for Creating Healthy Homes*. Point Roberts, WA: Hartley & Marks.

Note: All of the above listed books for chapter four are available through Terressentials, 2650 Old National Pike, Middletown, MD 21769-8817. Phone: 301-371-7333.

Bower, L. M. 1995. *The Healthy Household*.

Bower, J. 1997. *The Healthy House: How to Buy One, How to Build One, How to Cure a Sick One*.

Bower, J. 1997. *Healthy House Building: A Design and Construction Guide*.

Bower, J. *Understanding Ventilation: How to Design, Select, and Install Residential Ventilation Systems*.

"Your House, Your Health: A Non-Toxic Building Guide" (VHS video).

Note: The Bower books and the VHS video are available from The Healthy House Institute, 430 North Sewell Road, Bloomington, IN 47408. Phone: 812-332-5073; Website:http//:www.hhinst.com/
    A new magazine, *Natural Home*, is an ongoing source for environmentally friendly living. Debra Lynn Dadd is on the Editorial Advisory Board. Contact them at 201 E. Fourth St., Lovelend, CO 80537-5655. Phone: 800-272-2193; Fax: 970-667-8317; e-mail: naturalhome@interweave.com; Website: www.naturalhomemag.com

Personal Care:

Winter, R. 1989. *Consumer Dictionary of Cosmetic Ingredients. Third Revised Edition*. New York: Crown Publishing.

Cleaning and Household

Lynn Dadd, D. L. 1990. *Nontoxic, Natural, and Earthwise*. New York: Putnam.

Berthold-Bond, A. 1999. *Better Basics for the Home: Simple Solutions for Less Toxic Lifestyle*. New York: Three Rivers Press.

Berthold-Bond, A. 1990. *Clean & Green*. Woodstock, NY: Ceres Press.

These books along with Lynn Bower's book, *The Healthy Household* (listed above), could make you an expert on healthy products.

Water

Ingram, C. 1991. *The Drinking Water Book: A Complete Guide to Safe Drinking Water*. Berkeley, CA: Ten Speed Press. (Available through Terressentials.)

Pest Control

Olkowski, W., S. Daar, and H. Olkowski. 1991. *Common Sense Pest Control: Least Toxic Solutions for Your Home, Garden, Pets, & Community*. Newtown, CT: Taunton Press

Stein, D. 1994. *Least Toxic Home Pest Control*. Revised Edition. Summertown, TN: Book Publishing Co. (Available through Terressentials.)

Animals

Goldstein, M. 1999. *The Nature of Animal Healing*. New York: Alfred Knopf. This is an excellent book on animal care, feeding, and healing.

Schoen, A. M., and P. Proctor. 1995. *Love, Miracles, and Animal Healing*. New York: Fireside.

Environment in General

Harte, J., C. Holdren, R. Schneider, and C. Shirley. 1991. *Toxics A to Z: A Guide to Everyday Pollution Hazards*. Berkeley: University of California Press.
Very readable guide that discusses toxins in general and offers in laypersons' language some detailed information about 118 commonly used toxins.

Lappe, M. 1991. *Chemical Deception*. San Francisco: Sierra Club Books.

Lawson, L. 1994. *Staying Well in a Toxic World: Understanding Environmental Illness, Multiple Chemical Sensitivities, Chemical Injury, and Sick Building Syndrome*. Lynnword@aol.com
Lawson's book is an excellent overview of environmental hazards and has been referred to as "The Silent Spring of the 90s."

Wilson, C. 1993. *Chemical Exposure and Human Health*. Jefferson, NC: McFarland & Co., P.O. Box 611, Jefferson, NC 28640. Phone: 910-246-4460. Orders: 800-253-2187
An excellent reference to 314 chemicals. Information can be accessed by both symptom and chemical name.

Environmental Consultants

<u>Environmental Construction Outfitters of New York</u>, 190 Willow Ave., Bronx, NY 10454. Phone: 718-292-0626 or 800-238-5008; Website: http://www.EnvironProducts.com.

"State of the art building products, services, & technologies." ... "We can either discuss a particular category with you or help your designer write complete specifications for your project."

<u>Mary Oetzel</u>, Environmental Education and Health Services, Inc., P.O. Box 92004, Austin, TX 78709-2004. Phone: 512-288-2369.

Mary provides education and consultation, and recommends products that can be used in all phases of building construction. She has seventeen years of experience.

<u>Terressentials,</u> 2650 Old National Pike, Middletown, MD 21769-8817. Phone: 301-371-7333.

Has a Green Line consultation service that allows customers to speak, via telephone, to experienced architects and educated environmental professionals about safer environments at home, work, school, or in the garden. Cost is $3 per minute and calls usually last five to ten minutes. Green Line's phone number: 301-371-7333.

Chapter 5

Diet and Nutrition

Lynn Lawson (1994) traces the process of denaturing food in chapter eight of her book *Staying Well in a Toxic World*, and I highly suggest that you read this account.

Supplements

An excellent book to help you learn about nutrition and supplements is Michael Murray's *Encyclopedia of Nutritional Supplements* (1996) by Prima Publishing, Rocklin, CA.

Preservatives

For more information on food additives, see: R. Winter. 1994. *A Consumer Dictionary of Food Additives.* Fourth Edition. New York: Three Rivers Press.

For more scientific facts on MSG, see: www.inlabeling.org.

Pesticides

A Shopper's Guide to Pesticides in Produce. Environmental Working Group's summary of the FDA's data on forty-two fruits and vegetables. On the Web at www.ewg.org.

Indirect Contamination Through Animal Products

Lappe, F.M. 1975. *Diet For a Small Planet.* New York: Ballantine.

PETA and Ingrid Newkirk. *The Compassionate Cook,* Available through People for the Ethical Treatment of Animals (PETA), 501 Front St., Norfolk, VA 23510. Phone: 757-622-7382.

Robbins, J. 1987. *Diet for a New America.* Walpole, NH: Stillpoint.

To Learn More About Food

Lawson, L. 1994. *Staying Well in a Toxic World.* Lynnword Press. (e-mail: Lynnword@aol.com). Chapter 8: Factory Food.

Organic Gardening Magazine. P.O. Box 7752, Red Oak, IA 51591-0752. Printed on chlorine-free paper. Website: www.organicgardening.com

Rifkin, J. 1993. *Beyond Beef.* New York: NAL/Dutton.

Winter, R. 1991. *Poisons in Your Food: The Dangers You Face and What You Can Do About Them.* New York: Crown.

Winter, R. 1994. *A Consumer Dictionary of Food Additives.* Fourth Edition. New York: Three Rivers Press.

The Rotary Diversified Diet

Golos, N. 1983. *If It's Tuesday It Must Be Chicken.* Lincolnwood, IL: NTC/ Contemporary Publishing Co.

Rogers, S. 1986. *The EI Syndrome.* Prestige Publishers.

Anti-Candida Diet

Chaitow, L. 1985. *Candida Albicans.* New York: Thorsons.

Crook, W. G. 1986. *The Yeast Connection.* New York: Vintage.

Crook, W. G. 1996. *The Yeast Connection Handbook.* Jackson, TN: Professional Books.

Glassburn, V. 1991. *Who Killed Candida?* Brushton, NY: Teach Services. This book describes a comprehensive program for eliminating yeast. (This book is out of print, but you may be able to find it at your local library.)

Murray, M. T. 1997. *Chronic Candidiasis the Yeast Syndrome.* Rocklin, CA: Prima Publishing.

Trowbridge, J. P., and M. Walker. 1986. *The Yeast Syndrome.* New York: Bantam.

Truss, C. O. 1985. *The Missing Diagnosis.* Birmingham, AL: C. Orion Truss.

Chapter 6

Medical Help

Environmental Units:

Environmental Health Center—Dallas at 8345 Walnut Hill Lane, Suite 220, Dallas, TX 75231. Phone: 214-368-4132; Fax: 214-691-8432; e-mail: inform@ehcd.com; Website: http://www.ehcd.com (Practice of Dr. William Rea.)

Dr. Allan Lieberman, 7510 N. Forest Dr., N. Charleston, SC 29420. Phone: 803-572-1600.

Northeast Center for Environmental Medicine, P.O. Box 2716, Syracuse, NY 13220. Phone: 315-488-2856. (Practice of Dr. Sherry Rogers.)

For other practitioners of environmental medicine contact:

AAEM, American Financial Center, 7701 East Kellogg, Suite 625, Wichita, Kansas 67207. Phone: 316-684-5500.

Books on Environmental Medicine:

The basic tenets of Environmental Medicine are explained in T. G. Randolph, and R. W. Moss. 1982. *An Alternative Approach to Allergies.* New York: Harper & Row.
The book describes Randolph's work with chemically sensitive patients as early as the 1950s and includes many case studies.

Books by Dr. Sherry Rogers:

From Prestige Publishing, P.O. Box 3161, Syracuse, NY 13220:

Rogers, S. 1986. *The EI Syndrome.* Syracuse, NY: Prestige Publishing.

Rogers, S. 1990. *Tired or Toxic?* Syracuse, NY: Prestige Publishing.

From Phillips Publishing, Inc., 7811 Montrose Road, Potomac, MD 20854. 1-800-301-8970:

Rogers, S. 1997. *Are Chemicals Making Me Sick? A Primer on Chemical Sensitivity.*

Rogers, S. 1997. *Dr. Rogers' Solutions to Common Medical Problems.*

Rogers, S. 1997. *Why Am I So Tired? Dr. Rogers' 60-Day Plan to Boost Your Energy.*

From SK Publishing, P.O. Box 40104, Sarasota, FL 34242. Phone: 1-800-846-ONUS:

Rogers, S. 1994. *The Scientific Basis for Selected Environmental Medicine Techniques.*

Rogers, S. 1997. *Depression: Cured at Last.*

Detoxification:

The following book by an environmental physician is a comprehensive guide to detoxification:

Krohn, J., F. A. Taylor, and J. Prosser. 1996. *The Whole Way to Natural Detoxification.* Point Roberts, WA: Hartley & Marks.

EPD

See Johnson's 9/18/96 booklet for a six page discussion of EPD.

Neurontin

Johnson's newsletters from 3/20/97 and 9/19/97 contain more detailed information about neurontin with excerpts of testimonials from people who had tried it.

There is some question about receiving the needed help from Dr. Seastrunk if you need to withdraw from the drug. You can contact the office of Dr. Seastrunk for a packet of information that includes two of his articles, "Kindling, Focal Brain Injury and Chemical and Electrical Sensitivity in the Production of 'Environmental Disease'" and "Neurontin for Treatment of Focal Brain Injury."

Jay W. Seastrunk II, M.D., The Center for Adolescent and Family Care, Inc. 102 E. Freeman St., Duncanville, TX 75116. Phone: 972-709-4834; Fax: 972-709-1537.

Antibiotic Therapy for Mycoplama Fermentans

More detail about this microorganism is presented in a packet of information available from Sharon Briggs, R.N., Shasta CFIDS, 1780 Marlene Ave., Redding, CA 96002

e-mail: bandb@c-zone.net

Journal Articles on Mycoplasma Fermentans

Nicolson, G. L., E. Hyman, A. Korenyi-Both, D. A. Lopez, N. L. Nicolson, W. Rea, and H. Urnovitz. 1995. "Progress on Persian Gulf War Illness-Reality and Hypotheses." *International Journal of Occupation Medicine and Toxicology* 4(3):365–370.

Nicolson, G. L., and N. L. Nicolson. 1996. "Diagnosis and Treatment of Mycoplasmal Infections in Persian Gulf War Illness-CFIDS patients." *International Journal of Occupational Medical Immunology and Toxicology* 5:69–78, 83–86.

Mycoplasma: Testing Labs for Mycoplasma

The Institute for Molecular Medicine (Nicolsons' Lab), 15162 Triton Lane, Huntington Beach, CA 92649-1041. Phone: 714-903-2900.

Immunosciences Labs, Inc. (Dr. Aristo Vojdani), 8730 Wilshire Blvd. Ste 305, Beverly Hills, CA 90211. Phone: 800-950-4686.

Medical Diagnostic Laboratory, 133 Gaither Drive, Ste C, Mt. Laurel, NJ 08054. Phone: 609-608-1696.

Hospitalization

You can get *Healthier Hospitals* from Toni Temple, Ohio Network for the Chemically Injured, P.O. Box 29290, Parma, Ohio 44129. Cost is $8.50 + $1.50 postage.

Drs. Ann McCampbell and Erica Elliot have written a list of clear hospital guidelines for responding to an MCS patient. You may be able to use it to back up your requests for safer hospital treatment. To obtain a copy, write Dr. McCampbell at 13 Herrada Rd., Santa Fe, NM 87505.

Chapter Seven

Alternative Therapies

General Reading

Alternative Medicine: The Definitive Guide by the Burton Goldberg Group (1994). The book is expensive ($60), but is a comprehensive guide to natural therapies and the treatments for various health conditions.

Acupuncture

Resources

American Association of Acupuncture and Oriental Medicine, 4101 Lake Boone Trail, Suite 201, Raleigh, NC 27607. Phone: 919-787-5181.

Reading

Gleishman, G. F. 1988. *Acupuncture: Everything You Ever Wanted to Know*. Barrytown, NY: Barrytown.

Mitchell, E. R. 1987. *Plain Talk About Acupuncture*. New York: Whalehall, Inc.

Kaptchuk, T. 1992. *The Web That Has No Weaver: Understanding Chinese Medicine*. New York: Congdon and Weed.

Chiropractic and Kinesiology

Resources

American Chiropractic Association, 1701 Clarendon Boulevard, Arlington, VA 22209. Phone: 703-276-8800. Referrals and information.

International College of Applied Kinesiology, P.O. Box 905, Lawrence, KS 66044-0905. Phone: 913-542-1801. Referrals, newsletter, information.

Reading

Coplan-Griffiths, M. 1991. *Dynamic Chiropractic Today: The Complete and Authoritative Guide to This Major Therapy*. San Francisco, CA: HarperCollins.

Goodheart, G. *You'll Be Better, The Story of Applied Kinesiology*. Geneva, OH: AK Printing. Available from Dr. Goodheart: 313-881-0662.

Martin, R. 1992. *Today's Health Alternative*. Tehachapi, CA: America West Publishers.

Valentine, T., and C. Valentine. 1989. *Applied Kinesiology: Muscle Response in Diagnosis, Therapy and Preventative Medicine*. Rochester, VT: Inner Traditions.

Wilk, C. 1975. *Chiropractic Speaks Out*. Chicago: Wilk Publishing.
Concise guide available for $2.50 from Dr. Chester Wilk, 5130 West Belmont, Chicago, IL 60641

Massage

Resources

American Massage Therapy Association, 820 Davis Street, Suite 100, Evanston, IL 60201. Phone: 312-761-2682. Information, research, and *Massage Therapy Journal*.

Reading

Lidell, L. 1984. *The Book of Massage: The Complete Step-by-Step Guide to Eastern and Western Techniques.* New York: Simon & Schuster.

Massage Magazine, P.O. Box 1500, Davis, CA 95617. Phone: 916-757-6033. From NOAH Publishing Co. in Davis, CA.

Maxwell-Hudson, C. 1988. *The Complete Book of Massage.* New York: Random House.

Mumford, S. 1996. *The Complete Guide to Massage: A Step-by-Step Approach to Total Body Relaxation.* New York: Penguin.

Mitchell, S. 1997. *The Complete Illustrated Guide to Massage.* Boston, MA: Element Books.

Thompson, S. 1989. *Massage for Common Ailments.* New York: Fireside.

Rolfing

Resources

International Rolf Institute, P.O. Box 1868, Boulder, CO 80306. Phone: 303-449-5903. Information, training, certification.

Reading

Rolf, I. P. 1977. *Rolfing: The Integration of Human Structures.* New York: Harper and Row.

Alexander Technique

Resources

North American Society of Teachers of the Alexander Technique. Phone: 800-473-0620.

Reading

Barlow, W. 1991. *The Alexander Technique.* New York: Alfred A. Knopf.

Gray, J. 1991. *The Alexander Technique.* New York: St. Martin's Press.

Feldenkrais

Resources

Feldenkrais Guild, P.O. Box 489, Albany, OR 97321. Phone: 503-926-0981. Information, training, certification.

Reading

Feldenkrais, M. 1972. *Awareness through Movement: Health Exercises for Personal Growth*. New York: Harper & Row.

Feldenkrais, M., and M. Kimmey. 1992. *The Potent Self: A Guide to Spontaneity*. San Francisco, CA: Harper & Row.

Trager

Resources

Trager Institute, 33 Millwood, Mill Valley, CA 94941. Phone: 415-388-2688. Referral, information, training, certification.

Reading

Trager, M., and C. Guadagno. 1987. *Trager Mentastics: Movement as a Way to Agelessness*. Barrytown, NY: Station Hill Press.

Polarity

Reading

Seidman, M. 1991. *A Guide to Polarity Therapy: The Gentle Art of Hands-on-Healing*. Boulder, CO: Elan Press.

Stone, R. 1987. *Polarity Therapy: The Complete and Collected Works*. 2 vols. Sebastopol, CA: CRCS Publications.

Reflexology

Reading

Byers, D. 1987. *Better Health with Foot Reflexology*. St. Petersburg, FL: Ingham Publishing.

Carter, M. 1986. *Body Reflexology: Healing at Your Fingertips*. West Nyack, NY: Parker Publishing.

Dougans, I. 1996. *The Complete Illustrated Guide to Reflexology*. Rockport, MA: Element Books.

Dougans, I., with S. Ellis 1992. *The Art of Reflexology: A Step-by-Step Guide*. Rockport, MA: Element Books.

Gillanders, A. 1995. *The Joy of Reflexology: Healing Techniques for the Hands & Feet to Reduce Stress & Reclaim Health*. New York: Little, Brown, & Company.

Reiki

Reading

Stein, D. 1995. *Essential Reiki: A Complete Guide to an Ancient Healing Art*. Freedom, CA: The Crossing Press.

Therapeutic Touch

Reading

Krieger, D. 1993. *Accepting Your Power to Heal: Personal Practice of Therapeutic Touch*. Santa Fe: Bear and Company.

Krieger, D. *Living the Therapeutic Touch: Healing as Lifestyle*. Wheaton, IL: Quest Books.

Herbal Medicine

Resources

The approach that sees herbs as a holistic form of help in context with relationship to the earth can be found in writers such as David Hoffman, Susun Weed, Rosemary Gladstar, Juliet de Barclay Levy, and others.

David Hoffman's *The Herbal Handbook* (1988) is an excellent, concise, holistically oriented little manual that could be a good intro for you. David also has a correspondence course you can take for $400 or you can purchase the huge text for $150.

Herbalgram: The Journal of the American Botanical Council and the Herb Research Foundation. Published quarterly as an educational project by these nonprofits. Contact: American Botanical Council, P.O. Box 201660, Austin, TX 78720. Phone: 512-331-8868; Fax: 512-331-1924; Website: www.herbalgram.org. Subscriptions: $25/year.

Medical Herbalism. Newsletter by editor Paul Bergner. Box 20512, Boulder, CO 80308. Phone: 303-541-9552.

Reading

Arvigo, R., and M. Balick. 1993. *Rainforest Remedies: One Hundred Healing Herbs of Belize*. Second Edition. $15.95 Available from American Botanical Council Phone: 800-373-7105; e-mail: custserv@herbalgram.org.

Brown, D. J. 1996. *Herbal Prescriptions for Better Health: Your Everyday Guide to Prevention, Treatment, and Care*. Rockland, CA: Prima Publishing.

Foster, S. 1996. Herbs for Your Health. Loveland, CO: Interweave Press.

Gladstar, R. 1993. *Herbal Healing for Women: Simple Home Remedies for Women of All Ages*. New York: Fireside.

Hoffman, D. 1996. *The Complete Illustrated Holistic Herbal*. Rockport, MA: Element Books. $24.95.

Hoffman, D. 1988. *The Herbal Handbook: A User's Guide to Medicinal Herbalism*. Rochester, VT: Healing Arts Press.

Kloss, J. 1997. *Back to Eden*. Second Edition, revised and expanded. Loma Linda, CA: Back to Eden Books Publishing Co.

Mowrey, D. B. 1990. *Next Generation Herbal Medicine*. New Canaan, CT: Keats Publishing.

Mowrey, D. 1986. *The Scientific Validation of Herbal Medicine*. New Canaan, CT: Keats Publishing.

Murray, M. T. 1995. *The Healing Power of Herbs*. Rockland, CA: Prima Publishing.

Null, G. 1998. *Secrets of the Sacred White Buffalo: Native American Healing Remedies, Rites and Rituals*. Paramus, NJ: Prentice Hall.

Weed, S. S. 1989. *Wise Woman Herbal: Healing Wise*. Woodstock, NY: Ash Tree Publishing.

Weiss, R. 1988. *Herbal Medicine*. Beaconsfield, England: Beaconsfield Publishers.

Aromatherapy

Resources

The International Journal of Aromatherapy, P.O. Box 746, Hove, East Sussex, BN3 3XA, United Kingdom

Lotus Light, P.O. Box 1008, Wilmot, WI 53170. Phone: 414-889-8501. Mail order videos, books, materials.

Reading

Cooksley, V. G. 1996. *Aromatherapy: A Lifetime Guide to Healing with Essential Oils*. Paramus, NJ: Prentice Hall.

Fischer-Rizzi, S. 1990. *Complete Aromatherapy Handbook: Essential Oils for Radiant Health*. New York: Sterling Publishing.

Grace, U. 1996. *Aromatherapy for Practitioners*. Essex, United Kingdom: C.W. Daniel $17.95.

Jenney, D. 1997. *Aromatherapy: Essential Oils for Essential Health*. Pleasant Grove, UT: Woodland Publishing.

Rose, J. 1992. *The Aromatherapy Book: Applications & Inhalations*. San Francisco, CA: Herbal Studies Course; Berkeley, CA: North Atlantic Books.

Valnet, J. 1990. *The Practice of Aromatherapy*. Rochester, VT: Inner Traditions.

Walters, C. 1998. *Aromatherapy: An Illustrated Guide*. Boston, MA: Element Books.

Homeopathy

Reading

A very detailed discussion of the principles of homeopathy can be found in *The Science of Homeopathy* by George Vithoulkas (1979), New York, Grove Press. More user-friendly introductions that include photographs and advice for common problems are listed below.

Castro, M. 1990. *The Complete Homeopathy Handbook*. New York: St. Martin's Press. $15.95.

Hammond, C. 1995. *The Complete Family Guide to Homeopathy*. New York: Penguin.

Hayfield, R. 1994. *The Family Homeopath: Safe, Natural, and Effective Health Care for You and Your Children*. Rochester, VT: Healing Arts Press. $16.95. This book is excellent for a focus on children.

Lockie, A., and N. Geddes. 1995. *The Complete Guide to Homeopathy: The Principles and Practice of Treatment*. New York: Dorling Kindersley.

Panos, M. B., and J. Heimlich. 1980. *Homeopathic Medicine at Home*. New York: G.P. Putnam's Sons. $10.95.

Ullman, D. 1992. *Homeopathic Medicine for Children and Infants*. New York: G.P. Putnam's Sons. $12.95. Good focus on children.

Flower Essences

Reading

Bach, E., and F. J. Wheeler. 1952. *The Bach Flower Remedies*. New Canaan, CT: Keats Publishing.
(This book is three volumes in one and includes Bach's "Heal Thyself" and "The Twelve Healers," and Wheeler's "The Bach Remedies Repertory." Bach's "Heal Thyself" is one of the most spiritual and inspiring pieces I have ever read.)

Chancellor, P. M. 1971. *Handbook of the Bach Flower Remedies*. New Canaan, CT: Keats Publishing.

Kaminski, P. 1996. *Choosing Flower Essences: An Assessment Guide*. Nevada City, CA: Flower Essence Society.

Kaminski, P., and R. Katz. 1994. *Flower Essence Repertory*. Nevada City, CA: Flower Essence Society.

Kaslof, L. J. 1993. *The Traditional Flower Remedies of Dr. Edward Bach: A Self-Help Guide*. New Canaan, CT: Keats Publishing.

Chapter Eight

Chronic Illness

Compassionate Models

I recently wrote a review of three new books in psychology that represent a fair and compassionate look at the effects of illness on the lives of patients and their loved ones. Although they do not include MCS, two of these three books include CFS, and the discussion throughout is relevant to all health problems. It is heartening to see psychologists take a serious interest in chronic illness from the patient's point of view.

Jenny Altschuler (1997) has written *Working With Chronic Illness*, a book for professionals working with people with illness and their families. It is very sensitively and compassionately written, and may be helpful to you in understanding the impact of your MCS on your loved ones. It also may be useful to any therapist you might happen to see for help in coping with your health.

Books on Chronic Illness

Altschuler, J. 1997. *Working with Chronic Illness*. Hampshire, United Kingdom: MacMillan.

Goodheart, C. D., and M. H. Lansing. 1997. *Treating People with Chronic Disease: A Psychological Guide*. Washington, DC: American Psychological Association.

Rippere, V. 1983. *The Allergy Problem: Why People Suffer and What Should Be Done*. Wellingborough, Northamptonshire, United Kingdom: Thorsons Publishers Limited.

Strauss, A. 1984. *Chronic Illness and the Quality of Life*. St. Louis, MO: C.V. Mosby company
Strauss has an empathic understanding regarding the experience of people who cope with illness. (This book and Rippere's *The Allergy Problem* were my inspiration to study MCS.)

Chapter Ten

Identity

Inspirational Books

One very important spiritual book from the Christian perspective in my estimation is *The Little Notebook: The Journal of a Contemporary Woman's Encounters with Jesus* by Nicole Gausseron (1995). It is a French woman's story of her relationship and communication with Jesus Christ and its influence upon her social work with homeless men (referred to as the "companions"). It is one of the few spiritual books I have read where the author does not get caught up in their own ego, but simply tells what happened to her. She shares her struggles to cope, to develop, and to make a contribution, and receives spiritual experiences of Christ that are visual, tactile, and auditory. Although some may be reluctant to believe that Christ has ongoing dialogue with anyone, she is incredibly believable, and I recommend the book for anyone who is open to developing this relationship. The book addresses some of the difficult dilemmas that people with MCS face. Unfortunately, it has gone out of print and will be difficult to find.

Gausseron, N. 1995. *The Little Notebook: The Journal of a Contemporary Woman's Encounters with Jesus*. HarperSanFrancisco.

Kaplan A. 1985. *Jewish Meditation*. New York: Schocken Books.

St. John of the Cross. 1990. *Dark Night of the Soul*. New York: Bantam Doubleday Dell. (For those who are ready for complex Christian mysticism.)

The Upanishads (Any version, but my favorite is Juan Mascaro's translation.)

Chapter Twelve

Miscellaneous Pathways

Heartwarming and Inspiring Stories

Amory, C. 1997. *Ranch of Dreams: The Heartwarming Story of American's Most Unusual Animal Sanctuary*. New York: Viking Penguin.

Amory, C. 1987. *The Cat Who Came for Christmas*. New York: Penguin.

Laland, S. 1998. *Animal Angels: Amazing Acts of Love and Compassion*. Berkeley, CA: Conari Press.

Lasher, M. 1996. *And the Animals Will Teach You: Discovering Ourselves Through Our Relationships with Animals*. New York: Berkeley Publishing.

Masson. J. M. 1997. *Dogs Never Lie About Love: Reflections on the Emotional World of Dogs.* New York: Three Rivers Press.

McElroy, S. C. 1997. *Animals as Teachers and Healers: True Stories and Reflections.* New York: Ballantine.

Schoen, A. M., and P. Proctor. 1995. *Love, Miracles, and Animal Healing: A Heartwarming Look at the Spiritual Bond Between Animals and Humans.* New York: Fireside.

Von Kreisler, K. 1997. *The Compassion of Animals: True Stories of Animal Courage and Kindness.* Rocklin, CA: Prima Publishing.

Wylder, J. 1978. *Psychic Pets: The Secret Life of Animals.* New York: Random House.

Books on Animal Communication in the Psychic Sense

Boone, J. A. 1976. *Kinship with All Life.* New York: Harper Collins.

Fitzpatrick, S. 1997. *What the Animals Tell Me: Developing Your Innate Telepathic Skills to Understand and Communicate with Your Pets.* New York: Hyperion.

Myers, A. 1997. *Communicating with Animals: The Spiritual Connection Between People and Animals.* Chicago, IL: Contemporary Books.

Smith, P. 1993. *Animals, Our Return to Wholeness.* Point Reyes, CA: Pegasus.

Summers, P. 1998. *Talking with the Animals.* Charlottesville, VA: Hampton Roads.

Chapter Thirteen

Disability

Dubin, D. 1994. "What are You so Sensitive About? Accommodating Environmental Illness/Multiple Chemical Sensitivity." *The Disability Law Reporter Service* 3(9):8–40. September.

Warnings About Perfumes

The American Lung Association has advised while discussing childhood asthma on its Web site, that "perfume, room deodorizer, cleaning agents, paint, and even talcum powder can trigger an allergic reaction." Go to http://www.lungusa.org/, go to search, type in perfume, and choose tips for children with asthma (ALA and AMA 1998).

The American Medical Association's Web page cites perfumes as exposures that should be reduced to control asthma.

GAO Report

You can obtain the GAO report free of charge from the General Accounting Office, or read a summary of it in Volume 3, Number 3 (1997) of Medical & Legal Briefs from EARN. (See Appendix B.) To obtain the report from the GAO, write to U.S. GAO, P.O. Box 6015, Gaithersburg, MD 20884-6015 or phone: 202-512-6000. Ask for U.S. General Accounting Office GAO/HEHS-97-102 (August 1997) entitled "Social Security Disability: SSA Must Hold Itself Accountable for Continued Improvement in Decision-Making" from the General Accounting Office, Health, Education and Human Services Division. I received it rather quickly just by phoning.

Disability Issues and Disability Law

Newsletters such as *Our Toxic Times* from CIIN frequently discuss MCS disability issues.

U.S. Equal Employment Opportunity Commission, 1801 L Street NW, Washington, DC 20507. Phones: 800-669-3362 or 202-663-4264 (voice), 800-800-3302 or 202-663-7110 (TDD).

President's Committee on Employment of People with Disabilities Information Line: ADA Work: 800-232-9675 (voice and TDD)

Multiple Chemical Sensitivities at Work: A Training Workbook for Working People. 1993. New York: The Labor Institute. Available from The APEX Press, Publications Office, P.O. Box 337, Croton-On-Hudson, NY 10520. Also available is a half-hour videotape "MCS: An Emerging Occupational Hazard." Both are also available from ECHO, P.O. Box 0119, Hebron, CT 06248-1119. Phone/Fax: 860-228-2693.

Chapter Fourteen

Activism

See Appendix D: Organizations to join for ways of becoming involved with other MCS activists.

Appendix D

Organizational Support

Informational Sources

It can be tremendously helpful to belong to several of the MCS advocacy/support organizations. They publish excellent newsletters that include vital information for those confronting MCS. It can also be invaluable to belong to environmental organizations that deal with either general or specific environmental concerns, such as groups that focus on pesticides. Both types of organizations are listed below. If you have trouble tolerating inks and paper, you may need to use a reading box so that you can benefit from reading printed material about MCS. A reading box is a glass box that contains reading materials and vents to the outside so that vapors are not inhaled. You can wear gloves and turn pages without making contact with the ink. You can obtain reading boxes from The Safe Reading & Computer Box Company, 4407 Swinson-Neuman Rd., Rhodes, MI 48652. Phone: 517-689-6369.

Groups Offering Information, Support, and Advocacy

Chemical Injury Information Network (CIIN), P.O. Box 301, White Sulphur Springs, MT 59645. Phone: 406-547-2255
CIIN is a nonprofit organization dedicated to education regarding the negative effects of chemicals on health. The newsletter *Our Toxic Times* is published monthly by editor and director Cynthia Wilson. Special features of each issue include summaries of recent relevant research. There is no specified membership fee, but donations are requested and appreciated to fund the publication. CIIN reviews articles in its newsletter and also allows subscribers to purchase copies.

MCS: Health and Environment, P.O. Box 1732, Evanston IL 60201. Phone: 847-866-9630; e-mail: Lynnword@aol.com
Newsletter is *Canary News*, which is published monthly by Lynn Lawson, editor (also author of the book *Staying Well in a Toxic World*). Membership is $20 yearly for individuals or families. Send to John Truskowski, 251 Kimberly, Lake Forest, IL 60045. In cases of financial hardship, send a letter or card along with what you can afford. Special services of this group include "In Your Mailbox," which provides articles and resources to people for the cost of photocopying, and a lending library of books and tapes. When you join, you also receive a resource guide packed with helpful information about coping with MCS.

Ecological Health Organization and Action Coalition (ECHO), P.O. Box 0119, Hebron, CT 06248-1119. Phone/Fax: 860-228-2693. Web site: http://members.aol.com/ECHOMCST/home.html
ECHO is an affiliate of the National Center for Environmental Health Strategies (NCEHS), and "is a statewide nonprofit advocacy, support and referral organization for people who have Multiple Chemical Sensitivity (MCS) and others who care about preventing this illness." Newsletter is published bimonthly by editor Elaine Tomko. Membership is $15/$7 low income. Membership includes a copy of ECHO's very helpful resource guide, or you can purchase it separately for $5.

Environmental Health Network (EHN), P.O. Box 1155, Larkspur, CA 94977. Phone: 415-541-5075; e-mail: wilworks@lanminds.com; Website: http://users.lanminds.com/~wilworks/ehnindex.html
EHN focuses on "the issues and developments relating to the health and welfare of the environmentally sensitive." The newsletter *The New Reactor* is published bimonthly. Membership is $25/$15 low income/disability.

National Center for Environmental Health Strategies (NCEHS), 1100 Rural Avenue, Voorhees, NJ 08043. Phone: 856-429-5358; email:

ncehs@ncehn.org; Web site: www.ncehs.org. Mary Lamielle, director. NCEHS is a nonprofit organization committed to education, research, support, and advocacy services on environmental and public health issues including environmentally and occupationally induced illnesses. Lamielle published the excellent newsletter *The Delicate Balance*, but has been focusing recently on policy and visibility efforts. The center answers inquiries regarding MCS. Membership is $15/$10 low income.

National Coalition for the Chemically Injured (NCCI), 2400 Virginia Ave. NW Suite C-501, Washington, DC 20037. Contacts: Alice Osherman, 847-776-7792 (summer), 941-756-1606 (winter); and Larry Plumlee, M.D., 301-897-9614.
Coalition of MCS support and advocacy groups in the United States.

Ohio Network for the Chemically Injured, 6179 Stratford, Parma Hts., OH 44130. Headed by Toni Temple.
Regional group that is very active in sharing, support, community education, and advocacy. Has initiated a large number of projects.

Chemical Sensitivity Disorders Association (CSDA), 5717 Beech Ave., Bethesda, MD 20817. Phone/Fax: 301-897-9614
Newsletter: *The Chemical Sensitivity Connection*. This is the Baltimore Area EI/MCS Support/Advocacy Group. Larry Plumlee, M.D., president.

Health Coalition of Western MA, P.O. Box 61114, Leveratt, MA 01054. Statewide organization engaging in education, advocacy, and support. Headed by Peggy Wolff.

Groups Offering Primarily Information and Support

Human Ecology Action League, Inc. (HEAL), P.O. Box 29629, Atlanta, GA 30359-0629. Phone: 404-248-1898; e-mail: HEALNatnl@aol.com; Website: http://members.aol.com/HEALNatnl/index.html
HEAL is a nonprofit volunteer organization designed to serve and provide information to those whose health has been adversely affected by the environment. Emphasis is on support rather than advocacy. They publish *The Human Ecologist* quarterly. Membership is $26/$18 low income. HEAL can inform you of local HEAL support groups in your area.

The Jeremiah Project, HC 1 222 Soft Wind, Canyon Lake, TX 78133. Phone: 830-935-4618; e-mail: <jeremiah@texannet.net.>
The Jeremiah Project is an "interdenominational ministry with and for people who are chemically sensitive and/or have been chemically injured. We offer worship, support, and community for people with

MCS/EI." They are also an educational organization. The newsletter, *I Am Jeremiah*, is published bimonthly by Rev. Linda Reinhardt and includes discussions of faith and coping, book reviews, and updates. Donations are appreciated to cover costs.

Share Care & Prayer, P.O. Box 2080, Frazier Park, CA 93225.
This is a Christian organization that attempts to serve the needs of the chemically sensitive through prayer, provision of uncontaminated clothing, and other services. Contact is Janet Dauble.

The American Academy of Environmental Medicine (AAEM), Environmental Health Center—Dallas, 8345 Walnut Hill Lane, Suite 220, Dallas, TX 75231. Phone: 214-368-4132; Fax: 214-691-8432; e-mail: inform@ehcd. com; Website: http://www.ehcd.com
AAEM is a professional organization of practitioners of environmental medicine (previously referred to as Clinical Ecology). It sells tapes from their educational conferences.

Political/Legal/Access Issues Relating to MCS

Organizations

MCS Referral & Resources, 508 Westgate Road, Baltimore, MD 21207-6631. Phone: 410-362-6400; Fax: 410-362-6401. Albert Donnay, president.
This organization, founded by Grace Ziem, M.D., Dr.PH, focuses on "professional outreach, patient support, and public advocacy devoted to the prevention, diagnosis, treatment, and accommodation of Multiple Chemical Sensitivity Disorders (including porphyria) ... and offer[s] referral and research services and medical literature for MCS professionals (physicians, health educators, social workers, attorneys, etc.) as well as MCS patients, elected officials and the media."

EARN, CIIN, and **ECHO** (See above) also address disability/advocacy concerns in their newsletters.

Safe Schools, 8818 Sherman Mountain Rd, Cheyenne, WY 82009-8844. Phone: 307-772-0655; Fax: 307-772-0656. Irene Wilkenfeld, president.
Organization dedicated to improving the air quality in our children's schools.

Publications

The Environmental Protection Agency (EPA) has developed "Indoor Air Quality Tools for Schools," a user-friendly planning kit for locating, preventing, and resolving indoor air problems in the schools. It can be obtained from: ConnectiCOSH, 77 Huyshope Ave., Hartford, CT 06106. Phone: 860-549-1877.

Groups Focusing On Environmental Quality

Organizations

Center for Health Environment and Justice (Formerly, **Citizens Clearing House for Hazardous Waste**), P.O. Box 6806, Fall's Church, VA, 22040. Phone: 703-237-2249. Lois Marie Gibbs, executive director.

This organization has provided technical assistance to more than 10,000 community groups threatened by toxics. It aims to help people to "assess and clean up existing problems, prevent new ones, and develop sound economic and environmental health policies." They have written a wide variety of publications, including Gibbs' recent book *Dying from Dioxin: Reclaiming Our Health and Rebuilding Democracy*, and offer training in community organizing. Membership is $30; members receive the newsletter, *Everyone's Backyard*. Also available for an additional $35 is a subscription to *Environmental Health Monthly*, which reprints selected research on health and chemical exposures.

Environmental Research Foundation, P.O. Box 5036, Annapolis, MD 21403-7036. Phone: 410-263-1584.

Newsletter is *Rachel's Environment and Health Weekly*, Peter Montague Ph.D., editor. You can receive this weekly newsletter online by e-mailing: rachel-weekly-request@world.std.com with the word SUBSCRIBE in the message. Back issues are available by e-mailing: INFO@rachel.org with just the word HELP in the message area. This is an excellent exposé of the politics and facts regarding toxics. Montague can write them faster than I can read them, and all of them are packed with information and references.

Greenpeace USA, 1436 U. Street N.W., Washington, DC 20009. Phone: 202-462-1177.

Well-known, environmental activist group that addresses toxics, nuclear waste, and a host of serious issues relating to contaminants. Annual donation of $30 for membership and newsletter *Greenpeace Quarterly*.

National Coalition Against the Misuse of Pesticides (NCAMP), 701 E Street S.E., Suite 200, Washington, DC 20003. Phone: 202-543-5450.

NCAMP has the major goal of educating communities and individuals on the use and misuse of pesticides and on alternative methods of pest control. They also advocate for policies that protect the environment from harmful exposures. Newsletter is *Pesticides and You*. Also, *Technical Report* is a monthly bulletin that chronicles NCAMP's progress, tracks government agencies, and provides scientific reviews. Individual membership $25/family $50.

National Pesticide Telecommunications Network (NPTN), Phone: 800-858-7378; Fax: 541-737-0761; e-mail: nptn.@ace.orst.edu

NPTN offers free information on pesticides including what to do in a spill or emergency, proper use/cleanup, etc. Can also take reports of poisonings. Small charge for faxed or mailed information. Phone lines open daily, except holidays, 9:30 A.M. to 7:30 P.M. Eastern Standard Time.

New York Coalition for Alternatives to Pesticides (NYCAP), 353 Hamilton St., Albany, NY 12216-1709. Phone: 518-426-8246 or 518-426-9331. Pam Hadad Hurst, director.
NYCAP is a "citizens organization committed to public education and advocacy to reduce the pesticide hazards." *NYCAP News* is their quarterly newsletter edited by Tracy Frisch. Membership is $25 (suggested)/$6 to $10 minimum poverty.

Northwest Coalition for Alternatives to Pesticides (NCAP), P.O. Box 1393, Eugene, OR 97440. Phone: 541-344-5044. Norma Grier, executive director.
NCAP has a twenty-year history of providing information and assistance regarding prevention, policy, and victim assistance in relation to pesticides. Basic membership is $25 (limited income $15). Members receive the *Journal of Pesticide Reform.* Caroline Cox, editor.

Pesticide Action Network (PAN), 49 Powell St., 6th Floor, San Francisco, CA 94102. Phone: 415-981-1771; Fax: 415-981-1991. Monica Moore, director. Newsletter is *Global Pesticide Campaigner.*

Pesticide Education Center, P.O. Box 420870, San Francisco, CA 94142-0870. Phone: 415-391-8511; Fax: 415-391-9159
President: Marion Moses, M.D.

Pesticide Watch, 450 Geary St., Suite 500, San Francisco, CA 94102. Phone: 415-292-1486; Fax: 415-292-1497. Gregg Small, director.
Newsletter is *Pesticide Watch.* Engages in community organizing in California, working with agricultural workers, people with MCS, and others.

Public Citizen, 1600 20th Street, N.W., Washington, DC 20009. Phone: 202-588-1000. Founder: Ralph Nader.

Rachel Carson Council Inc., 8940 Jones Mill Road, Chevy Chase, MD 20815. Phone: 301-652-1877; e-mail: rccounsil@aol.com. Dr. Diana Post, director. This is a nonprofit, independent, scientific organization dedicated to protection of the environment from the threat of pesticides and other chemicals. Provides resources including pamphlets and books on pesticides. For a $25 membership, you receive the newsletter *Rachel Carson Council News*, two other papers, and help with inquiries.

Appendix E

Toxicology Readings

Abou-Donia, M. B., K. F. Jensen, F. W. Oehme, and T. L. Kurt. 1996. "Neuro-toxicity Resulting From Coexposure to Pyridostigmine Bromide, DEET, and Permethrin: Implications of Gulf War Chemical Exposures." *Journal of Toxicology and Environmental Health* 48:35–56.

Amdur, M. O., J. Doull, and C. D. Klaassen (Eds.) 1991. *Casarett and Doull's Toxicology: The Basic Science of Poisons.* Fourth Edition. New York: Pergamon Press.

Ammann, H. M. 1987. Effects of Indoor Air Pollution on Sensitive Populations. *Clinical Ecology* V(1):15–21.

Aschengrau, A., A. Beiser, D. Bellinger, D. Copenhafer, and M. Weitzman. 1997. "Residential Lead Based Paint Hazard Remediation and Soil Abatement: Their Impact Among Children with Mildly Elevated Blood Lead Levels." *American Journal of Public Health* 87(10):1698–1702.

Baker, E. L. 1994. "A Review of Recent Research on Health Effects of Human Occupational Exposure to Organic Solvents: A Critical Review." *Journal of Occupational Medicine* 36(10):1079–1092.

Bang, K. M. 1984. "Health Effects of Common Organic Solvents in the Workplace." *Family and Community Health* 7(3):15–29.

Banks, E. C., L. E. Ferretti, and D. W. Shucard. 1997. "Effects of Low-level Lead Exposure on Cognitive Function in Children: A Review of Behavioral, Neuropsychological and Biological Evidence." *Neurotoxicology* 18(1): 237–281.

Brewster, M. A., B. S. Hulka, and T. L. Lavy. 1992. "Biomarkers of Pesticide Exposure." *Reviews of Environmental Contamination and Toxicology* 128: 17–42.

Briggs, S. A. 1992. *Basic Guide to Pesticides*. Rachel Carson Council. Chevy Chase, MD: Taylor & Francis.

Broughton, A., J. D. Thrasher, and R. Madison. 1990. "Chronic Health Effects and Immunological Alterations Associated with Exposure to Pesticides." *Comments Toxicology* 4(1):59–71.

Bryce-Smith, D. 1986. "Environmental Chemical Influences on Behavior, Personality, and Mentation." *Journal of Biosocial Research* 8(12):115–150.

Callender, T. J., L. Morrow, K. Subramanian, D. Duhon, and M. Ristovv. 1993. "Three-Dimensional Brain Metabolic Imaging in Patients with Toxic Encephalopathy." *Environmental Research* 60:295–319.

Carson, R. 1962. *Silent Spring*. Boston: Houghton Mifflin.

Cernichiari, E., R. Brewer, G. J. Myers, D. O. Marsh, L. W. Lapham, C. Cox, C. F. Shamlaye, M. Berlin, P. W. Davidson, and T. W. Clarkson. 1995. "Monitoring Methylmercury During Pregnancy: Maternal Hair Predicts Fetal Brain Exposure." *Neurotoxicology* 16(4):705–710.

Chaiklin, H. 1979. "The Treadmill of Lead." *American Journal of Orthopsychiatry* 49(4):571–573.

Colburn, T., D. Dumanoski, and J. P. Myers. 1996. *Our Stolen Future: Are We Threatening Our Fertility, Intelligence, and Survival? A Scientific Detective Story*. New York: Penguin Books.

Collins, J. J., J. F. Acquavella, and N. A. Esmen. 1997. "An Updated Meta-Analysis of Formaldehyde Exposure and Upper Respiratory Tract Cancers." *Journal of Occupational and Environmental Medicine* 39:639–651.

The Commonwealth of Massachusetts Special Legislative Commission on Indoor Air Pollution. 1989. *Indoor Air Pollution In Massachusetts, Final Report*.

Conservation Foundation. 1987. *State of the Environment: A View Toward the Nineties*. Washington, DC: Library of Congress Cataloging-in-Publication Data.

Dager, S. R., J. P. Holland, D. S. Cowley, and D. L. Dunner. 1987. "Panic Disorder Precipitated by Exposure to Organic Solvents in the Work Place." *American Journal of Psychiatry* 144(8):1056–1058.

David, O., S. Hoffman, J. Sverd, J. Clark, and K. Voeller. 1976. "Lead and Hyperactivity. Behavioral Response to Chelation: A Pilot Study." *American Journal of Psychiatry* 133(10):1155–1158.

David, O. J., G. Grad, B. McGann, and A. Koltun. 1982. "Mental Retardation and 'Nontoxic' Lead Levels." *American Journal of Psychiatry* 139(6): 806–809.

Davis, J. R., R. C. Brownson, R. Garcia, B. J. Bentz, and A. Turner. 1993. "Family Pesticide Use and Childhood Brain Cancer." *Archives of Environmental Contamination and Toxicology* 24:87–92.

Dibb, S. 1995. "Swimming in a Sea of Oestrogens: Chemical Hormone Disrupters." *The Ecologist* 25(1):27–31.

Dick, R. B. 1988. "Short Duration Exposures to Organic Solvents: The Relationship Between Neurobehavioral Test Results and Other Indicators." *Neurotoxicology and Teratology* 10(1):39–50.

Dudley, D. L. 1993. "Chemical Toxicity: A Neurometric Study of Changes in the Auditory and Visual Cognitive Evoked Potential in Response to Olfaction." Abstract in *AFCR Clinical Research* 41:383A.

Duehring, C. 1993. "Immune Alteration Associated with Exposure to Toxics." *Environmental Access Profiles* 3(6):1–2.

Duehring, C., and Wilson, C. 1994. *The Human Consequences of the Chemical Problem*. White Sulphur Springs, MT: T T Publishing.

Freeza, M., C. di Padova, G. Pozzato, M. Terpin, E. Baraona, and C. Lieber. 1990. "High Blood Alcohol Levels in Women: The Role of Decreased Gastric Alcohol Dehydrogenase Activity and First-Pass Metabolism." *New England Journal of Medicine* 322(2):95–99.

Gibbons, A. 1993. "Dioxin Tied to Endometriosis." *Science* 262:1373.

Godish, T. 1990. "Residential Formaldehyde: Increased Exposure Levels Aggravate Adverse Health Effects." *Journal of Environmental Health* 53(3):34–37.

Gold, E., L. Gordis, J. Tonascia, and M. Szklo. 1979. "Risk Factors for Brain Tumors in Children." *American Journal of Epidemiology* 109:309–319.

Goldblum, R. M., R. P. Relley, and A. A. O'Donnell. 1992. "Antibodies to Silicone Elastomers and Reactions to Ventriculoperitoneal Shunts." *Lancet* 340:510–513.

Hansen, T. C., and J. Lurie. 1995. "Ecocide in Indian Country." *News from Indian Country: The Nations Native Newspaper* Vol. IX(14):14–15.

Hartman, D. E. 1987. "Neuropsychological Toxicology: Identification and Assessment of Neurotoxic Syndromes." *Archives of Clinical Neuropsychology* 2:45–65.

Henry, T. K. 1995. "Pesticide Exposure Seen in Primary Care." *Nurse Practitioner Forum* 8(2):50–58.

Hoffman, D. A., S. Stockdale, L. L. Hicks, and J. E. Schwaninger. 1995. "Neurocognitive Symptoms and Quantitative EEG Results in Women Presenting with Silicone-Induced Autoimmune Disorder." *International Journal of Occupational Medicine and Toxicology* 4(1):91–98.

Hooisma, J., H. Hanninen, H. H. Emmen, and B. M. Kulig. 1994. "Symptoms Indicative of the Effects of Organic Solvent Exposure in Dutch Painters." *Neurotoxicology and Teratology* 16(6):613–622.

Hudson, D., K. Miller, and J. Briggs. 1995. "The Tiny Victims of Desert Storm." *Time*, November, 46–62.

Huggins, H. A. 1982. "Mercury: A Factor in Mental Disease?" *Journal of Orthomolecular Psychiatry* 11(1):3–16.

Iregren, A. 1982. "Effects on Psychological Test Performance of Workers Exposed to a Single Solvent (Toluene): A Comparison with Effects of Exposure to a Mixture of Organic Solvents." *Neurobehavioral Toxicology and Teratology* 4:695–701.

Jarvis, S., S. Chinn, C. Luczynska, and P. Burney. 1996. "Association of Respiratory Symptoms and Lung Function in Young Adults with Use of Domestic Gas Appliances." *The Lancet* 347:426–431.

Juntunen, J., M. Antti-Poika, S. Tola, and T. Partanen. 1982. "Clinical Prognosis of Patients with Diagnosed Chronic Solvent Intoxication." *Acta Neurologica Scandinavica* 65:488–503.

Kaplan, J. G., J. Kessler, N. Rosenberg, D. Pack, and H. H. Schaumberg. 1993. "Sensory Neuropathy Associated with Dursban (Chlorpyrifos) Exposure." *Neurology* 43:2193–2196.

Kelly, S .S., E. Mutch, F. M. Williams, and P. G. Blain. 1994. "Electrophysiological and Biochemical Effects Following Single Doses of Organophosphates in the Mouse." *Archives of Toxicology* 68:459–466.

Kingman, A., T. Albertini, and L. J. Brown. 1998. "Mercury Concentrations in Urine and Whole Blood Associated with Amalgam Exposure in a U.S. Military Population." *Journal of Dental Research* 77(3):461–471.

Krzyzanowski, M., J. J. Quackenboss, and M. D. Lebowitz. 1990. "Chronic Respiratory Effects of Indoor Formaldehyde Exposure." *Environmental Research* 52:117–125.

Landrigan, P. J. 1983. "Toxic Exposures and Psychiatric Disease—Lessons from the Epidemiology of Cancer." *Acta Psychiatrica Scandinavica* 67 (suppl 303): 6–15.

Landrigan, P. J. 1985. "The Uses of Epidemiology in the Study of Neurotoxic Pollutants: Lessons from the Workplace." *International Journal of Mental Health* 14(3):44–63.

Lanphear, B. P., M. Weitzman, N. L. Winter, S. Eberly, B. Yakir, M. Tanner, M. Emond, and T. D. Matte. 1996. "Lead Contaminated House Dust and Urban Children's Blood Lead Levels." *American Journal of Public* 86(10):1416–1421.

Lappe, M. 1991. *Chemical Deception: The Toxic Threat to Health and the Environment.* San Francisco, CA: Sierra Club.

Lave, L. B., and F. K. Ennever. 1990. "Toxic Substances Control in the 1990s: Are We Poisoning Ourselves with Low-Level Exposures?" *Annual Review of Public Health* 11:68–87.

Lawson, L. 1994. *Staying Well in a Toxic World.* Chicago: Lynnword Press.

Levenson, T., P. A. Greenberger, and R. Murphy. 1996. "Peripheral Blood Eosinophilia, Hyperimmunoglobulinemia A and Fatigue: Possible Complications Following Rupture of Silicone Breast Implants." *Annals Allergy Asthma Immunology* 77(2):119–122.

Lindelof, B., O. Almkvist, and C. J. Gothe. 1992. "Sleep Disturbances and Exposure to Organic Solvents." *Archives of Environmental Health* 47(2): 104–106.

Lindstrom, K. 1973. "Psychological Performances of Workers Exposed to Various Solvents." *Work-Environment-Health* 10:151–155.

Lorig, T. S. 1994. "EEG and ERP Studies of Low-Level Odor Exposure in Normal Subjects." [Special Issue]. Proceedings of the Conference on Low-Level Exposure to Chemicals and Neurobiologic Sensitivity. *Toxicology and Industrial Health* 10:579–586.

Lorig, T. S., K. B. Herman, and G. E. Schwartz. 1990. "EEG Activity During Administration of Low-Concentration Odors." *Bulletin of the Psychonomic Society* 28(5):405–408.

Lorig, T. S., E. Huffman, A. DeMartino, and J. DeMarco. 1991. "The Effects of Low Concentration Odors on EEG Activity and Behavior." *Journal of Psychophysiology* 5:68–77.

Lorig, T. S., A. C. Sapp, and J. Campbell. 1993. "Event-Related Potentials to Odor Stimuli." *Bulletin of the Psychonomic Society* 31(2):131–134.

Lorig, T. S., and G. E. Schwartz. 1988. "Brain and Odor: I. Alteration of Human EEG Odor Administration." *Psychobiology* 16(3):281–284.

Lundberg, A. 1996. "Psychiatric Aspects of Air Pollution." *Otolaryngology, Head and Neck Surgery* 114(2):227–231.

Mackert, J. R., and A. Berglund. 1997. "Mercury Exposure from Dental Amalgam Fillings: Absorbed Dose and the Potential for Adverse Health Effects." *Critical Review of Oral Biological Medicine* 8(4):410–436.

Marlowe, M. 1986. "Metal Pollutant Exposure and Behavior Disorders: Implications for School Practices." *Journal of Special Education* 20(2): 251–264.

Marlowe, M., A. Cossairt, C. Moon, J. Errera, A. MacNeel, R. Peak, J. Ray, and C. Schroeder. 1985. "Main and Interaction Effects of Metallic Toxins on Classroom Behavior." *Journal of Abnormal Child Psychology* 13(2): 185–198.

Marlowe, M., A. Cossairt, K. Welch, and J. Errera. 1984. "Hair Mineral Content as a Predictor of Learning Disabilities." *Journal of Learning Disorders* 17(7):418–421.

Marlowe, M., and J. Errera. 1982. "Low Lead Levels and Behavior Problems in Children." *Behavior Disorders* 7:163–172.

Marlowe, M., J. Errera, T. Ballowe, and J. Jacobs. 1983. "Low Metal Levels in Emotionally Disturbed Children." *Journal of Abnormal Psychology* 92(3): 386–389.

Marlowe, M., R. Folio, D. Hall, and J. Errera. 1982. "Increased Lead Burdens and Trace-Mineral Status in Mentally Retarded Children." *Journal of Special Education* 16(1):87–99.

McCaffrey, R. J., T. S. Lorig, D. L. Pendrey, N. B. McCutcheon, and J. C. Garrett. 1993. "Odor-Induced EEG Changes in PTSD Veterans." *Journal of Traumatic Stress* 6(2):213–225.

Miller, D. B. 1982. "Neurotoxicity of the Pesticidal Carbamates." *Neurobehavioral Toxicology and Teratology* 4:779–787.

Montague, P. 1997a. "The Truth About Breast Cancer"—Parts 1–5. http://www.monitor.net/rachel/

Montague, P. 1997b. "Diabetes Is Increasing." *Rachel's Environment & Health Weekly*, 558, August 14.

Morrow, L. A., T. Callender, S. Lottenberg, M. S. Buchsbaum, J. J. Hodgson, and N. Robin. 1990. "PET and Neurobehavioral Evidence of Tetrabromoethane Encephalopathy." *Journal of Neuropsychiatry and Clinical Neurosciences* 2:431–435.

Morrow, L. A., C. M. Ryan, G. Goldstein, and M. J. Hodgson. 1989. "A Distinct Pattern of Personality Disturbance Following Exposure to Mixtures of Organic Solvents." *Journal of Occupational Medicine* 31:743–748.

Morrow, L. A., C. M. Ryan, M. J. Hodgson, and N. Robin. 1990. "Alterations in Cognitive and Psychological Functioning After Organic Solvent Exposure." *Journal of Occupational Medicine* 32(5):444–450.

Morrow, L. A., C. M. Ryan, M. J. Hodgson, and N. Robin. 1991. "Risk Factors Associated with Persistence of Neuropsychological Deficits in Persons with Organic Solvent Exposure." *The Journal of Nervous and Mental Disease* 179(9):540–545.

Morrow, L. A., S. R. Steinhauer, and M. J. Hodgson. 1992. "Delay in P300 Latency in Patients with Organic Solvent Exposure." *Archives of Neurology* 49:315–320.

Morrow, L. A., S. R. Steinhauer, and C. M. Ryan. 1994. "The Utility of Psychophysiologic Measures in Assessing the Correlates and Consequences of Organic Solvent Exposure." [Special Issue]. Proceedings of the Conference on Low-Level Exposure to Chemicals and Neurobiologic Sensitivity. *Toxicology and Industrial Health* 10:537–544.

Moses, M., E. S. Johnson, W. K. Anger, W. W. Burse, W. W. Horstman, and R. J. Jackson. 1993. "Environmental Equity and Pesticide Exposure." *Toxicology and Industrial Health* 9(5):913–959.

Muldoon, S. B., J. A. Cauley, L. H. Kuller, L. Morrow, H. L. Needleman, J. Scott, and F. J. Hooper. 1996. "Effects of Blood Lead Levels on Cognitive Function of Older Women." *Neuroepidemiology* 15(2):62–72.

Muto, M. A., F. Lobelle, J. H. Bidanset, and J. Wurpel. 1992. "Embrotoxicity and Neurotoxicity in Rats Associated with Prenatal Exposure to Dursban." *Veterinary and Human Toxicology* 34(6):498–501.

National Institutes of Health Technology Assessment Workshop Statement. 1994. *The Persian Gulf Experience and Health.* April 27–29.

National Research Council. 1993. *Pesticides in the Diets of Infants and Children.* Washington, DC: Academy Press.

Needleman, H. L., J. A. Riess, M. J. Tobin, G. E. Biesecker, and J. B. Greenhouse. 1996. "Bone Lead Levels and Delinquent Behavior." *Journal of the American Medical Association* 7:363–369.

Nolan, K. R. 1983. "Copper Toxicity Syndrome." *Journal of Orthomolecular Psychiatry* 12(4):270–282.

Nriagu, J., and M. Simmons. 1990. *Food Contamination from Environmental Sources*. New York: John Wiley.

Odkvist, L. M., L. M. Bergholtz, B. Larsby, R. Tham, B. Eriksson, and C. Edling. 1985. "Solvent-Induced Central Nervous System Disturbances Appearing in Hearing and Vestibulo-Culomotor Tests." *Clinical Ecology* III(3):149–153.

O'Malley, M. 1997. "Clinical Evaluation of Pesticide Exposure and Poisonings." *The Lancet* 349:1161–1166.

Partanen, T. 1993. "Formaldehyde Exposure and Respiratory Cancer: A Meta-Analysis of the Epidemiologic Evidence." *Scandinavian Journal of Work Environmental Health* 19:8–15.

Perez-Comas, A. 1991. "Mercury Contamination in Puerto Rico: the Ciudad Cristiana Experience." *Bol. Assoc. Med. Puerto Rico* 83:296–299.

Perfecto, I., and B. Velasquez. 1992. "Farm Workers: Among the Least Protected." *EPA Journal*, March-April:13–14.

"Pesticides May Affect Mental Health." 1996. *Solutions* 1(1):27. Spring.

Pimentel, D., and H. Lehman. 1993. *The Pesticide Question: Environment, Economics, and Ethics*. New York: Chapman & Hall.

Regenstein, L. 1982. *America the Poisoned: How Deadly Chemicals Are Destroying Our Environment, Our Wildlife, Ourselves, and How We Can Survive*. Washington, DC: Acropolic Books, Ltd.

Reidy, T. J., R. M. Bowler, S. S. Rauch, and G. I. Pedroza. 1992. "Pesticide Exposure and Neuropsychological Impairment in Migrant Farm Workers." *Archives of Clinical Neuropsychology* 7:85–95.

Rios, R., G. V. Poje, and R. Detels. 1993. "Susceptibility to Environmental Pollutants Among Minorities." *Toxicology and Industrial Health* 9(5):797–820.

Rogers, S. A. 1989. "Diagnosing the Tight Building Syndrome or Diagnosing Chemical Hypersensitivity." *Environment International* 15:75–79.

Rogers, S. A. 1990. *Tired or Toxic*. Syracuse, NY: Prestige Publishers.

Rosen, J. F. 1995. "Adverse Health Effects of Lead at Low Exposure Levels: Trends in the Management of Childhood Lead Poisoning." *Toxicology* 97(1-3):11–17.

Schottenfeld, R. S., and M. Cullen. 1984. "Organic Affective Illness Associated with Lead Intoxication." *American Journal of Psychiatry* 141(11):1423–1426.

Seeber, A., K. Blaszkewicz, K. Golka, and E. Kiesswetter. 1997. "Solvent Exposure and Ratings of Well-Being: Dose-Effect Relationships and Consistency of Data." *Environmental Research* 73:81–91.

Semchuk, K. M., E. J. Love, and R. G. Lee. 1992. "Parkinson's Disease and Exposure to Agricultural Work and Pesticide Chemicals." *Neurology* 42:1328–1335.

Setlow, V. P., C. E. Lawson, and N. F. Woods, eds. 1998. *Gender Differences in Susceptibility to Environmental Factors: A Priority Assessment.* Workshop Report of the Committee on Gender Differences in Susceptibility to Environmental Factors. Division of Health Sciences Policy, Institute of Medicine. Washington, DC: National Academy Press.

Sharpe, R., and N. Shakkebaek. 1993. "Are Estrogens Involved in Falling Spermcounts and Disorders of the Male Reproductive Tract?" *Lancet* 341:1392–95.

Sherman, J. 1995. "Chlorpyrifos (Dursban) Associated Birth Defects: Report of Four Cases." *Archives of Environmental Health* 51:5–8.

Simcox, N. J., R. A. Fenske, S. A. Woiz, I. Lee, and D. A. Kalman. 1995. "Pesticides in Housedust and Soil: Exposure Pathways for Agricultural Families." *Environmental Health Perspectives* 103(12):1126–1134.

Simons, S. S. 1996. "Environmental Estrogens: Can Two 'Alrights' make a Wrong?" *Science* 272:1451.

Soine, L. 1995. "Sick Building Syndrome and Gender Bias: Imperiling Women's Health." *Social Work in Health Care* 20(3):51–64.

Spiera, H., and R. F. Spiera. 1997. "Silicone Breast Implants and Connective Tissue Disease: An Overview." *Mt. Sinai Journal of Medicine* 64 (6): 363–371.

Steingraber, S. 1997. *Living Downstream: An Ecologist Looks at Cancer and the Environment.* Reading, MA: Addison-Wesley.

Thornton, J. 1993. *Chlorine, Human Health, and the Environment: The Breast Cancer Warning.* Washington, DC: Greenpeace.

Thrasher, J. D., A. Broughton, and R. Madison. 1990. "Immune Activation and Autoantibodies in Humans with Long-Term Inhalation Exposure to Formaldehyde." *Archives of Environmental Health* 45:217–223.

Travis, C. B., B. E. McLean, and C. Ribar, eds. 1989. *Environmental Toxins: Psychological, Behavioral, and Sociocultural Aspects, 1973-1989.* Bibliographies in

Psychology No. 5. Washington, D.C.: American Psychological Association.

Vimy, M. J., D. E. Hooper, W. W. King, and F. L. Lorscheider. 1997. "Mercury from Maternal 'Silver' Tooth Fillings in Sheep and Human Breast Milk: A Source of Neonatal Exposure." *Biological Trace Elements Research* 56(2):143–152.

Walsh, F. W., D. A. Solomon, and L. R. Espinoza. 1989. "Human Adjuvant Disease: A New Cause of Chylous Effusions." *Archives of Internal Medicine* 149:1194–1196.

Wantke, F., C. M. Demmer, P. Tappler, M. Gotz, and R. Jarisch. 1996. "Exposure to Gaseous Formaldehyde Induces IgE-Mediated Sensitization to Formaldehyde in School Children." *Clinical and Experimental Allergy* 26:276–280.

Weiss, B. 1983. "Behavioral Toxicology and Environmental Health Science: Opportunity and Challenge for Psychology." *American Psychologist* 38:1174–1187.

Weiss, R. 1991. "Breast Implant Fears Put Focus On Biomaterial." *Science* 252:1059–1160.

Welsh, L., H. Kirshner, A. Heath, R. Gilliland, and S. Broyles. 1991. "Chronic Neuropsychological and Neurological Impairment Following Acute Exposure to a Solvent Mixture of Toluene and Methyl Ethyl Ketone (MEK)." *Clinical Toxicology* 29(4):435–445.

White, R. F., S. P. Proctor, D. Echeverria, J. Schweikert, and R. G. Feldman. 1995. "Neurobehavioral Effects of Acute and Chronic Mixed-Solvent Exposure in the Screen Printing Industry." *American Journal of Industrial Medicine* 28:221–231.

Wilson, C. 1995, *Chemical Sensitivities: A Global Problem*. Prepared at the request of the U.S. Interagency Taskforce on Multiple Chemical Sensitivities.

Wilson, C. 1993. *Chemical Exposure and Human Health*. Jefferson, NC: McFarland.

Wolff, M. S., P. G. Toniolo, E. W. Lee, M. Rivera, and N. Dubin. 1993. "Blood Levels of Organochlorine Residues and Risk of Breast Cancer." *Journal of the National Cancer Institute* 85:648–652.

References

ABC News. 1997. *20/20*. January 3.

ALA and AMA. "Fragrances Do Trigger Asthma." 1998, March-April. *The New Reactor* 8(2):1-2.

Altschuler, J. 1997. *Working with Chronic Illness*. Hampshire, England: MacMillan.

Americans with Disabilities Act of 1990. 1990. (Public Law 101-336.) July 26.

Anderson, J. H. 1997. "Reactions to Carpet Emissions: A Case Series." *Journal of Nutritional and Environmental Medicine* 7:177-185.

Anderson, R. C., and J. H. Anderson. 1998. "Acute Toxic Effects of Fragrance Products." *Archives of Environmental Health* 53(2):138-146.

Arnold, K. 1997. "Psychological Help for Toxic Chemical Injuries." *Our Toxic Times* 8(6):1, 3-7.

Ashford, N., B. Heinzow, K. Lutjen, C. Marouli, L. Molhave, B. Monah, S. Papadopoulos, K. Rest, D. Rosdahl, P. Siskos, and E. Velonakis. 1995. *Chemical Sensitivity in Selected European Countries: An Exploratory Study*. Athens, Greece: LTD.

Ashford, N. A., and C. S. Miller. 1998. *Chemical Exposures: Low Levels and High Stakes*. Second Edition. New York: Van Nostrand Reinhold.

Baiz, T. A. 1997. "Documenting a Personal Injury Claim." *Our Toxic Times* 8(3):5-7. March.

Baker, G. P. 1994. "Porphyria and MCS Overlap Symptoms: Another Chemical Connection." *Our Toxic Times* 5(8):1, 3-5. August.

Barrera, M. 1986. "Distinctions Between Social Support Concepts, Measures, and Models." *American Journal of Community Psychology* 14:413-445.

Barshay, J. M. 1993. "Another Strand of Our Diversity: Some Thoughts from a Feminist Therapist with Severe Chronic Illness." *Women and Therapy* 14: 159-169. Also printed as a chapter in M. E. Willmuth and L. Holcomb, eds. 1993. *Women with Disabilities: Found Voices*. New York: Haworth Press.

Bell, I. R. 1994. "White Paper: Neuropsychiatric Aspects of Sensitivity to Low-Level Chemicals: A Neural Sensitization Model." [Special Issue]. Proceedings of the Conference on Low-Level Exposure to Chemicals and Neurobiologic Sensitivity." *Toxicology and Industrial Health* 10:277-312.

Bell, I. R., C.S. Miller, and G. E. Schwartz. 1992. "An Olfactory-Limbic Model of Multiple Chemical Sensitivity Syndrome: Possible Relationship to Kindling and Affective Spectrum Disorders." *Biological Psychiatry* 32:218-242.

Bell, I. R., J. M. Peterson, and G. E. Schwartz. 1995. "Medical Histories and Psychological Profiles of Middle-Aged Women with and without Self-Reported Illness from Environmental Chemicals." *Journal of Clinical Psychiatry* 56(4):151-160.

Bell, I. R., G. E. Schwartz, J. M. Peterson, and D. Amend. 1993. "Self-Reported Illness from Chemical Odors in Young Adults Without Clinical Syndromes or Occupational Exposures." *Archives of Environmental Health* 48(1):6-13.

Bergner, M., R. A. Bobbitt, S. Kressel, W. E. Pollard, B. S. Gilson, and J. R. Morris, J.R. 1976. "The Sickness Impact Profile: Conceptual Formulation and Methodology for the Development of a Health Status Measure." *International Journal of Health Services* 6(3):393-415.

Bergner, M., R. A. Bobbitt, W. E. Pollard, D. P. Martin, and B. S. Gilson. 1976. "The Sickness Impact Profile: Validation of a Health Status Measure." *Medical Care* 14(1):57-67.

Berkson, J. B. 1996. *A Canary's Tale*. Baltimore, MD: Jacob Berkson.

Bertschler, J., J. R. Butler, G. F. Lawlis, W. J. Rea, and A. R. Johnson. 1985. "Psychological Components of Environmental Illness: Factor Analysis of Changes During Treatment." *Clinical Ecology* 3(2)85-94.

Black, D. W. 1996. "Psychiatric Perspective of Persons with 'Environmental Illness'". *Clinical Reviews in Allergy and Immunology* 14:337-355.

Bloom, J. B., and L. Kessler. 1994. "Emotional Support Following Cancer: A Test of the Stigma and Social Activity Hypotheses." *Journal of Health and Social Behavior* 35:118-133.

Bolla-Wilson, K., R. J. Wilson, and M. L. Bleecker. 1988. "Conditioning of Physical Symptoms After Neurotoxic Exposure." *Journal of Occupational Medicine* 30(9):684-687.

Bower, J. 1997a. *The Healthy House*. Bloomington, IN: The Healthy House Institute, 430 North Sewell Road, Bloomington, IN 47408.

Bower, J. 1997b. *Healthy House Building*. Second Edition. Bloomington, IN: The Healthy House Institute, 430 North Sewell Road, Bloomington, IN 47408.

Bower, L. 1995. *The Healthy Household*. Bloomington, IN: The Healthy House Institute, 430 North Sewell Road, Bloomington, IN 47408.

Brodsky, C. M. 1983. "Psychological Factors Contributing to Somatoform Diseases Attributed to the Workplace." *Journal of Occupational Medicine* 25(6):459-464.

Brodsky, C. M., M. A. Green, and E. S. Ogrod. 1989. "Environmental Illness: Does it Exist?" *Patient Care*, November 15, 41-59.

Bryce-Smith, D. 1986. "Environmental Chemical Influences on Behavior, Personality, and Mentation." *Journal of Biosocial Research* 8(12):115-150.

Buchwald, D., and D. Garrity. 1994. "Comparison of Patients with Chronic Fatigue Syndrome, Fibromyalgia, and Multiple Chemical Sensitivities." *Archives of Internal Medicine* 154:2049-2053.

Burton Goldberg Group. 1994. *Alternative Medicine: The Definitive Guide*. Fife, WA: Future Medicine Publishing, Inc.

Bury, M. 1982. "Chronic Illness as Biographical Disruption." *Sociology of Health & Illness* 4(2):167-182.

Chatfield, K. B. 1985. "The Treatment of Pesticide Poisoning with Traditional Acupuncture." *American Journal of Acupuncture* 13(4):339-345.

Cohen, J. 1997. "The Effects of Different Storage Temperatures on the Taste and Chemical Composition of Diet Coke." *The New Reactor*, May/June, 11-13.

Colborn, T., D. Dumanoski, and J. P. Myers. 1997. *Our Stolen Future: Are We Threatening Our Fertility, Intelligence, and Survival? A Scientific Detective Story.* New York: Penguin.

Conneley, W. 1998. Personal communication. Summer.

Crook, W. G. 1986. *The Yeast Connection.* New York: Vintage Press.

Cullen, M. R. 1987. "The Worker with Multiple Chemical Sensitivities: An Overview." In *Workers with Multiple Chemical Sensitivities,* M. R. Cullen, ed. *Occupational Medicine: State of the Art Reviews* 2(4): 655-666.

Dager, S. R., J. P. Holland, D. S. Cowley, and D. L. Dunner. 1987. "Panic Disorder Precipitated by Exposure to Organic Solvents in the Work Place." *American Journal of Psychiatry* 144(8):1056-1058.

Davidoff, L. L. 1989. "Multiple chemical sensitivities" *The Amicus Journal* Winter, 13-23.

Davidoff, A. L., and L. Fogarty. 1994. "Psychogenic Origins of Multiple Chemical Sensitivities Syndrome: A Critical Review of the Research Literature." *Archives of Environmental Health* 49:316-325.

Davis, J. R., R. C. Brownson, R. Garcia, B. J. Bentz, and A. Turner. 1993. "Family Pesticide Use and Childhood Brain Cancer." *Archives of Environmental Contamination and Toxicology* 24:87-92.

De-Nour, A. K. 1982. "Psychosocial Adjustment to Illness Scale (PAIS): A Study of Chronic Hemodialysis Patients." *Journal of Psychosomatic Research* 26(1):11-22.

Derogatis, L. R. 1986. "The Psychosocial Adjustment to Illness Scale (PAIS)." *Journal of Psychosomatic Research* 30(1):77-91.

Diagnostic and Statistical Manual of the American Psychiatric Association. Fourth Edition. 1994. Washington, DC: American Psychological Association.

Diener, E., R. A. Emmons, R. J. Larsen, and S. Griffin. 1985. "The Satisfaction With Life Scale." *Journal of Personality Assessment* 49:71-75.

Donnay, A. 1997. "Somatization Disorder, Organophosphate Poisoning or Overlapping Syndromes of Chronic Fatigue, Fibromyalgia and Multiple Chemical Sensitivity?" Information for Presentation to the VA Persian Gulf Expert Scientific Committee. From MCS Referral & Resources, 508 Westgate Rd., Baltimore, MD 21229. June 13.

Donnay, A. 1999. Personal Communication. July 23.

Dougans, I., with S. Ellis. 1992. *The Art of Reflexology: A Step-by-Step Guide.* Rockport, MA: Element Books.

Dubin, D. 1994. "What Are You So Sensitive About? Accommodating Environmental Illness/Multiple Chemical Sensitivity." *The Disability Law Reporter Service* 3(9):8-40. September.

Dudley, D. L. 1993. "Chemical Toxicity: A Neurometric Study of Changes in the Auditory and Visual Cognitive Evoked Potential in Response to Olfaction." *Clinical Research* 41(2):383A.

Duehring, C. 1993a. "Immune Alteration Associated with Exposure to Toxics." *Environmental Access Profiles* 3(6):1-2.

Duehring, C. 1993b. "Carpet—Part One: EPA Stalls and Industry Hedges While Consumers Remain at Risk." *Informed Consent* 1(1):6-11, 30-32.

Edelson, S., and J. Statman. 1998. *Living with Environmental Illness: A Practical Guide to Multiple Chemical Sensitivity.* Dallas, TX: Taylor Publishing.

Ehrenreich, B., and D. English. 1973. *Complaints and Disorders: The Sexual Politics of Sickness.* New York: The Feminist Press.

Engel, L.R., P. R. Gibson, M. E. Adler, and V. M. Rice. 1996. "Unmet Medical Needs in Persons with Self-Reported Multiple Chemical Sensitivity." Poster delivered at the Annual Meeting of the Southeastern Psychological Association, Norfolk, Virginia, March 20-23. March.

Esten, G., and L. Willmott. 1993. "Double Bind Messages: The Effects of Attitude Towards Disability on Therapy." *Women and Therapy* 14:29-41. Also printed as a chapter in M. E. Willmuth and L. Holcomb, eds. 1993. *Women with Disabilities: Found Voices.* New York: Haworth Press.

Estes, C. P. 1992. *Women Who Run with the Wolves.* New York: Ballantine.

Fishbain, D. A., and M. Goldberg. 1991. "The Misdiagnosis of Conversion Disorder in a Psychiatric Emergency Service." *General Hospital Psychiatry* 13:177-181.

Foote, A. W., D. Piazza, J. Holcombe, P. Paul, and P. Daffin. 1990 "Hope, Self-Esteem and Social Support in Persons with Multiple Sclerosis." *Journal of Neuroscience Nursing* 22(3):155-159.

Freeza, M., C. di Padova, G. Pozzato, M. Terpin, E. Baraona, and C. Lieber. 1990. "High Blood Alcohol Levels in Women: The Role of Decreased Gastric Alcohol Dehydrogenase Activity." *New England Journal of Medicine* 322(2):95-99.

Friedman, L. 1993. "Survival." *Women and Therapy* 14:19-27. Also printed as a chapter in M. E. Willmuth and L. Holcomb, eds. 1993. *Women with Disabilities: Found Voices.* New York: Haworth Press.

General Accounting Office. 1997. *Social Security Disability: SSA Must Hold Itself Accountable for Continued Improvement in Decision*. Gaithersburg, MA.: General Accounting Office

Gibson, P. R. 1999. "Social Support and Attitude Toward Health Care Delivery as Predictors of Hope in Persons with Multiple Chemical Sensitivity." *Journal of Clinical Nursing* 8:(3)275–283.

Gibson, P. R., J. Cheavens, and M. L. Warren. 1998. "Social Support in Persons with Self-Reported Sensitivity to Chemicals." *Research in Nursing & Health* 21(2):103-115.

Gibson, P. R., J. Cheavens, and M. L. Warren. 1996. "Multiple Chemical Sensitivity/Environmental Illness and Life Disruption." *Women & Therapy* 19:63–79.

Gibson, P. R., V. M. Rice, E. Dowling, D. B. Stables, and M. Keens. 1997. "The Phenomenology of Multiple Chemical Sensitivity at Four Levels of Severity." In P. Gibson, chair, "Multiple Chemical Sensitivity: An Emerging Social, Environmental and Medical Issue." Symposium delivered at the 105th Annual Convention of the American Psychological Association, August 15-19, Chicago, IL. August.

Gibson, P. R., M. A. White, and V. M. Rice. 1997. "Life Satisfaction in Persons with Invisible Disabilities: Chemical Sensitivity/Chemical Injury." Poster delivered at the 21th National Conference, Association for Women in Psychology, March 6-9, Pittsburgh, PA. March.

Glassburn, V. 1991. *Who Killed Candida?* Brushton, NY: Teach Services.

Glendinning, C. 1990. *When Technology Wounds*. London: Taylor & Francis.

Gold, E., L. Gordis, J. Tonascia, and M. Szklo. 1979. "Risk Factors for Brain Tumors in Children." *American Journal of Epidemiology* 109:309-319.

Goldman, L. 1997. EPA Memorandum to Dow Elanco. January 14.

Goodheart, C. D., and M. H. Lansing. 1997. *Treating People with Chronic Disease: A Psychological Guide*. Washington, DC: American Psychological Association.

Gomez, R. L., R. W. Schvaneveldt, and H. Staudenmayer. 1996. "Assessing Beliefs About 'Environmental Illness/Multiple Chemical Sensitivity'". *Journal of Health Psychology* 1(1):107-123.

Guranathan, S., M. Robson, N. Freeman, B. Buckley, A. Roy, R. Meyer, J. Bukowski, and P. Lioy. 1998. "Accumulation of Chlorpyriphos on Residential Surfaces and Toys Accessible to Children." *Environmental Health Perspectives 106*, 9-16.

Hall, K. 1994. "Impacts of the Energy Industry on the Navajo and Hopi." In R. Bullard, ed., *Unequal Protection: Environmental Justice and Communities of Color*. 130–154. San Francisco, CA: Sierra Club Books.

Hansen, T. C., and J. Lurie. 1995.. "Ecocide in Indian Country." *News from Indian Country: The Nations Native Newspaper* 9(14):14-15. July

Harte, J., C. Holdren, R. Schneider, and C. Shirley. 1991. *Toxics A to Z: A Guide to Everyday Pollution Hazards*. Berkekey, CA: University of California Press.

Haveman, R., B. Wolfe, L. Buron, and S. C. Hill. 1995. "The Loss of Earnings Capability from Disability/Health Limitations: Toward a New Social Indicator." *Review of Income and Wealth* 41:289-308.

Herth, K. 1991. "Development and Refinement of an Instrument to Measure Hope." *Scholarly Inquiry for Nursing Practice* 5(1):39-51.

Heuser, G., A. Wojdani, and S. Heuser. 1992. "Diagnostic Markers of Multiple Chemical Sensitivity." In National Research Council *Multiple Chemical Sensitivities: Addendum to Biologic Markers in Immunotoxicology*. Washington, D.C.: National Academy Press. 117-138.

Hirzy, J., and R. Morison. 1989. 4-Phenylcyclohexane/Carpet Toxicity: The EPA Headquarters Case. Paper presented at the Annual Meeting of the Society for Risk Analysis, San Francisco, CA. October.

Hooisma, J., H. Hanninen, H. H. Emmen, and B. M. Kulig. 1994. "Symptoms Indicative of the Effects of Organic Solvent Exposure in Dutch Painters." *Neurotoxicology and Teratology* 16(6):613-622.

House Government Reform and Oversight Subcommittee, hearings on Gulf War Illness. Sept. 19, 1996. Subcommittee Chair Rep. Christopher Shays.

Ingram, C. 1991. *The Drinking Water Book: A Complete Guide to Safe Drinking Water*. Berkeley, CA: Ten Speed Press.

Interagency Workgroup on Multiple Chemical Sensitivity. 1998. *A Report on Multiple Chemical Sensitivity*. Predecisional Draft. August 24.

Jarvis, S., S. Chinn, C. Luczynska, and P. Burney. 1996. "Association of Respiratory Symptoms and Lung Function in Young Adults with Use of Domestic Gas Appliances." *The Lancet* 347:426-431.

Jenney, D. 1997. *Aromatherapy: Essential Oils for Essential Health*. Pleasant Grove, VY: Woodland Publishing.

Johnson, A. 1996-1998. *MCS Information Exchange Newsletter*. November 8, 1996; March 20, 1997; September 19, 1997; February 13, 1998. Brunswick, ME: MCS Information Exchange.

Johnson, A. 1998. "Multiple Chemical Sensitivity: How Chemical Exposures May be Affecting Your Health." Videotape. MCS Infomation Exchange, 2 Oakland Street, Brunswick, ME 04011.

Kaminski, P., and R. Katz. 1996. *Choosing Flower Essences: An Assessment Guide.* Nevada City, CA: Flower Essence Society.

Kidner, D. W. 1994. "Why Psychology is Mute about the Environmental Crisis." *Environmental Ethics* 16:359-376.

Killian, S., S. D. Fretwell, and J. McMichael. 1997. "Antigenic Cross-Reactivity Suggested by Intradermal Skin Test Correlations." *Journal of Nutritional & Environmental Medicine* 7:237-251.

Klonoff E., and H. Landrine. 1997. *Preventing the Misdiagnoses of Women.* Newbury Park, CA: Sage Publications.

Krebaum, S. 1998. Personal communication.

Kreutzer, R. 1999. "Prevalence of People Reporting Sensitivities to Chemicals in a Population-Based Survey." *American Journal of Epidemiology* 150(1):1-11.

Krohn, J. 1996. *Natural Detoxification: The Complete Guide to Clearing Your Body of Toxins.* Point Roberts, WA: Hartley & Marks.

Labor Institute. 1993. *Multiple Chemical Sensitivities at Work: A Training Workbook for Working People.* New York: The Labor Institute.

Lawson, L. 1994. *Staying Well in a Toxic World: Understanding Environmental Illness, Multiple Chemical Sensitivities, Chemical Injury, and Sick Building Syndrome.* Chicago: Noble Press.

Lawrence, L., and B. Weinhouse. 1994. *Outrageous Practices: The Alarming Truth about how Medicine Mistreats Women.* New York: Fawcett Columbine.

Lax, M. B. 1998. "Multiple Chemical Sensitivities: The Social Construction of an Illness." *International Journal of Health Services* 28(4):725-745.

Leroy, J., T. H. Davis, and L. A. Jason. 1996. Treatment Efficacy: A Survey of 305 MCS Patients. The CFIDS Chronicle: Winter, 52–53.

Lester, S. 1998. "Biological Warfare: Experimenting at Home." *Everyone's Backyard* 16(2):6-8. From Center for Health, Environment, and Justice.

Levin, A. S., and V. S. Byers. 1992. "Multiple Chemical Sensitivities: A Practicing Clinician's Point of View—Clinical and Immunologic Research Findings." [Special issue]. Proceedings of the Association of Occupational and Environmental Clinics (AOEC) Workshop on Multiple Chemical Sensitivity. *Toxicology and Industrial Health* 8(4):95-109.

Lieberman, A. D., M. R. Craven, H. A. Lewis, and J. H. Nemenzo. 1998. "Genotoxicty from Domestic Use of Organophosphate Pesticides." *Journal of Occupational and Environmental Medicine* 40(11):954-957.

Lorig, T. S., and G. E. Schwartz. 1988. "Brain and Odor: I. Alteration of Human EEG Odor Administration." *Psychobiology* 16(3):281-284.

Louden, J. 1992. *The Women's Comfort Book: A Self-Nurturing Guide for Restoring Balance in Your Life.* HarperSan Francisco.

Louden, J. 1997. *The Woman's Retreat Book: A Guide to Restoring, Rediscovering, and Reawakening Your True Self—in a Moment, an Hour, a Day, or a Weekend.* Harper SanFrancisco.

MacDonald, W. 1998. Personal communication. September 16.

Mander, J. 1991. *In the Absence of the Sacred: The Failure of Technology & the Survival of the Indian Nations.* San Francisco: Sierra Club Books.

Manzo, L. C., and M. D. Weinstein. 1987. "Behavioral Commitment to Environmental Protection: A Study of Active and Nonactive Members of the Sierra Club." *Environment and Behavior* 19:673-694.

Marinelli, J., and P. Bierman-Lytle. 1995. *Your Natural Home.* New York: Little, Brown & Co.

McFadden, S. 1996. "Phenotypic Variation in Xenobiotic Metabolism and Adverse Environmental Response: Focus on Sulfur-Dependent Detoxification Pathways." *Toxicology* 111:43-65.

Meadow, H. L., J. T. Mentzer, D. R. Rahtz, and M. J. Sirgy. 1992. "A Life Satisfaction Measure Based on Judgement Theory." *Social Indicators Research* 26:23-59.

Meggs, W. J. 1992a. "Multiple Chemical Sensitivities and the Immune System." [Special issue]. Proceedings of the Association of Occupational and Environmental Clinics (AOEC) Workshop on Multiple Chemical Sensitivity. *Toxicology and Industrial Health* 8(4):203-214.

Meggs, W. J. 1992b. "Immunological Mechanisms of Disease and the Multiple Chemical Sensitivity Syndrome." In National Research Council, *Multiple Chemical Sensitivities: Addendum to Biologic Markers in Immunotoxicology.* 155-168 Washington, D.C.: National Academy Press.

Meggs, W. J. 1995a. "Multiple Chemical Sensitivities: Chemical Sensitivity as a Symptom of Airway Inflammation." *Clinical Toxicology* 33(2):107-110.

Meggs, W. J. 1995b. "Neurogenic Switching: A Hypothesis for a Mechanism for Shifting the Site of Inflammation in Allergy and Chemical Sensitivity." *Environmental Health Perspectives* 103(1):2-4.

Meggs, W. J., and C. H. Cleveland. 1993. "Rhinolaryngoscopic Examination of Patients with the Multiple Chemical Sensitivity Syndrome." *Archives of Environmental Health* 48(1):14-18.

Meggs, W. J., K. A. Dunn, R. M. Bloch, P. E. Goodman, and A. L. Davidoff. 1996. "Prevalence and Nature of Allergy and Chemical Sensitivity in a General Population." *Archives of Environmental Health* 51(4):75-82.

Mies, M. 1993. "Who Made Nature Our Enemy?" In M. Mies and V. Shiva, *Ecofeminism*. Atlantic Highlands, NJ: Zed Books.

Miller, C. S. 1992. "Possible Models for Multiple Chemical Sensitivity: Conceptual Issues and Role of the Limbic System." [Special issue]. Proceedings of the Association of Occupational and Environmental Clinics (AOEC) Workshop on Multiple Chemical Sensitivity. *Toxicology and Industrial Health* 8(4):181-202.

Miller, C. S. 1994. "Chemical Sensitivity: History and Phenomenology. White Paper." [Special Issue]. Proceedings of the Conference on Low-Level Exposure to Chemicals and Neurobiologic Sensitivity. *Toxicology & Industrial Health* 10(4/5):253-276.

Morrow, L. A., C. M. Ryan, G. Goldstein, and M. J. Hodgson. 1989. "A Distinct Pattern of Personality Disturbance Following Exposure to Mixtures of Organic Solvents." *Journal of Occupational Medicine* 13:743-748.

Morrow, L. A., C. M. Ryan, M. J. Hodgson, and N. Robin. 1991. "Risk Factors Associated with Persistence of Neuropsychological Deficits in Persons with Organic Solvent Exposure." *Journal of Nervous and Mental Disease* 179(9):540-545.

Morrow, L. A., S. R. Steinhauer, and M. J. Hodgson. 1992. "Delay in P300 Latency in Patients with Organic Solvent Expsoure." *Archives of Neurology* 49:315-320.

Moses, M., E. S. Johnson, W. K. Anger, W. W. Burse, W. W. Horstman, R. J. Jackson, et al. 1993. "Environmental Equity and Pesticide Exposure." *Toxicology and Industrial Health* 9(5):913-959.

"Multiple Chemical Sensitivity: A 1999 Consensus." 1999. *Archives of Environmental Health* 54(3):147-149.

Nethocott, J. R., L. L. Davidoff, B. Curbow, and H. Abbey. 1993. Multiple Chemical Sensitivities Syndrome: Toward a Working Case Definition. *Archives of Environmental Health* 48:19–26.

Nevid, J. S., S. A. Rathus, and B. Greene. 1997. *Abnormal Psychology in a Changing World*. Third Edition. Englewood Cliffs, NJ: Prentice Hall.

NIH Consensus Statement: Acupuncture. 1997. National Institutes of Health Continuing Medical Education 15(5). November 3-5.

Neugarten, B. L., R. J. Havighurst, and S. S. Tobin. 1961. "The Measurement of Life Satisfaction." *Journal of Gerontology* 16:134-143.

Nicolson, G., and N. Nicolson. 1995. "Chronic Illness of Operation Desert Storm: The Presence of Stealth Microorganisms in Gulf War Veterans' Blood Suggests that Biological Warfare May Have Been Used in Desert Storm." *Extraordinary Science* Volume and page numbers to come from author.

Nicolson, G., and N. Nicolson. 1996. "Diagnosis and Treatment of Mycoplasmal Infections in Persian Gulf War Illness CFIDS Patients." *International Journal of Occupational Medicine, Immunology, and Toxicology* 5(1):69-78, 83-86.

Nutrition Action Healthletter. 1997. June.

Patrick D., and R. A. Deyo. 1989. Generic and Disease-Specific Measures in Assessing Health Care Status and Quality of Life." *Medical Care* 27: S217–S232.

Pennebaker, J. W. 1994. "Psychological Bases of Symptom Reporting: Perceptual and Emotional Aspects of Chemical Sensitivity." Proceedings of the Conference on Low-Level Exposure to Chemicals and Neurobiologic Sensitivity. *Toxicology & Industrial Health* [Special Issue] 10(4/5):497-511.

Perez-Comas, A. 1991. "Mercury Contamination in Puerto Rico: The Ciudad Cristiana Experience." *Bol. Assoc. Med. Puerto Rico* 83:296-299.

Peters-Golden, H. 1982. "Breast Cancer: Varied Perceptions of Social Support in the Illness Experience." *Social Science and Medicine* 16:483-491.

Pinsky, M. 1995. *What You Should Know About Electromagnetic Fields, Electromagnetic Radiation, and Your Health.* New York: Warner Books.

Plunkett, S. P. 1993. "Indoor Air Pollution: Sick Building Syndrome, Multiple Chemical Sensitivity and the Courts." *Journal of Environmental Law & Practice* 4(1):1-58.

Raleigh, E. 1992. "Sources of Hope in Chronic Illness." *Ontological Nursing Forum* 19:443–448

Randolph, T. G., and R. W. Moss. 1982. *An Alternative Approach to Allergies"* New York, New York: Harper & Row.

Report of the Ad Hoc Committee on Environmental Hypersensitivity Disorders. 1985. Toronto, Ontario: Canadian Ministry of Health. *August.*

Rest, K. M. 1992. "Advancing the Understanding of Multiple Chemical Sensitivity (MCS): Overview and Recommendations from an AOEC Workshop." [Special issue]. Proceedings of the Association of Occupational and Environmental Clinics (AOEC) Workshop on Multiple Chemical Sensitivity. *Toxicology and Industrial Health* 8(4):1-13.

Rios, R., G. V. Poje, and R. Detels. 1993. "Susceptibility to Environmental Pollutants Among Minorities." *Toxicology and Industrial Health* 9(5): 797-820.

Rippere, V. 1983. *The Allergy Problem: Why People Suffer and What Should Be Done.* Wellingborough, Northamptonshire, United Kingdom: Thorsons Publishers Limited.

Root, M. P. P. 1992. "Reconstructing the Impact of Trauma on Personality." In L. S. Brown and M. Ballou, eds., *Personality and Psychopathology: Feminist Reappraisals.* New York: Guilford.

Rogers, S. A. 1986. *The EI Syndrome.* Syracuse, NY: Prestige Publishers.

Rogers, S. A. 1990. *Tired or Toxic.* Syracuse, NY: Prestige Publishers.

Rosenberg, S. J., M. R. Freedman, K. B. Schmaling, and C. Rose. 1990. "Personality Styles of Patients Asserting Environmental Illness." *Journal of Occupational Medicine* 32(8):678-679.

Ross, G. H. 1992. "Treatment Options in Multiple Chemical Sensitivity." Proceedings of the Association of Occupational and Environmental Clinics (AOEC) Workshop on Multiple Chemical Sensitivity. *Toxicology and Industrial Health* [special issue] 8(4):87-94.

Rossi, J. 1996. "Sensitization Induced by Kindling and Kindling-Related Phenomena as a Model for Multiple Chemical Sensitivity." *Toxicology* 111:87-100.

Roy, R. 1994. "Influence of Chronic Pain on the Family Relations of Older Women." In K. A. Roberto, ed., *Older Women with Chronic Pain.* New York: Haworth. 73-88.

Schottenfeld, R. S., and M. Cullen. 1984. "Organic Affective Illness Associated with Lead Intoxication." *American Journal of Psychiatry* 141(11):1423-1426.

Seastrunk, J. W. No Date. "Neurontin for the Treatment of Focal Brain Injury." Unpublished handout from the office of D. Jay Seastrunk, The Center for Adolescent and Family Care, Inc., 102 E. Freeman St., Duncanville, TX 7516.

Selner, J. C. 1988. "Chemical Sensitivity." In B.C. Decker, ed., *Current Therapy in Allergy, Immunology and Rheumatology* 3:48-52.

Selner, J. C., and H. Staudenmayer. 1992. "Neuropsychophysiolologic Observations in Patients Presenting with Environmental Illness." [Special issue]. Proceedings of the Association of Occupational and Environmental Clinics (AOEC) Workshop on Multiple Chemical Sensitivity. *Toxicology and Industrial Health* 8(4):145-155.

Sherman, J. 1995. "Chlorpyrifos (Dursban) Associated Birth Defects: Report of Four Cases." *Archives of Environmental Health* 51:5-8.

Shumaker, S. A., and D. R. Hill. 1991. "Gender Differences in Social Support and Physical Health." *Health Psychology* 10:102-111.

Simon, G. 1994. "Psychiatric Symptoms in Multiple Chemical Sensitivity." [Special Issue]. Proceedings of the Conference on Low-Level Exposure to Chemicals and Neurobiologic Sensitivity. *Toxicology & Industrial Health* 10(4/5):487-496.

Simon, G. E., W. J. Katon, and P. J. Sparks. 1990. "Allergic to Life: Psychological Factors in Environmental Illness." *American Journal of Psychiatry* 147(7):901-906.

Stein, D. 1995. *Essential Reiki: A Complete Guide to an Ancient Healing Art.* Freedom, CA: The Crossing Press.

Strauss, A. 1984. *Chronic Illness and the Quality of Life.* St. Louis, MO: C.V. Mosby Company.

Svoboda, T. 1997. "EPA Poisons EPA: My Sister's Story." New York: Svoboda/Bull Productions. Videotape available from Terese Svoboda, 56 Ludlow Street, New York, NY 10002. sbull@el.net

Temple, T. 1996. *Healthier Hospitals: A Comprehensive Guide to Assist in the Medical Care of the Patient with Multiple Chemical Sensitivity.* Parma, Ohio: Toni Temple and the Ohio Network for the Chemically Injured.

Thoits, P. A. 1995. "Stress, Coping and Social Support Processes: Where Are We? What Next?" *Journal of Health and Social Behavior* 36(suppl):53-79.

Thornton, J. 1993. *Chlorine, Human Health, and the Environment: The Breast Cancer Warning.* Washington, DC: Greenpeace.

Toxic Secrets: Inert Ingredients in Pesticides 1987–1997. 1998. National Coalition for Alternatives to Pesticides and Californians for Pesticide Reform.

Uchino, B. N., J. T. Cacioppo, and J. K. Kiecolt-Glaser. 1996. "The Relationship Between Social Support and Physiological Processes: A Review with Emphasis on Underlying Mechanisms and Implications for Health." *Psychological Bulletin* 119:488-531.

Versendaal, D. A. 1993. Contact Reflex Analysis and Designed Clinical Nutrition. Hoezee Marketing. (No city given.)

Voorhees, R. 1999. "Results of Analysis of Multiple Chemical Sensitivities Questions, 1997." Behavioral Risk Factor Surveillence System, New Mexico Department of Health, Feb. 8.

Ware, N. C. 1992. "Suffering and the Social Construction of Illness: The Delegitimation of Illness Experience in Chronic Fatigue Syndrome." *Medical Anthropology Quarterly* 6:347-361.

Weed, S. S. 1989. Wise *Woman Herbal: Healing Wise.* Woodstock, NY: Ash Tree Publishing.

Weinert, C. 1987. "A Social Support Measure: PRQ85." *Nursing Research* 36:273-277.

White, N. E., J. M. Richter, and C. Fry. 1992. "Coping, Social Support, and Adaptation to Chronic Illness." *Western Journal of Nursing Research* 14(2):211-224.

Wilkinson, S., and C. Kitzinger. 1994. "Towards a Feminist Approach to Breast Cancer." In S. Wilkinson and C. Kitzinger, eds., *Women and Health: Feminist Perspectives.* London: Taylor & Francis.

Wilson, C. 1993. *Chemical Exposure and Human Health.* Jefferson, HC: MacFarland.

Wilson, C. 1995. *Chemical Sensitivities: A Global Problem.* Report prepared at the request of the U.S. Interagency Taskforce on Multiple Chemical Sensitivities.

Wilson, C. 1997. "Chemical Injury as a Women's Health Issue." *Our Toxic Times* 8(9):1, 3.

Wilson, C. 1999. "MCS Treatments are Plentiful but Still No Cure in Sight." *Our Toxic Times* 10(3):3-4.

Winter, R. 1994. *A Consumer's Dictionary of Food Additives.* Fourth Edition. New York: Three Rivers Press.

Wittenberg, J. S. 1996.*The Rebellious Body: Reclaim your Life From Environmental Illness or Chronic Fatigue Syndrome.* New York: Insight Books.

Wood, V., M. L. Wylie, and B. Sheafor, B. 1969. "An Analysis of a Short Self-Report Measure of Life Satisfaction: Correlation with Rater Judgements." *Journal of Gerontology* 24:465-469.

Ziem, G. E. 1992. "Multiple Chemical Sensitivity: Treatment and Follow-Up with Avoidance and Control of Chemical Exposures." [Special issue]. Proceedings of the Association of Occupational and Environmental Clinics (AOEC) Workshop on Multiple Chemical Sensitivity. *Toxicology and Industrial Health* 8(4):73-86.

Zwillinger, R. 1997. *The Dispossessed: Living with Multiple Chemical Sensitivities.* Paulden, AZ: The Dispossessed Project.

Index

planning, 170, 171

plants: medicinal, 124, 126-128; nurturing quality of, 224

pleasure program, 217

Poe, Edgar Allen, 23

polarity therapy, 123, 125

political involvement, 172

positive affirmations, 218-219

positive self-attribute list, 217

prayer, 187-188

preservative-free testing, 104-105

preservatives in foods, 78, 79

pressure-treated lumber, 73; source for obtaining, 310

privacy issues, 153

private disability insurance, 235

procrastination, 148-149

product sources, 301-312; air purifiers, 310-311; bedding, 303; building products, 303; carpeting, 304; children's products, 304-305; cleaning products, 305-306; clothing, 306; EMF meters, 306; flooring, 306; furniture, 307; gardening supplies, 307; hair products, 307-308; heaters, 308; macrobiotic foods, 308; makeup, 308-309; multiple product companies, 301-303; paints, 309; pellet stoves, 309; personal care products, 309-310; pest control, 307, 310; pet products, 310; pressure-treated wood, 310; reading boxes, 311; saunas, 311; solar energy, 311; wall coverings, 311-312; water purifiers, 310-311; water testing products, 312

propane, 48-49

propylene glycol, 56

Protecto-Zone accommodation booth, 269

provocation/neutralization (P/N) testing, 103-104

psychiatric symptoms, 169

psychological causes of MCS, 24-28; disability compensation and, 238-239; problems with research on, 157-162; treatment controversy and, 28-29

psychological challenges: assertiveness, 146-147; attitudes and beliefs about MCS, 163-164; discontinuous sense of identity, 154-155, 171-172, 175-176; emotional reactions, 149-155, 176-177; feelings of loss, 152, 169, 178-179; inappropriate labeling by therapists, 155-157, 161; overachievement, 148; personality style, 149; procrastination, 148-149; self-esteem and self-worth, 147-148; working with therapists, 164-165

psychological tests, 161

psychologists: guidelines for working with, 164-165; inappropriate labeling by, 155-157, 161; roles performed by, 155; treatment suggestions for, 166-173

Psychosocial Adjustment to Illness Scale (PAIS), 161, 196-197, 282

public access issues, 37

publications: inspirational, 225; research, 298-300

purifiers: air, 61-64; product sources for, 310-311; water, 66-68

treatments for MCS: alternative therapies, 117-131; controversy surrounding, 28-29; dietary, 83-92; environmental medicine, 100-107, 115; experimental, 107-110; medical, 93-116; psychotherapeutic, 166-173

triggering, 12

V

Versendaal, D. A., 121

vinegar, 54, 59

VOCs (volatile organic compounds): in carpets, 50; in water, 65

W

wall coverings, 51-52; product sources for, 311-312

water: contaminants found in, 64-66; filters for treating, 66-68, 310-311; products for testing, 312

Weed, Susun, 127

Who Killed Candida? (Glassburn), 86

Wilkenfeld, Irene Ruth, 262-266

Wilson, Cynthia, 13, 15, 22, 106, 111, 252-253

Winter, Ruth, 78

Wittenberg, Janet Strubbe, 123, 163-164

Wolff, Peggy, 266-268

women: cultural stereotypes of, 216; health diagnoses and, 156-157; multiple chemical sensitivity and, 14-15

Women and Aging journal, 137

Women Who Run with the Wolves (Estes), 183

Women's Retreat Book, The (Louden), 225

wood, pressure-treated, 73, 310

wood stoves, 49, 309

workers' compensation, 237

Working with Chronic Illness (Altschuler), 139

workplace: accommodating MCS in, 74, 230-234; chemical injury in, 32-34, 290-291

World Health Organization, 118, 126, 130

Wysocki, Carolyn, 258

Y

Yeast Connection, The (Crook), 85

yeasts: anticandida diets and, 85-89; candidiasis and, 23

Z

Zwillinger, Rhonda, 36, 261, 275

More New Harbinger Titles

HEALTHY BABY, TOXIC WORLD

This practical guide helps new and expectant parents understand the threat of scores of potentially harmful chemicals and take steps to detoxify their child's home environment.   *Item BABY $15.95*

THE CHRONIC PAIN CONTROL WORKBOOK

A team of specialists in all areas of pain management detail the treatment strategies for managing and recovering from chronic pain.
Item PN2 Paperback $17.95

FIBROMYALGIA & CHRONIC MYOFASCIAL PAIN SYNDROME

This survival manual is the first comprehensive patient guide for managing these conditions. Readers learn how to identify trigger points, cope with chronic pain and sleep problems, and deal with the numbing effects of "fibrofog."   *Item FMS Paperback, $19.95*

OVERCOMING REPETITIVE MOTION INJURIES THE ROSSITER WAY

This system of easy-to-learn stretches has brought pain relief to thousands who suffer from carpal tunnel syndrome and other repetitive motion injuries and from everyday aches and pains.   *Item ROSS Paperback, $15.95*

PERIMENOPAUSE

Beginning with subtle changes in the mid-thirties and forties, perimenopause can encompass a bewildering array of symptoms. This self-care guide helps women assure health and vitality in the years ahead.
Item PERI Paperback, $16.95

Call **toll-free 1-800-748-6273** to order. Have your Visa or Mastercard number ready. Or send a check for the titles you want to New Harbinger Publications, 5674 Shattuck Avenue, Oakland, CA 94609. Include $3.80 for the first book and 75¢ for each additional book to cover shipping and handling. (California residents please include appropriate sales tax.) Allow four to six weeks for delivery.

Prices subject to change without notice.

Some Other New Harbinger Self-Help Titles

Virtual Addiction, $12.95
After the Breakup, $13.95
Why Can't I Be the Parent I Want to Be?, $12.95
The Secret Message of Shame, $13.95
The OCD Workbook, $18.95
Tapping Your Inner Strength, $13.95
Binge No More, $14.95
When to Forgive, $12.95
Practical Dreaming, $12.95
Healthy Baby, Toxic World, $15.95
Making Hope Happen, $14.95
I'll Take Care of You, $12.95
Survivor Guilt, $14.95
Children Changed by Trauma, $13.95
Understanding Your Child's Sexual Behavior, $12.95
The Self-Esteem Companion, $10.95
The Gay and Lesbian Self-Esteem Book, $13.95
Making the Big Move, $13.95
How to Survive and Thrive in an Empty Nest, $13.95
Living Well with a Hidden Disability, $15.95
Overcoming Repetitive Motion Injuries the Rossiter Way, $15.95
What to Tell the Kids About Your Divorce, $13.95
The Divorce Book, Second Edition, $15.95
Claiming Your Creative Self: True Stories from the Everyday Lives of Women, $15.95
Six Keys to Creating the Life You Desire, $19.95
Taking Control of TMJ, $13.95
What You Need to Know About Alzheimer's, $15.95
Winning Against Relapse: A Workbook of Action Plans for Recurring Health and Emotional Problems, $14.95
Facing 30: Women Talk About Constructing a Real Life and Other Scary Rites of Passage, $12.95
The Worry Control Workbook, $15.95
Wanting What You Have: A Self-Discovery Workbook, $18.95
When Perfect Isn't Good Enough: Strategies for Coping with Perfectionism, $13.95
Earning Your Own Respect: A Handbook of Personal Responsibility, $12.95
High on Stress: A Woman's Guide to Optimizing the Stress in Her Life, $13.95
Infidelity: A Survival Guide, $13.95
Stop Walking on Eggshells, $14.95
Consumer's Guide to Psychiatric Drugs, $16.95
The Fibromyalgia Advocate: Getting the Support You Need to Cope with Fibromyalgia and Myofascial Pain, $18.95
Healing Fear: New Approaches to Overcoming Anxiety, $16.95
Working Anger: Preventing and Resolving Conflict on the Job, $12.95
Sex Smart: How Your Childhood Shaped Your Sexual Life and What to Do About It, $14.95
You Can Free Yourself From Alcohol & Drugs, $13.95
Amongst Ourselves: A Self-Help Guide to Living with Dissociative Identity Disorder, $14.95
Healthy Living with Diabetes, $13.95
Dr. Carl Robinson's Basic Baby Care, $10.95
Better Boundries: Owning and Treasuring Your Life, $13.95
Goodbye Good Girl, $12.95
Fibromyalgia & Chronic Myofascial Pain Syndrome, $19.95
The Depression Workbook: Living With Depression and Manic Depression, $17.95
Self-Esteem, Second Edition, $13.95
Angry All the Time: An Emergency Guide to Anger Control, $12.95
When Anger Hurts, $13.95
Perimenopause, $16.95
The Relaxation & Stress Reduction Workbook, Fourth Edition, $17.95
The Anxiety & Phobia Workbook, Second Edition, $18.95
I Can't Get Over It, A Handbook for Trauma Survivors, Second Edition, $16.95
Messages: The Communication Skills Workbook, Second Edition, $15.95
Thoughts & Feelings, Second Edition, $18.95
Depression: How It Happens, How It's Healed, $14.95
The Deadly Diet, Second Edition, $14.95
The Power of Two, $15.95
Living Without Depression & Manic Depression: A Workbook for Maintaining Mood Stability, $18.95
Couple Skills: Making Your Relationship Work, $14.95
Hypnosis for Change: A Manual of Proven Techniques, Third Edition, $15.95
Letting Go of Anger: The 10 Most Common Anger Styles and What to Do About Them, $12.95
Infidelity: A Survival Guide, $13.95
When Anger Hurts Your Kids, $12.95
Don't Take It Personally, $12.95
The Addiction Workbook, $17.95
It's Not OK Anymore, $13.95
Beyond Grief: A Guide for Recovering from the Death of a Loved One, $14.95

Call **toll free, 1-800-748-6273,** or log on to our online bookstore at **www.newharbinger.com** to order. Have your Visa or Mastercard number ready. Or send a check for the titles you want to New Harbinger Publications, Inc., 5674 Shattuck Ave., Oakland, CA 94609. Include $3.80 for the first book and 75¢ for each additional book, to cover shipping and handling. (California residents please include appropriate sales tax.) Allow two to five weeks for delivery.

Prices subject to change without notice.